Supervision
in
Communication Disorders

Supervision in Communication Disorders

Stephen S. Farmer

Judith L. Farmer
New Mexico State University

MERRILL PUBLISHING COMPANY
A Bell & Howell Information Company
Columbus Toronto London Melbourne

Published by Merrill Publishing Company
A Bell & Howell Information Company
Columbus, Ohio 43216

This book was set in Usherwood.

Administrative Editor: Vicki Knight
Production Coordinator: Carol Driver
Cover Designer: Brian Deep

Copyright © 1989 by Merrill Publishing Company. All rights reserved. No part of this book may be reproduced in any form, electronic or mechanical, including photocopy, recording, or any information storage and retrieval system, without permission in writing from the publisher. "Merrill Publishing Company" and "Merrill" are registered trademarks of Merrill Publishing Company.

Library of Congress Catalog Card Number: 88-61041
International Standard Book Number: 0-675-20963-3
Printed in the United States of America
1 2 3 4 5 6 7 8 9 — 92 91 90 89

To Christopher and Bethany

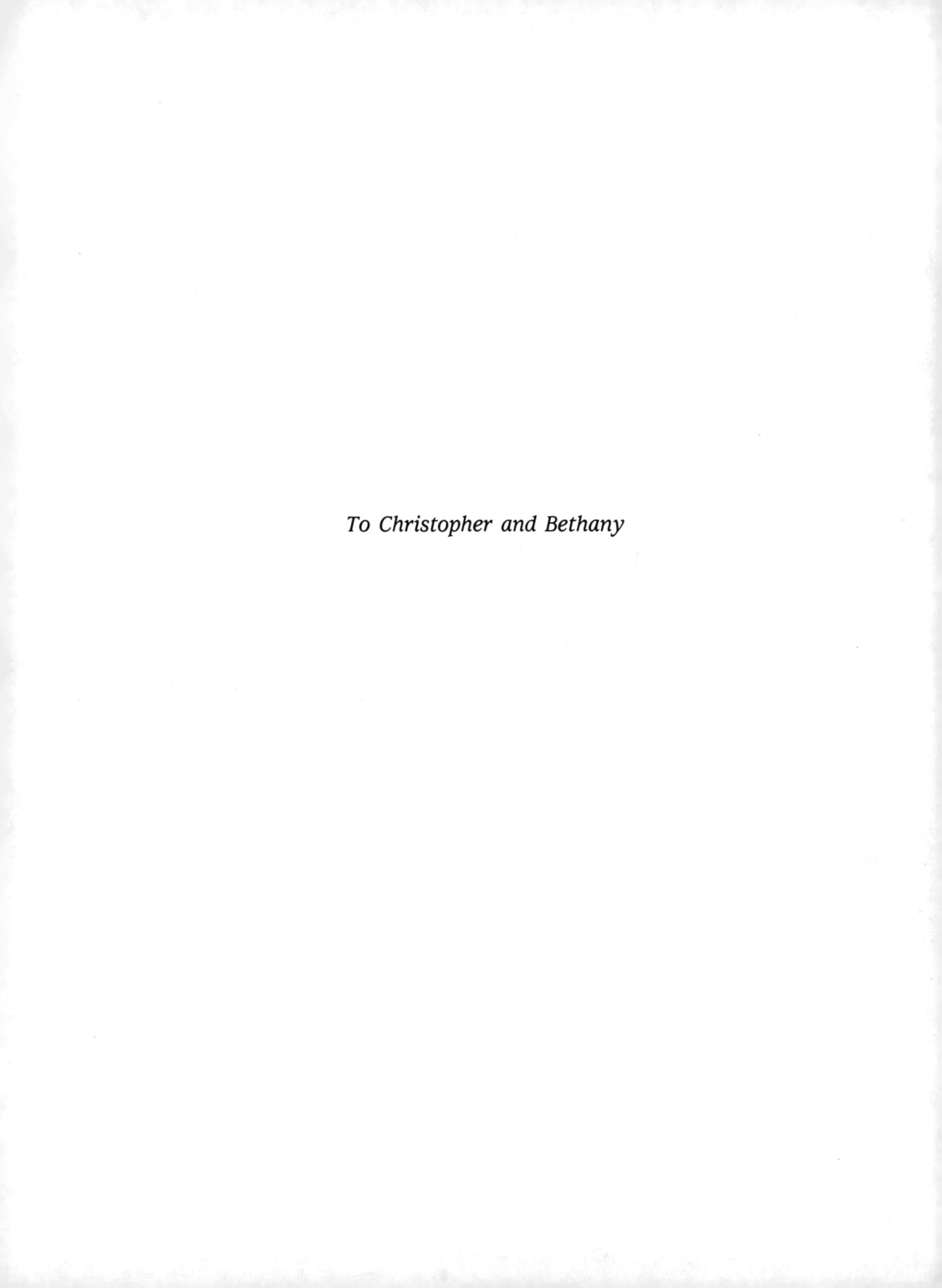

Preface

Supervision in Communication Disorders is the process of people (supervisors) helping people (speech-language pathologists and audiologists) to help people (clients or patients) who have problems communicating. Recognition of the importance of supervision has led to an increasing sense of the importance of training in the supervision process. Although a number of Speech-Language Pathology and Audiology training programs have developed courses in supervision, and continuing education workshops about supervision are increasingly common, more institutions and organizations would offer such training if guidelines for it were available. The question often arises, "What do Communication Disorders supervisors need to be prepared to do?" This book addresses that question; it is a resource to be used in preparing supervisors at preservice (undergraduate and graduate) and service levels. It can also be used to supplement related undergraduate and graduate courses (e.g., courses in observation, administration, or clinical procedures). Although primarily intended for preparing untrained personnel to supervise productively, this textbook includes material useful to experienced supervisors as well.

We believe that supervisees, as well as supervisors, benefit from preparation to participate in the supervision process. We also believe that supervision procedures in Speech-Language Pathology and in Audiology are more similar than different and therefore that the basic competencies of supervision can be developed and then adapted to either area and to specific contexts. To that end, this book includes synthesized theoretical and applied information that focuses on the development of interpersonal and technological supervisor competencies in professional, research, education, administration, and clinical areas.

The text is organized into four parts containing a total of 12 chapters. Part I, "Supervision in Communication Disorders: An Overview," describes the history and development of supervision in Communication Disorders. Eight assumptions that culminate in an operational definition of Communication Disorders supervision set the stage for the rest of the book.

Part II, "Composition of the Supervision Process," presents the *Trigonal Model* of Communication Disorders supervision. Because supervision is a human endeavor, we provide in chapter 2 information about the people, or *Constituents,* involved in the supervision process as the first dimension of the model. Theories, ideas, and issues provide material for chapter 3, which covers the *Concepts* dimension of the model. We complete the Trigonal Model in chapter 4 with a discussion of supervision in five basic worksites, or *Contexts*.

The skills important for competent supervisors are considered in the seven chapters of part III, "Supervisor Development." Chapter 5 reviews verbal and nonverbal dimensions of communication: intrapersonal, interpersonal, conflict, small-group, organizational, professional, and nontraditional (e.g., multicultural). Systems of critical observation and recording are presented in chapter 6. The science of decision making, or vertical, logical thinking, is a highly technical topic never before presented in the literature of Communication Disorders supervision. The topic becomes comprehensible in chapter 7 through the conversational presentation of Edgar Garrett. In chapter 8 we present the companion topic of problem managing, offering creative approaches based on the concept of lateral thinking to complement the scientific aspect of supervisory decision making. Clinical literacy, including the skills of setting goals and objectives, reporting, and editing, is explained in chapter 9. Electronic technology is applied for the first time to the Communication Disorders supervision process in chapter 10. Regrettably, this chapter is the only contribution to the field of supervision that Gary Rushakoff, a leader in applying microcomputer technology to Speech-Language Pathology and Audiology, had the opportunity to make before his death in 1987. He has laid the groundwork for a rapidly changing specialty that will have a strong impact on supervision. Chapter 11, on assessment in supervision, covers evaluation instruments, special situations such as evaluating marginal personnel, peers, or supervisees who exhibit a communication impairment, and generic versus categorical evaluation.

In Part IV, "Research," Susann Dowling presents a historical view of the formal study of Communication Disorders supervision. She encourages future research in supervision by analyzing a variety of research designs, summarizing the work that has been done, and suggesting areas where future research is needed.

Each of the 12 chapters begins with a brief outline and a list of critical concepts to prepare the reader for the content of the chapter. Discussion topics, laboratory experiences, suggested research projects, and a list of references conclude each chapter. Two appendices ("Competencies for Effective Clinical Supervision" and "Characteristics of Communication Disorders Supervision STYLES"), a glossary of supervision terms, and extensive subject and author indexes complete the text.

We appreciate the people who contributed their knowledge and expertise to this project. Vicki Knight, the administrative editor, provided just the right amount of guidance and support. Carol Driver, production editior, coordinated our project expertly. Margaret Conable, copyeditor, helped us clarify our ideas and express them more efficiently. The contributing authors, Edgar Garrett, Gary Rushakoff, and Susann Dowling, met every deadline with quality work. Our many supervisees provided the foundation for the book. Our clients at the New Mexico State University Speech and Hearing Center and our students and colleagues in the Department of Special Education/Communication Disorders allowed our camera to record their activities. We also wish to thank the professionals who provided helpful suggestions in their reviews of our manuscripts: Debra R. Suffolk, Pennsylvania State Univeristy; Mary Ellen Brandell, Central Michigan University; Lou Echols-Chambers, University of Illinois at Urbana-Champaign; Brenda Y. Terrell, Case Western Reserve University; Jeniece Nelson, Western Kentucky University; Marsha Hershman, Stockton State College; Nancy Creaghead, University of Cincinnati; and Stephanie Martin, University of Oregon.

Our understanding of supervision in Communication Disorders continues to grow. It is our intent that this textbook stimulate supervisors and supervisees to further explore the development of supervision competence as they use their knowledge of the process in their various employment contexts.

Contents

PART ONE
Supervision in Communication Disorders: An Overview 1

Chapter 1
Supervision in Communication Disorders: Evaluation of a Profession 2
Stephen S. Farmer

INTRODUCTION   3
HISTORY   3
ASSUMPTIONS   7
DEFINITION   9
SUMMARY   10
APPLICATIONS   10

PART TWO
Composition of the Supervision Process 15

Chapter 2
The Trigonal Model of Communication Disorders Supervision: Constituents 16
Stephen S. Farmer

INTRODUCTION   17
SUPERVISORS   17
SUPERVISEES   46
OTHERS   47
SUMMARY   48
APPLICATIONS   48

Chapter 3
The Trigonal Model of Communication Disorders Supervision: Concepts 54
Stephen S. Farmer

INTRODUCTION   55
IDEAS AND ISSUES   55
SUMMARY   79
APPLICATIONS   79

Chapter 4
The Trigonal Model of Communication Disorders Supervision: Contexts 84
Stephen S. Farmer

INTRODUCTION   85
WORKSITE PROFILES   85
SUPERVISION TASKS RELATIVE TO WORKSITES   89
SUMMARY   90
APPLICATIONS   91

PART THREE
Supervisor Development 93

Chapter 5
Communication Competence 94
Stephen S. Farmer

INTRODUCTION 96
COMMUNICATION CONCEPTS 96
COMMUNICATION CATEGORIES 114
COMMUNICATION ANALYSIS 135
COMMUNICATION COMPETENCE AND
   INCOMPETENCE 142
DEVELOPMENT OF COMMUNICATION
   COMPETENCE 142
SUMMARY 145
APPLICATIONS 145

Chapter 6
Observation Competence 154
Judith L. Farmer

INTRODUCTION 155
VISUAL LITERACY 158
OBSERVING NONVERBAL BEHAVIOR 165
OBSERVING VERBAL BEHAVIOR 167
MODES 168
SYSTEMATIC OBSERVATION 172
OBSERVATION RECORDING
   SYSTEMS 175
SUMMARY 178
APPLICATIONS 178

Chapter 7
Decision Making: The Science 182
Edgar R. Garrett

INTRODUCTION 183
DECISION ANALYSIS 185
DECISION MAKING 198
SUMMARY 200
APPLICATIONS 201

Chapter 8
Creative Problem Managing: The Art 204
Stephen S. Farmer

INTRODUCTION 205
PROBLEMS 206
PROBLEM MANAGING 206
THEORIES OF PROBLEM MANAGING 207
OBSTACLES TO PRODUCTIVE PROBLEM
   MANAGEMENT 214
PROBLEM MANAGING PROGRAMS 217
SUSTAINING PRODUCTIVE PROBLEM
   MANAGING 221
SUMMARY 222
APPLICATIONS 223

Chapter 9
Clinical Literacy 229
Judith L. Farmer

INTRODUCTION 229
DEVELOPING COMPETENCE IN CLINICAL
   REPORTING 231
DEVELOPING COMPETENCE IN WRITING
   GOALS AND OBJECTIVES 236
EDITING 245
SUMMARY 246
APPLICATIONS 246

Chapter 10
Supervision Applications of Microcomputer Technology 250
*Gary E. Rushakoff and
Stephen S. Farmer*

INTRODUCTION 251
RECORD KEEPING 252
TELECOMMUNICATIONS 264
OTHER APPLICATIONS 265
CONCERNS 268
SUMMARY 269
APPLICATIONS 270

Chapter 11
Assessment in Supervision 274
Stephen S. Farmer

INTRODUCTION   275
THE ASSESSMENT SYSTEM   276
SPECIAL CONSIDERATIONS   304
SUMMARY   306
APPLICATIONS   307

PART FOUR
Research 313

Chapter 12
Research: Past, Present, Future 314
Susann S. Dowling

INTRODUCTION   515
RESEARCH METHODOLOGY AND DESIGN   316
WHAT WE KNOW ABOUT THE SUPERVISORY PROCESS IN SPEECH-LANGUAGE PATHOLOGY AND AUDIOLOGY   324
RESEARCH CONSIDERATIONS   331
SUPERVISION RESEARCH AND THE FUTURE   333
SUMMARY   340
APPLICATIONS   340

Appendix A
Competencies for Effective Clinical Supervision 351

Appendix B
Characteristics of Communication Disorders Supervision Styles 356

Glossary 364

Author Index 371

Subject Index 378

PART ONE
Supervision in Communication Disorders: An Overview

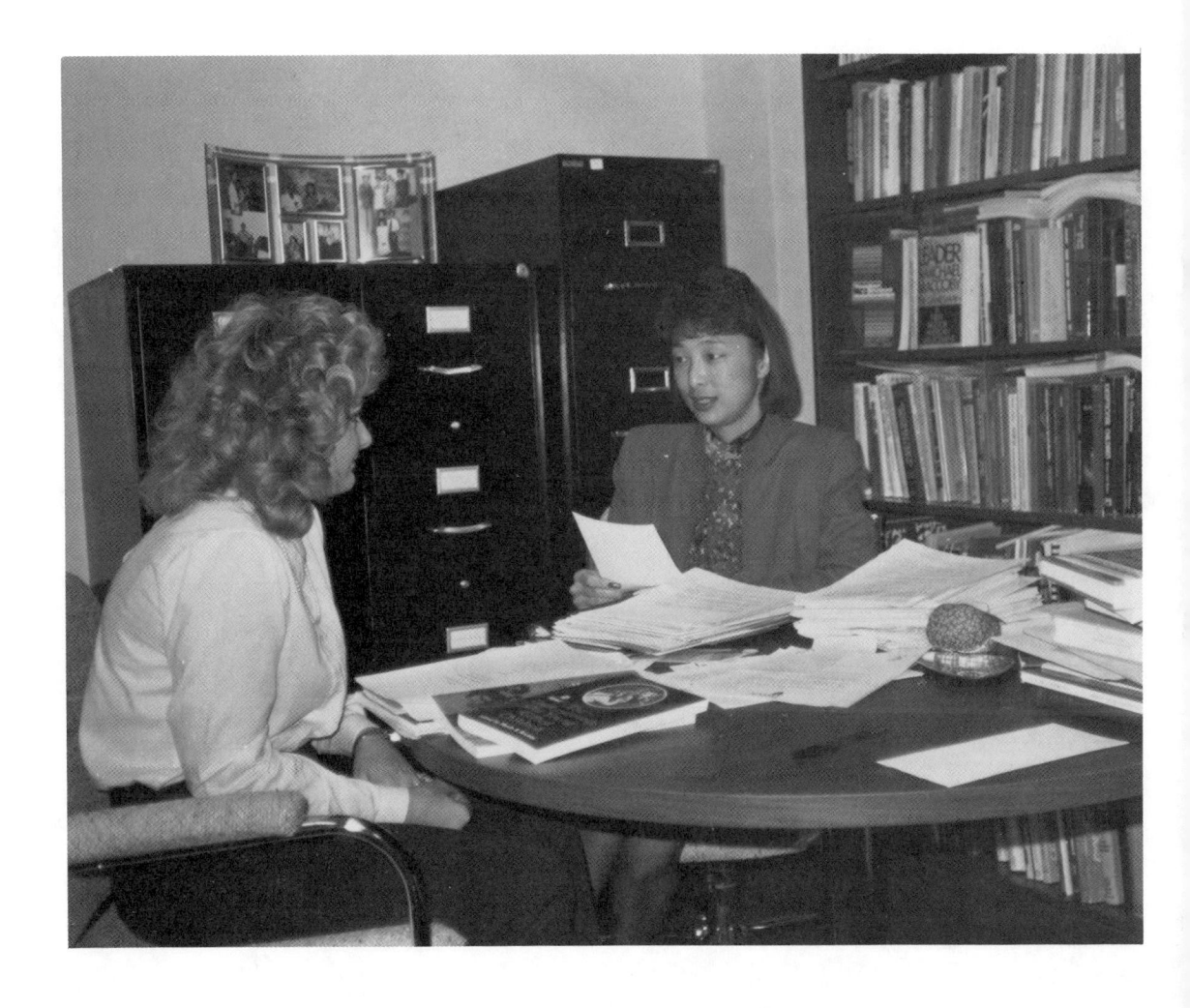

1
Supervision in Communication Disorders: Evolution of a Profession

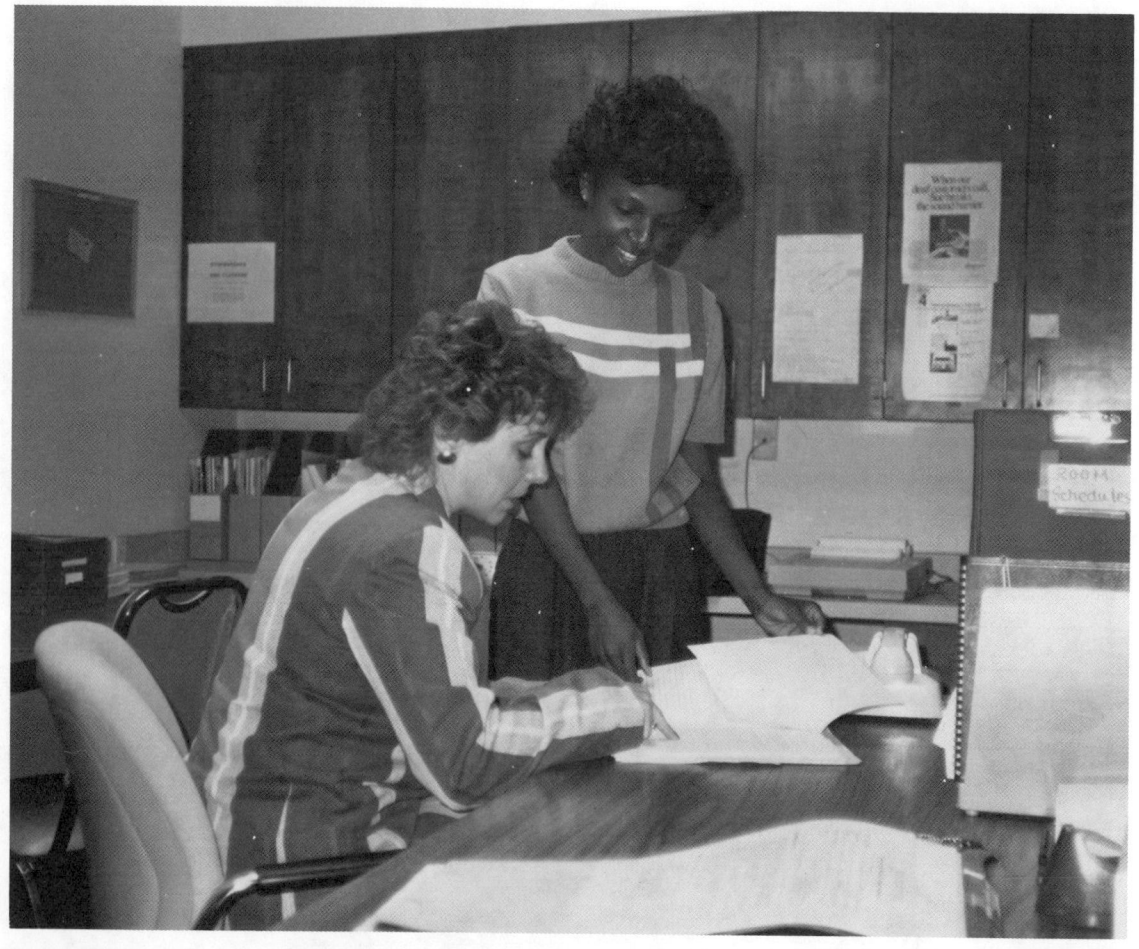

CRITICAL CONCEPTS

- *Supervision in Communication Disorders has evolved through developmental stages.*
- *Supervision in Communication Disorders is based on eight assumptions.*
- *The Trigonal Model of supervision in Communication Disorders is composed of Constituents, Concepts, and Contexts.*
- *The Constituents, Concepts, and Contexts components combined with the Professional, Research, Education, Administration, and Clinical domains form the Pentagonal Model of supervision in Communication Disorders.*
- *An operational definition of supervision in Communication Disorders has evolved from the 50-year developmental process.*

OUTLINE

INTRODUCTION
HISTORY
ASSUMPTIONS
DEFINITION
SUMMARY
APPLICATIONS

INTRODUCTION

Supervision in Communication Disorders has come of age. After more than half a century, the concept of supervision has developed to the point where it commands serious attention. The intent of this chapter is threefold: first, to summarize the major historic milestones of supervision in Communication Disorders (Speech-Language Pathology and Audiology); second, to present eight assumptions about supervision that have evolved from the past 50 years of study; and third, to provide an operational definition of supervision that forms a philosophical, theoretical, and conceptual framework for studying the phenomenon.

HISTORY

The Communication Disorders profession relies heavily on information about human growth (an increase in size) and development (an increase in complexity). The familiar stages of human growth and development can be used as a metaphor for the historical maturation of supervision in Communication Disorders. Figure 1–1 plots the stages and major events of supervision growth and development.

The field of Communication Disorders emerged in the early 1900s primarily from two sources, medical and educational. The people who were first interested in impaired communication were members of the National Association of the Teachers of Speech (NATS). On December 19, 1925, eleven people created a subgroup of NATS called the American Academy of Speech Correction. In 1935, the *Journal of Speech Disorders* was first published. In 1947, the name of the organization was changed to the American Speech and Hearing Association and the journal title was changed to *Journal of Speech and Hearing Disorders* shortly thereafter. The present name of the organization, the American Speech-Language-Hearing Associa-

This chapter was contributed by Stephen S. Farmer, New Mexico State University.

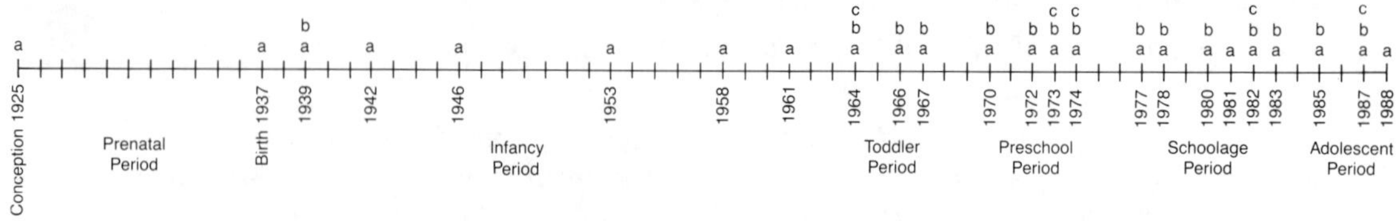

SUPERVISION IN COMMUNICATION DISORDERS: AN OVERVIEW

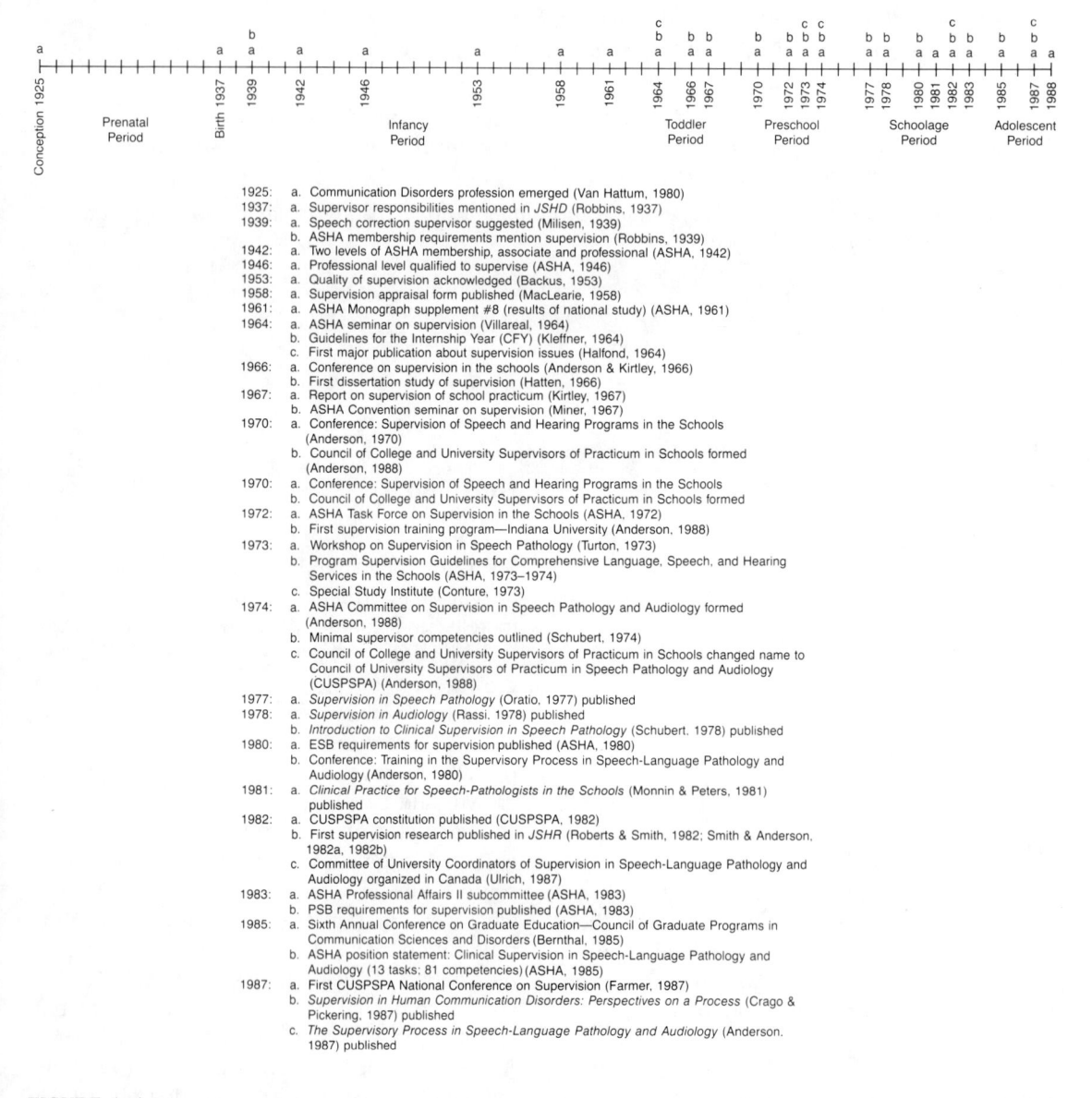

1925: a. Communication Disorders profession emerged (Van Hattum, 1980)
1937: a. Supervisor responsibilities mentioned in *JSHD* (Robbins, 1937)
1939: a. Speech correction supervisor suggested (Milisen, 1939)
b. ASHA membership requirements mention supervision (Robbins, 1939)
1942: a. Two levels of ASHA membership, associate and professional (ASHA, 1942)
1946: a. Professional level qualified to supervise (ASHA, 1946)
1953: a. Quality of supervision acknowledged (Backus, 1953)
1958: a. Supervision appraisal form published (MacLearie, 1958)
1961: a. ASHA Monograph supplement #8 (results of national study) (ASHA, 1961)
1964: a. ASHA seminar on supervision (Villareal, 1964)
b. Guidelines for the Internship Year (CFY) (Kleffner, 1964)
c. First major publication about supervision issues (Halfond, 1964)
1966: a. Conference on supervision in the schools (Anderson & Kirtley, 1966)
b. First dissertation study of supervision (Hatten, 1966)
1967: a. Report on supervision of school practicum (Kirtley, 1967)
b. ASHA Convention seminar on supervision (Miner, 1967)
1970: a. Conference: Supervision of Speech and Hearing Programs in the Schools (Anderson, 1970)
b. Council of College and University Supervisors of Practicum in Schools formed (Anderson, 1988)
1970: a. Conference: Supervision of Speech and Hearing Programs in the Schools
b. Council of College and University Supervisors of Practicum in Schools formed
1972: a. ASHA Task Force on Supervision in the Schools (ASHA, 1972)
b. First supervision training program—Indiana University (Anderson, 1988)
1973: a. Workshop on Supervision in Speech Pathology (Turton, 1973)
b. Program Supervision Guidelines for Comprehensive Language, Speech, and Hearing Services in the Schools (ASHA, 1973–1974)
c. Special Study Institute (Conture, 1973)
1974: a. ASHA Committee on Supervision in Speech Pathology and Audiology formed (Anderson, 1988)
b. Minimal supervisor competencies outlined (Schubert, 1974)
c. Council of College and University Supervisors of Practicum in Schools changed name to Council of University Supervisors of Practicum in Speech Pathology and Audiology (CUSPSPA) (Anderson, 1988)
1977: a. *Supervision in Speech Pathology* (Oratio, 1977) published
1978: a. *Supervision in Audiology* (Rassi, 1978) published
b. *Introduction to Clinical Supervision in Speech Pathology* (Schubert, 1978) published
1980: a. ESB requirements for supervision published (ASHA, 1980)
b. Conference: Training in the Supervisory Process in Speech-Language Pathology and Audiology (Anderson, 1980)
1981: a. *Clinical Practice for Speech-Pathologists in the Schools* (Monnin & Peters, 1981) published
1982: a. CUSPSPA constitution published (CUSPSPA, 1982)
b. First supervision research published in *JSHR* (Roberts & Smith, 1982; Smith & Anderson, 1982a, 1982b)
c. Committee of University Coordinators of Supervision in Speech-Language Pathology and Audiology organized in Canada (Ulrich, 1987)
1983: a. ASHA Professional Affairs II subcommittee (ASHA, 1983)
b. PSB requirements for supervision published (ASHA, 1983)
1985: a. Sixth Annual Conference on Graduate Education—Council of Graduate Programs in Communication Sciences and Disorders (Bernthal, 1985)
b. ASHA position statement: Clinical Supervision in Speech-Language Pathology and Audiology (13 tasks; 81 competencies) (ASHA, 1985)
1987: a. First CUSPSPA National Conference on Supervision (Farmer, 1987)
b. *Supervision in Human Communication Disorders: Perspectives on a Process* (Crago & Pickering, 1987) published
c. *The Supervisory Process in Speech-Language Pathology and Audiology* (Anderson, 1987) published

FIGURE 1–1
Developmental timeline of supervision in Communication Disorders

tion, was adopted in 1978, but the acronym ASHA was retained (Van Hattum, 1980).

Since the beginning of the profession, its members have recognized the need for clinical practice. Inherent in that recognition was the sense of a need for someone to oversee the work of novice clinicians, although the terms *supervision* and *supervisor* were not used and guidelines for supervision consequently did not exist. As Figure 1–1 shows, supervision was "conceived" as an integral part of Communication Disorders, which became established as an ancillary health profession in 1925. After a 12-year prenatal period, supervision's "birth" was recorded in the *Journal of Speech and Hearing Disorders* (Robbins, 1937). According to Anderson (1988), the word *supervisor* first appeared in a Senate bill that would have authorized the U.S. Commissioner of Education to provide money to states for educating the physically handicapped (including the communicatively disordered) and to develop the qualifications of "teachers, supervisors, and directors . . . thus assuring adequately trained teachers for physically handicapped children" (Robbins, 1937, p. 34). The bill did not pass. During the succeeding 27-year "infancy" period of supervision, the following milestones occurred.

Milisen (1939) suggested that a "speech correction supervisor" might train and monitor classroom teachers to provide help to students with speech problems. Also in 1939, ASHA membership required "active, present participation in actual clinical work in speech correction or in administrative duties immediately concerned with the supervision and direction of such work" (Robbins, 1939, p. 78).

In 1942, ASHA defined two levels of membership, associate and professional. The professional members were credited with the ability to "instruct" others in the art and science of Speech Pathology and Audiology. In 1946, the membership guidelines specifically stated that professional members were considered "qualified to supervise others in the correction of defects" (ASHA, 1946, p. 55).

Backus (1953) asserted that more attention needed to be paid to supervising clinical work and to the qualifications of those doing the supervision. MacLearie (1958) stated that improvements in Communication Disorders programming in the schools must come primarily from the improvement of clinicians and that clinician improvement grew from supervision. To formalize that stand, she published an assessment tool for speech and hearing personnel, to be used by supervisors and administrators.

In 1961, a nationwide study of speech and hearing services in the schools raised concern about the content and supervision of clinical practicum in university training programs (ASHA, 1961).

Supervision entered the "toddler" period in 1964 through an ASHA seminar that recognized supervision as a viable entity (Villareal, 1964). In the same year, guidelines for the Clinical Fellowship Year (CFY) were reported by Kleffner (1964); they included supervision requirements. Kleffner argued that supervision must be an ongoing part of any comprehensive clinical service program. Also during this year, the first major article devoted to issues of supervision was published (Halfond, 1964). Halfond argued for the importance of supervision, stating that "supervision, which serves in the transition from academic proficiency to professional application, is either downgraded or neglected. There is evidence that supervision is a stepchild of the educative process" (p. 441).

Conferences and seminars in supervision were held in the 1960s (Anderson & Kirtley, 1966; Kirtley, 1967; Miner, 1967). The first dissertation study of supervision was completed (Hatten, 1967). In addition, the Research Committee of the California Speech and Hearing Association conducted the first major research study of supervision (Flower, 1969; Rees & Smith, 1967, 1968).

Although many consider supervision in Communication Disorders to have been delayed in development, the delay ceased in 1970, and healthy growth and development ensued during the "preschool" years; supervision events began to increase in number and sophistication and so did supervisors. During the first half of the 1970s three conferences on supervision were held and their proceedings published (Anderson, 1970; Conture, 1973; Turton, 1973). A peer group for supervisors (the Council of College and University Supervisors of Practicum in Schools) was established. An ASHA task force on supervision in schools (ASHA, 1972) created the *Program Supervision Guidelines for Comprehensive Language, Speech, and Hearing Services in the Schools* (ASHA 1973–1974). The first supervisor training program was integrated into a Communication Disorders program at Indiana University. Minimal competencies for supervisors were suggested (Schubert, 1974), and the ASHA Committee on Supervision in Speech-Language Pathology and Audiology was formed.

The "school-age" period (1977–1983) brought supervision into an age of literacy and formal operations. Three supervision textbooks in Speech-Language Pathology (Monnin & Peters, 1981; Oratio, 1977; Schubert, 1978) and one in Audiology (Rassi, 1978) were published. The first published supervision research appeared in the *Journal of Speech and Hearing Research* (Roberts & Smith, 1982; Smith & Anderson, 1982a, 1982b). Also during this 6-year period, the ASHA Educational Services Board (ESB) and Professional Services Board (PSB) requirements validated the need for supervision in training and professional service programs. Supervisors expanded their peer group, whose name had changed in 1974 to Council of University Supervisors of Practicum in Speech Pathology and Audiology (CUSPSPA), and ratified a constitution. The newly developed ASHA Professional Affairs II subcommittee, which selects proposals to be presented at annual ASHA conventions, allowed supervision to be more visible professionally at a national level. In 1982, the Committee of University Coordinators of Supervision in Speech-Language Pathology and Audiology was formed by members of the Canadian Association of Speech-Language Pathologists and Audiologists (CASLPA), thus moving Communication Disorders supervision to an international level (Ulrich, 1987).

In human growth and development, the period of puberty or adolescence is a time of major change requiring revisions in management. Such a period came, too, for supervision. In 1985, a majority of the Sixth Annual Conference on Graduate Education in Communication Sciences and Disorders programs was devoted to the past, present, and projected status of supervision (Bernthal, 1985). Perhaps the two events that mark the maturity of supervision in Communication Disorders are the first national conference on supervision sponsored by CUSPSPA (Farmer, 1987) and the list of 13 tasks and 81 competencies developed by the ASHA Committee on Supervision in Speech-Language Pathology and Audiology and published in *Asha* in 1985 (see appendix A).

The growth and development of supervision in Communication Disorders is obvious from the timeline, from the changes documented in two books, *Supervision in Human Communication Disorders: Perspectives on a Process* (Crago & Pickering, 1987) and *The Supervisory Process in Speech-Language Pathology and Audiology* (Anderson, 1988), and from the information contained in this text.

If the analogy to human growth and development is accurate, and supervision in Communication Disorders has come of age, then certain predictions can be made about future changes. As Ulrich (1987) stated in her closing remarks at the first CUSPSPA-sponsored national conference on supervision,

> Supervision in Human Communication Disorders will assert its uniqueness as a specialty area. It will seek, discard, modify, and adapt the thinking of others and will generate ideas of its own. It will move from a position of dependence on its progenitors, both within and outside the profession, to one of looking to its peer groups across disciplines for substantial portions of nurturing and validation. It will become socialized within the institutional and organizational structures where it exists. And it will mature from a largely egocentric beginning to a stage in which it contributes to others and demonstrates its competence to self-analyze and self-direct. (p. 238)

Using the knowledge gleaned during the 50-year developmental history of supervision in Communication Disorders, we have formulated eight assumptions to be used as focal points for this text.

ASSUMPTIONS

Assumption 1: Supervision in Communication Disorders is necessary.

To assure quality service to the communication impaired population, a number of regulating and accrediting bodies have set standards that include aspects of supervision. ASHA emphasizes the importance of supervision in two ways. First, it requires supervision in the initial training of speech-language pathologists and audiologists and later during the Clinical Fellowship Year (CFY) as one step toward attaining the Certificate of Clinical Competence (CCC) (ASHA, 1982). Second, the ASHA Council on Professional Standards has adopted supervision requirements in its standards and guidelines for both educational and professional services programs (ASHA, 1980, 1983). In addition to ASHA, other organizations emphasize the need for supervision. Laws regulating state licensing and school certification consistently specify the need for supervision of practicum experiences and of initial work performance. Finally, accrediting and regulating bodies such as the Joint Commission on Accreditation of Hospitals (JCAH) and the Commission on Accreditation of Rehabilitation Facilities (CARF) require a system of continuous supervision throughout professional careers.

Assumption 2: Supervision in Communication Disorders has three components—*Constituents, Concepts,* and *Contexts*—that form the theoretical *Trigonal Model.*

The *Constituents* component of the Trigonal Model of Communication Disorders supervision includes the *people* involved in the supervision process: supervisors, supervisees, clients/patients, families/primary caregivers/significant others, and ancillary personnel. (The Constituents component is described in chapter 2.)

The *Concepts* component is made up of the *ideas* being explored to define various aspects and structures of supervision. From the literature, we have identified many topics as contributing substantially to the developing identity of supervision. (The salient topics are discussed in chapter 3.)

The *Contexts* component involves the *sites* where supervision takes place. Five broad categories of context are college and university training programs; schools (public, private, institutional); medical settings (hospitals, extended care facilities, nursing homes, rehabilitation centers); community speech, language, and hearing centers; and businesses (private practices, hearing aid dealerships, contractual agencies). (The Contexts of supervision are explored in detail in chapter 4.)

The Constituents, Concepts, and Contexts components juxtapose to form the *Trigonal Model* of Communication Disorders supervision, shown in Figure 1–2.

Assumption 3: Supervision in Communication Disorders includes five domains: *Professional, Research, Educational, Administrative, Clinical.*

A major step in understanding Communication Disorders supervision has been the identification of multiple domains in which supervisors are involved (Farmer, 1985). Supervisors must function actively in as many as five different roles. The *Professional* role involves participation in professional groups, whether disciplinary

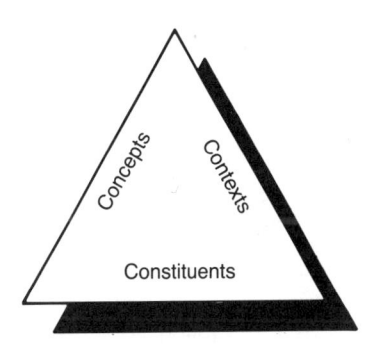

FIGURE 1–2
The Trigonal Model of Communication Disorders supervision

(Speech-Language Pathology and/or Audiology) or supervision-related organizations such as ASHA, CUSPSPA, or state, regional, and local groups.

The *Researcher* role includes applying methods of inquiry to the clinical and/or supervision processes; disseminating, interpreting, evaluating, and applying results; and encouraging colleagues and supervisees to participate in research at some level.

The *Educator* role is the largest responsibility for most supervisors and consists of work in the academic and/or clinical teaching-learning process. Supervisors help supervisees to develop knowledge and skills in speech-language pathology or audiology in either the classroom or the clinic. Classroom education requires skill in the formal teaching of information to groups of people; clinical education is often more informal and more interpersonal. Supervisors teach about diagnostic and therapeutic methods, materials, and equipment; communication competence, critical observation, clinical literacy, decision making, and creative problem managing. A supervisor may function as a "master clinician" and teach supervisees by modeling clinical work. The role of Educator also includes evaluating and grading student or personnel performance.

The *Administrator* role brings a variety of tasks associated with program management, such as program development, monitoring, maintenance, and evaluation; and personnel employment, evaluation, and termination.

The *Clinician* role includes the assessment, treatment, and case management of clients (a personal caseload). The role of Clinician in this domain differs from the educational role of "master clinician" in that its purpose does not include teaching supervisees about the clinical process; the sole purpose is service delivery.

Combining the Trigonal Model with the five domains produces the *Pentagonal Model* of Communication Disorders supervision (see Figure 1–3).

Assumption 4: Supervision in Communication Disorders is a process.

Supervision consists of a series of actions or operations marked by gradual, continuous, transacted changes that lead to particular results.

Assumption 5: Supervision in Communication Disorders is an art and a science.

An *art* is an activity in which knowledge is applied creatively using a complex of skills of perception and judgment that can be refined with practice. A *science* is any skill that reflects a precise application of facts or principles (*Random House College Dictionary*, rev. ed.). Because communication and management require creative application of knowledge and the use of skills that are continually refined, supervision, which is management through communication, is by definition art. The application of facts or principles from areas such as computer science, education, electronics, mathematics, physics, psychology, and statistical and natural inquiry qualifies supervision as a science. Our understanding of supervision as a process comes from recognizing the evolutionary nature of art and science.

Assumption 6: Supervision in Communication Disorders will change.

Supervision is an evolutionary process. Some of what is known and believed about supervision today will be rethought tomorrow. Supervisors are expected to do the best job possible at the time, and most people involved in the supervision process are comfortable knowing that supervision is less fully developed than it can become. In time, through continued experience and research, supervision will evolve into more and more mature forms.

Assumption 7: Competency standards for supervision exist, and supervisors should receive training to develop competence.

FIGURE 1-3
The Pentagonal Model of Communication Disorders supervision

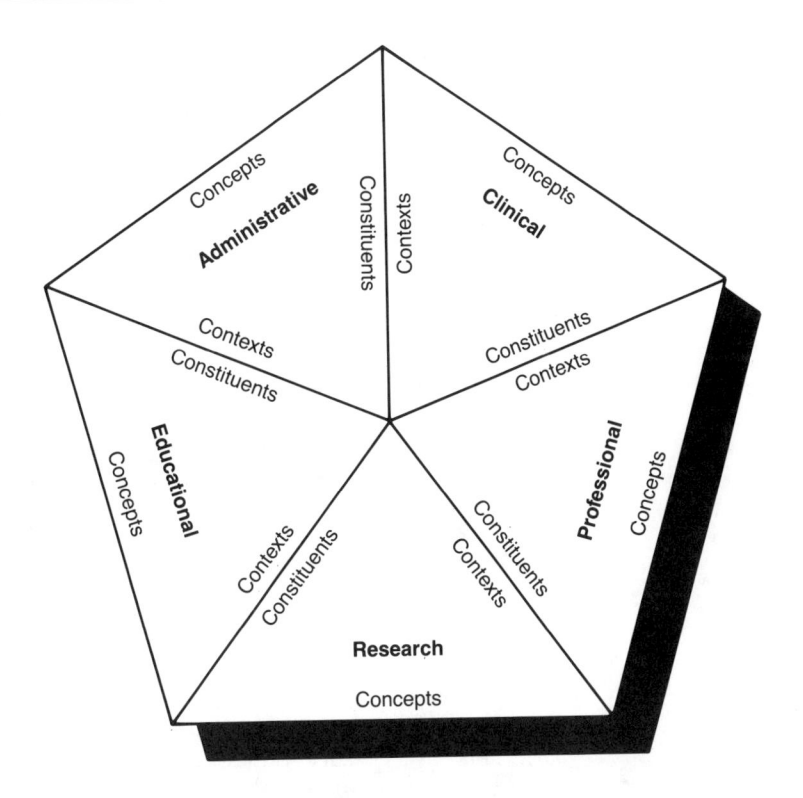

The ASHA Committee on Supervision listed 13 tasks and 81 competencies as guidelines for training and evaluating supervisors (ASHA, 1985). The competencies can be acquired through academic training, continuing education, or research activities.

Assumption 8: Supervision is a specialty area within the Communication Disorders profession.

Supervision in Communication Disorders is a special area requiring competencies that differ from, but complement, the clinical competencies for which all speech-language pathologists and audiologists receive training. The additional training supervisors need should be recognized as constituting a special branch of the Communication Disorders profession adaptable equally to Speech-Language Pathology and to Audiology.

The eight assumptions integrate salient information from half a century of supervision experience and research in Communication Disorders. They culminate in the operational definition used in this text.

DEFINITION

Supervision in Communication Disorders is a necessary, artistic/scientific, and changing process composed of three *components* (Constituents, Concepts, and Contexts) that function in the Professional, Research, Educational, Administrative, and Clinical *domains* of Speech-Language Pathology and Audiology to assure initial and continuing training of competent professionals who can provide quality services for education or health care consumers. Supervisors, who are specialists in the Communication Disorders profession, require training to meet the standards of quality set by the ASHA Committee on Supervision.

SUMMARY

Supervision in Communication Disorders has over 50 years of history. Through stages of growth and development, supervision has come of age. It has evolved to the point where our knowledge can be synthesized into eight assumptions, the scaffolding for the remainder of this text. Supervision in Communication Disorders

- is necessary.
- has three components: Constituents, Concepts, and Contexts.
- includes five domains: Professional, Research, Educational, Administrative, and Clinical.
- is a process.
- is an art and a science.
- will change.
- is guided by competencies that require training.
- is a specialty area of the Communication Disorders profession.

Supervisors are proud of the growth and development of supervision in Communication Disorders to this point but recognize the need and have the desire to facilitate its future evolution.

APPLICATIONS

Discussion Topics

1. Discuss the assumption that supervision in Communication Disorders is necessary. Should accrediting agencies set specific supervision standards?
2. Discuss the assumption that supervision in Communication Disorders is made up of three components: Constituents, Concepts, and Contexts.
3. Discuss the assumption that supervision in Communication Disorders occurs in five domains: Professional, Research, Educational, Administrative, and Clinical. As a supervisor, how many of these domains do you work in? As a supervisee, do you see your supervisors operating in the different domains?
4. Discuss the assumption that supervision in Communication Disorders is evolving and will have changed 5 years from now.
5. Discuss the assumption that supervision is a blend of art and science. What concrete conceptualizations of supervision are possible other than the Trigonal and Pentagonal Models?

Laboratory Experiences

1. Illustrate or dramatize the concept of Communication Disorders supervision as a scientific art form.
2. Illustrate or demonstrate the definition of Communication Disorders supervision presented in this chapter.

3. Develop a set of requirements for specialty certification in Communication Disorders supervision.

4. Using the competencies for supervision (see appendix A), list competencies for supervisees. Are they interchangeable?

5. Develop a speech for the board of directors of your community speech, language, and hearing center that will demonstrate the need for the supervision staff to be trained in the supervisory process. Propose a plan for having all supervisors trained within a 2-year period.

Research Projects

1. Develop an in-depth oral or written history of supervision in Communication Disorders.

2. Design a study to provide empirical data that could support or refute the assumption that supervision makes a difference.

3. Design a study to validate the 13 tasks and accompanying competencies (see appendix A).

4. Develop a videotape to recruit personnel into Communication Disorders supervision.

5. Write a proposal for a paper to explore some aspect of Communication Disorders supervision discussed in chapter 1. Put the proposal into a format that would be appropriate to submit for presentation at an ASHA convention.

REFERENCES

American Speech and Hearing Association. (1946). Membership requirements. *Journal of Speech and Hearing Disorders, 11,* 54–55.

American Speech and Hearing Association. (1961). Public school speech and hearing services (S. Darley, Ed.). *Journal of Speech and Hearing Disorders* Monograph Supplement 8.

American Speech and Hearing Association. (1972). Supervision in the schools. Report of task force on supervision. *Language, Speech, and Hearing Services in the Schools, 3,* 4–10.

American Speech and Hearing Association. (1973–1974). *Program Supervision Guidelines for Comprehensive Language, Speech, and Hearing Programs in the Schools* (pp. 6–8). Washington, DC: Author.

American Speech-Language-Hearing Association. (1980). *Standards for accreditation by the Education and Training Board.* Rockville, MD: Author.

American Speech-Language-Hearing Association. (1982). *Requirements for the certificates of clinical competence* (rev. ed.). Rockville, MD: Author.

American Speech-Language-Hearing Association. (1983). New standards for accreditation by the Professional Services Board. *Asha, 6,* 51–58.

American Speech-Language-Hearing Association. (1985). Committee on Supervision of Speech-Language Pathology & Audiology. Clinical supervision in speech-language pathology and audiology (position statement). *Asha, 27,* 57–60.

Anderson, J. (Ed.). (1970). *Conference on supervision of speech and hearing programs in the schools.* Bloomington: Indiana University Press.

Anderson, J. (1988). *The supervisory process in speech-language pathology and audiology.* Boston: Little, Brown/College-Hill Press.

Anderson, J., & Kirtley, D. (Eds.). (1966). *Institute on Supervision of Speech and Hearing Programs in the Public Schools.* Indianapolis, IN: Department of Public Instruction.

Backus, O. (1953). Letter to the editor. *Journal of Speech and Hearing Disorders, 18,* 193–203.

Bernthal, J. (Ed.). (1985). *Proceedings of the Sixth Annual Conference on Graduate Education.* Lincoln: University of Nebraska, Department of Special Education and Communication Disorders.

Conture, E. (1973). *Special study institute: Management and supervision of programs for speech and hearing handicapped.* Syracuse, NY: Syracuse University.

Crago, M., & Pickering, M. (Eds.). (1987). *Supervision in human communication disorders: Perspectives on a process.* Boston: Little, Brown/College-Hill Press.

Farmer, S. (1985, November). *Supervision in communicative disorders: Metalinguistic analysis of assumptions and predictions. Phase I.* Paper presented at the annual convention of the American Speech-Language-Hearing Association, Washington, DC.

Farmer, S. (Ed.). (1987). *Clinical supervision: A coming of age. Proceedings of a national conference on supervision.* Las Cruces: New Mexico State University.

Flower, R. (Ed.). (1969). *Conference on standards for supervised experience for speech and hearing specialists in public schools.* Los Angeles, CA: Department of Education.

Halfond, M. (1964). Clinical supervision: Stepchild in training. *Asha, 6,* 441–444.

Hatten, J. (1966). A descriptive and analytic investigation of speech therapy supervisors-therapist conferences. *Dissertation Abstracts International, 26,* 5595–5596. (University Microfilms No. 71-18, 014)

Kirtley, D. (Ed.). (1967). *Supervision of student teaching in speech and hearing therapy.* Indianapolis, IN: Department of Public Instruction.

Kleffner, F. (Ed.). (1964). *Seminar on guidelines for the internship year.* Washington, DC: American Speech and Hearing Association.

MacLearie, E. (1958). Appraisal form for speech and hearing therapists. *Journal of Speech Disorders, 12,* 612–614.

Milisen, R. (1939). Speech correction in the schools. *Journal of Speech Disorders, 4,* 241–245.

Miner, A. (1967). A symposium: Improving supervision of clinical practicum. *Asha, 9,* 471–482.

Monnin, L., & Peters, K. (1981). *Clinical practice for speech pathologists in the schools.* Springfield, IL: Charles C. Thomas.

Oratio, A. (1977). *Supervision in speech pathology.* Baltimore, MD: University Park Press.

Rassi, J. (1978). *Supervision in audiology*. Baltimore, MD: University Park Press.

Rees, M., & Smith, J. (1967). Supervised school experience for student clinicians. *Asha, 9,* 251–257.

Rees, M., & Smith, J. (1968). Some recommendations for supervised school experience for student clinicians. *Asha, 10,* 93–103.

Robbins, S. (1937). Federal aid for speech defectives near. *Journal of Speech and Hearing Disorders, 2,* 78.

Robbins, S. (1939). Changes in election of new members. *Journal of Speech Disorders, 4,* 78.

Roberts, J., & Smith, K. (1982). Supervisor-supervisee role differences and consistency of behavior in supervisory conferences. *Journal of Speech and Hearing Research, 25,* 428–434.

Schubert, G. (1974). Suggested minimum requirements for clinical supervisors. *Asha, 16,* 10.

Schubert, G. (1978). *Introduction to clinical supervision in speech pathology*. St. Louis: Warren H. Green.

Smith, K., & Anderson, J. (1982a). Development and validation of an individual supervisory conference rating scale for use in speech-language pathology. *Journal of Speech and Hearing Research, 25,* 252–261.

Smith, K., & Anderson, J. (1982b). Relationship of perceived effectiveness to content in supervisory conferences in speech-language pathology. *Journal of Speech and Hearing Research, 25,* 243–251.

Turton, L. (Ed.). (1973). *Proceedings of a workshop on supervision in speech pathology*. Ann Arbor: University of Michigan, Institute for the Study of Mental Retardation and Related Disabilities.

Ulrich, S. (1987). Coming of age: The future of supervision. In S. Farmer (Ed.), *Clinical supervision: A coming of age. Proceedings of a national conference on supervision* (pp. 237–238). Las Cruces: New Mexico State University.

Van Hattum, R. (Ed.). (1980). *Communication disorders*. New York: Macmillan.

Villareal, J. (Ed.). (1964). *Seminar on guidelines for supervision in clinical practicum*. Washington, DC: American Speech and Hearing Association.

PART TWO
Composition of the Supervision Process

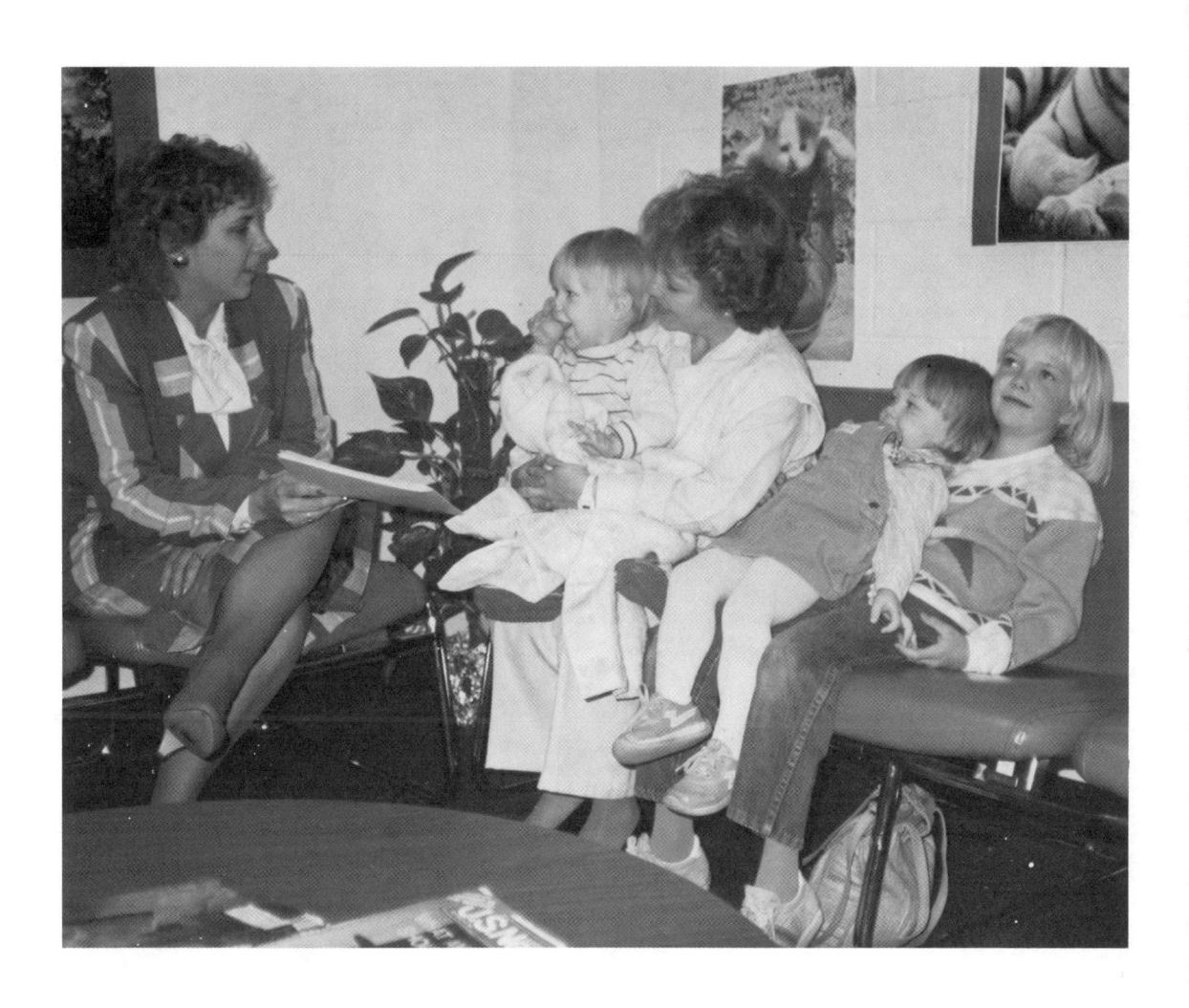

2
The Trigonal Model of Communication Disorders Supervision: Constituents

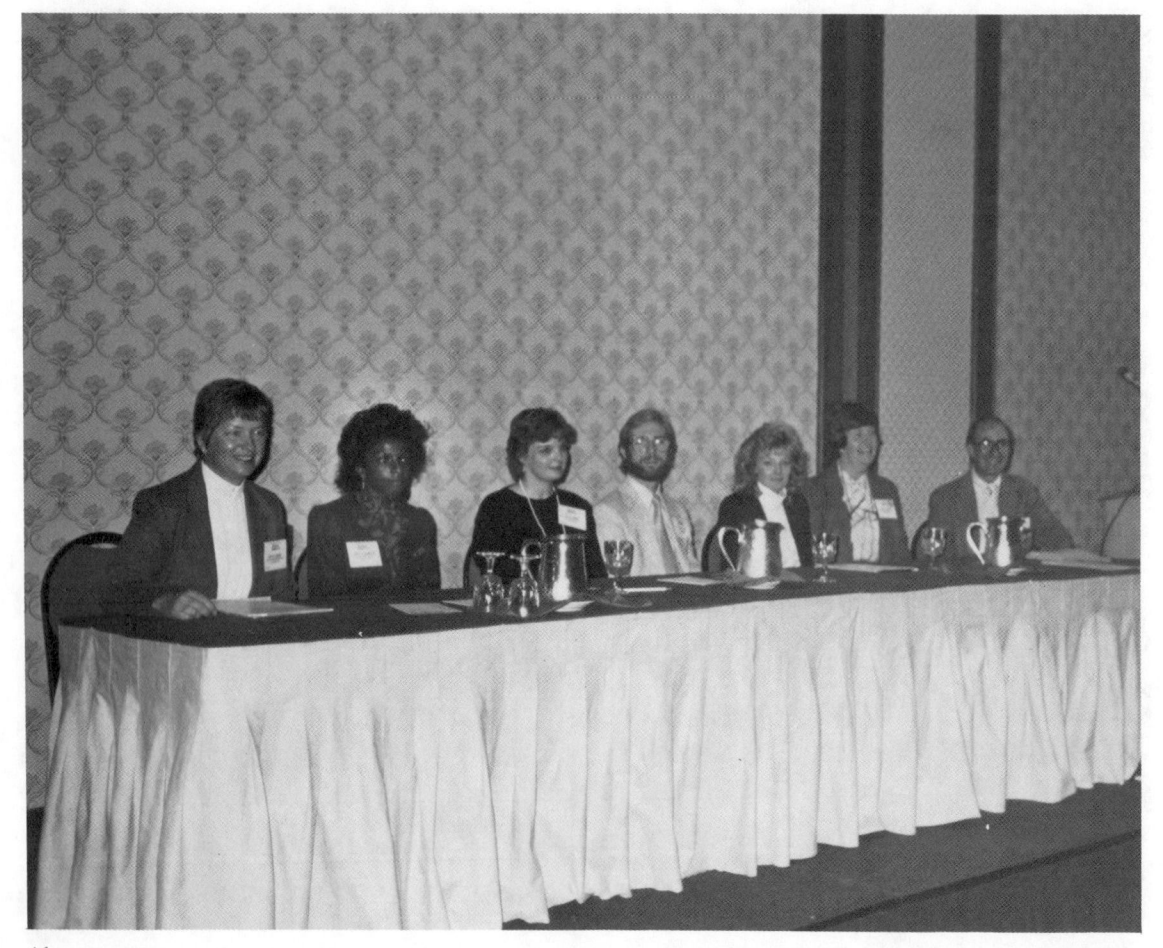

CRITICAL CONCEPTS

- ☐ Four groups of people are involved in the supervision process.
- ☐ Supervisors operate in five domains and develop five corresponding roles.
- ☐ Supervisors are classified in four ways.
- ☐ Guidelines for supervisor competence are emerging.
- ☐ Constituents need preparation to participate in the supervision process.

OUTLINE

INTRODUCTION
SUPERVISORS
    Demographics
    CUSPSPA
    Roles
    Classifications
    Supervisor Competence
    Education and Training in Supervision
    Career Development
    Stress and Burnout
SUPERVISEES
    Types
    Levels
    Differential Supervision
OTHERS
    Clients/Patients
    Other Constituents
SUMMARY
APPLICATIONS

INTRODUCTION

The premise of this textbook is that supervision training programs and continuing education planners need guidelines for designing courses to prepare speech-language pathologists and audiologists for supervision. Chapters 2, 3, and 4 discuss in detail topics that should be included in such supervision preparation.

The Trigonal Model of Communication Disorders supervision offered in chapter 1 is composed of Constituents, Concepts, and Contexts. In the next three chapters, the components are presented as separate entities (i.e., as individual sides of a triangle). In reality, they form a single, collective unit of interconnecting components, just as the triangle is a unit whose structure is formed by the sides when they connect.

Because supervision is a human endeavor, it is logical to begin part II by discussing the people who may be involved in the supervision process. These Constituents include supervisors, supervisees, clients or patients, their families and significant others, and ancillary personnel.

SUPERVISORS

The generic term *supervisor* does not in itself describe the person who holds such a title. Therefore, the ensuing paragraphs provide

---

This chapter was contributed by Stephen S. Farmer, New Mexico State University.

descriptive information, specific to the field of Communication Disorders, about supervisor demographics, competence, training, responsibilities and roles, classifications, career development, stress, and burnout.

Demographics

Supervisors in the profession cluster into at least three groups: (a) supervisors of undergraduate and graduate students in speech-language pathology and audiology, (b) supervisors of clinical peers or colleagues, and (c) supervisor trainees. Some demographic data exist to help describe supervisors. In 1988, it was reported that approximately 4.2% of the 50,000 members of ASHA devote the major part of their work to activities associated with supervision (Shewan, 1988). Of these supervisors, the large majority are women who hold master's degrees and who have had no formal training in the supervisory process. The majority of supervisors work in school settings. The second largest percentage supervise in college or university training programs. The third largest supervise in nonuniversity clinical settings such as hospitals, rehabilitation centers, and community speech and hearing centers. As summarized by Anderson (1987), all the surveys that have been done suggest a need for additional, qualified supervisors.

Supervisors have a professional organization of colleagues, the Council of University Supervisors of Practicum in Speech-Language Pathology and Audiology (CUSPSPA).

CUSPSPA

In 1970, the Council of College and University Supervisors of Practicum in the Schools was founded to bring together those interested in supervision within school programs. Later the organization changed its name to the Council of University Supervisors of Practicum in Speech-Language Pathology and Audiology (CUSPSPA), thereby allowing a broader cadre of individuals to become involved. In 1982, the CUSPSPA Constitution was adopted (CUSPSPA, 1982). The document (pp. 8-10) lists as the organization's purposes:

1. To promote cooperation among persons engaged in supervision of students dealing with communication disorders (Speech-Language Pathology and Audiology) as exemplified in educational, clinical, and rehabilitation settings.
2. To support and promote the development of adequacy of supervision of practicum.
3. To encourage and implement standards for practicum and practicum supervision.
4. To encourage research and innovation in the process of supervision.
5. To stimulate the exchange and dissemination of information among those engaged in practicum supervision.

To help unify supervisors all over the country into a functioning unit, SUPERNET (Supervision of University Practicum: Education and Research NETwork) was created as a way for members of CUSPSPA to pool their expertise and interest to meet the needs of supervisors in all geographic locations and workplaces.

The strongest link among CUSPSPA members is *SUPERvision*, a quarterly digest that is a forum for the exchange of ideas, concerns, and issues about supervision. A high priority of CUSPSPA and SUPERNET members has been to address the issues involved in training supervisors.

CUSPSPA continues to grow annually. During 1987, CUSPSPA registered 312 members, 270 women and 42 men; it adds 15 to 25 new members each year. Of the female members, 75% hold master's degrees and 20% hold doctorates, whereas 54% of the males hold doctorates and 45% have master's degrees (Langellier & Natalle, 1987). As it grows, CUSPSPA continues to develop a more complete understanding of what supervisors in Communication Disorders do. For example, research has found that supervisors in Communication Disorders work within five roles (Farmer, 1985).

According to Ulrich (1987), supervision within

Canada is reflected in national, provincial, and regional activities of the Committee of University Coordinators of Supervision in Speech-Language Pathology and Audiology, a related committee of the Canadian Association of Speech-Language Pathologists and Audiologists (CASLPA). Canadian supervision publications are disseminated primarily through CASLPA's publication *Human Communication Canada*. Supervision topics are presented at CASLPA conventions.

Roles

Supervisors in Communication Disorders are active to different degrees in five roles, which can be remembered by the acronym PREAC: Professional, Researcher, Educator (academic and clinical), Administrator, and Clinician. Supervisors become competent to work in the roles that are germane to their specific job descriptions.

Professional. The Professional role requires having the desire, competence, and dedication necessary to participate in disciplinary (Speech-Language Pathology and/or Audiology) or supervision-related organizations such as ASHA, CUSPSPA, and state, regional, and local groups. Rassi (1987) suggested that one way to demonstrate the importance of the Professional role is by comparing the benefits of CUSPSPA service with the 13 tasks of supervision put forth by the ASHA Committee on Supervision (ASHA, 1985). (See appendix A.) Through minor editing and slight shifts of reference. Rassi (pp. 2-3) revised the tasks in this way:

1. Establishing and maintaining an effective working relationship with others.
2. Assisting others in developing goals and objectives.
3. Assisting others in developing and refining problem assessment skills.
4. Assisting others in developing and refining group management skills.
5. Demonstrating for and participating with others in the organizational process.
6. Assisting others in observing and analyzing meetings and planning sessions.
7. Assisting others in the development and maintenance of the organization's records.
8. Interacting with others in planning, executing, and analyzing group conferences.
9. Assisting others in self-evaluation of performance.
10. Assisting others in applying skills of verbal reporting and writing for the purpose of disseminating information.
11. Sharing information regarding political, regulatory, and institutional aspects of the profession as they relate to supervision.
12. Modeling and facilitating professional-group conduct.
13. Promoting research in the clinical and supervisory processes.

It can be said that a profession is only as vital as its governing organization. If this is so, supervision organizations must have active participants and guidelines to direct their growth. CUSPSPA, for example, has broadened its membership to include supervisors who are not affiliated with university programs but are still active and interested in supervision. Rassi's revised tasks have the latitude necessary for developing professionals in that population; ASHA, Communication Disorders training programs, and worksites should provide the incentive for supervisors to join supervision organizations.

Researcher. Although some supervisors may have had opportunities to conduct, critique, apply, and disseminate research during their clinical training, few have participated in research as supervisors. Perhaps this role has not been stressed enough in the past because of the strong emphasis on the supervisor's role as clinical educator. Some supervisors, too, may have research expertise but may not be able to use it because of time constraints or lack of administrative support. Until the Researcher role is established as an integral part of the Communication Disorders supervisor's employment responsibilities, and is understood as such by supervisors and employers, needed research will remain unconducted, and what does emerge will come from the core of individual supervisors (usually university affiliates) who already include research in their supervision profile.

Educator. The Educator role has been predominant throughout the history of Communication Disorders supervision. However, preparation for it has been minimal, based on the notion that the only prerequisite for teaching was participation in the clinical process. Two distinct aspects of the Educational domain are now evident: clinical education (i.e., applying classroom knowledge to the clinical process), and academic education (i.e., formal teaching in the classroom). Clinical education occurs when the supervisor demonstrates diagnostic and therapeutic procedures and strategies, observes supervisees in clinical work and then discusses their performance in conferences and in writing. Clinical education generally includes evaluation or grading. To assume that even a master clinician is qualified to perform the tasks of clinical education for diverse groups of supervisees without further training does not seem reasonable. Therefore, supervisors must prepare to be clinical educators so that future speech-language pathologists and audiologists will be supervised well. A parallel case can be made for academic instruction: classroom educators need sound theories and techniques to guide their students' learning. Supervision training programs should teach these methods so as to prepare supervisors to teach academic courses.

Administrator. The Administrator role is fast becoming one of the most important of the five. In an attempt to unify overlapping areas of professional service, schools and medical facilities are seeking personnel who are multi-competent. Administrative skill is one of the most useful competencies to add to existing professional preparation. Supervisors often are required to perform the tasks of program management. Therefore, we need to view administration as part of a supervisor's role and prepare supervision personnel to do it effectively. Program management can include such diverse tasks as program development, budget development and maintenance, grant writing and other forms of fund-raising, community public relations, and interviewing, employing, training, monitoring, evaluating, and deploying personnel. These tasks require preparation in areas such as business, management, and communication. Supervision preparation programs, both in universities and in continuing education, must meet this need. ASHA has helped prepare speech-language pathologists and audiologists to fulfill administration duties by developing prototypic management systems. Three such tools that can assist supervisors in program management are the Comprehensive Assessment and Service Evaluation (CASE) system, the Child Services Review System (CSRS), and the Program Planning Evaluation (PPE) system.

The CASE information system (ASHA, 1976) organizes data at two levels: case level and program level. The case level includes the information required to document screening, assessment, placement, and intervention services for individual clients. The program level includes information needed to summarize the nature and scope of all client services, to implement cost analysis, and to complete reports to local, state, or federal agencies. Although developed for the management of children in school programs, CASE can be easily adapted to all types of programs and all age levels.

ASHA developed CSRS in response to the need for quality assurance in school programs (ASHA, 1982; Barnes & Pines, 1982). CASE is primarily an organizing system in program development; CSRS is a client-audit system to ensure that quality services are being delivered. With modifications, CSRS is applicable to adults as well as children, and in all settings.

The PPE was created by Dublinske and Grimes (1971) as a prototype for developing new programs or modifying existing ones. The model contains an ongoing evaluation component, an element critical to the success of program development.

ASHA has sponsored workshops and seminars on these systems, as well as on other areas of program management, during annual directors' conferences. In addition to preparing for the Administrator role in supervision training programs, supervisors who work as administrators could benefit from the directors' conferences.

Clinician. The Clinician role needs minimal discussion; all supervisors have clinical expertise because they hold ASHA certification. Two aspects of a supervisor's clinical role, however, are (a) keeping current with advances in the clinical process, and (b) balancing the requirements of a clinical caseload with the other duties of supervision.

If supervisors devote time, on the job, to learning about the supervision process, the clinical process may be neglected. Supervisors need planning, organization, and management abilities in order to balance multiple roles.

Classifications

Supervisors are referred to by different titles depending on what their jobs involve, who they supervise, and where they do their supervision. The different kinds of supervisor jobs can be classified according to four distinct criteria: (a) whether the supervisor supervises Communication Disorders students or professional clinical staff members, (b) the domains of a supervisor's responsibilities and the percentage of time devoted to each, (c) whether the supervision is intra- or interdisciplinary, and (d) in what context the supervision takes place.

The first classification is based on whether the supervisees are at preservice or service level. *Clinical supervisors* work in college and university training programs where the emphasis is on developing student clinical competence; *staff supervisors* work in service delivery sites where the focus is on monitoring and maintaining professional staff competence.

The categories of *primary supervisor* (who works full-time in clinical education) and *secondary supervisor* (part-time in clinical education and part-time in administration, academic teaching, clinical service delivery, and/or research) make up the second classification, which distinguishes the supervisor working in a single domain from one with multiple responsibilities.

The third type of differentiation is *generic* versus *categorical* supervision. A generic supervisor may be a Communication Disorders professional who supervises staff from other disciplines in addition to speech-language pathologists and audiologists, or else a supervisor from another discipline, such as a Special Education administrator in the schools or a physiatrist in a hospital, who has the responsibility for overseeing the Communication Disorders staff. A categorical supervisor is a speech-language pathologist or audiologist who supervises in the area(s) of his or her ASHA certification.

The last classification defines supervisors in relation to a college or university Communication Disorders training program, and the dichotomy is *on-campus* and *off-campus* (or *field*). The on-campus supervisor (also called a clinical supervisor) works in the training site clinic; the field supervisor is generally employed as a clinician, or a staff supervisor, in another setting such as a school or hospital, but supervises student clinicians who are completing off-campus practicum assignments in affiliation with the college or university Communication Disorders program.

All supervisors, no matter what their classification, need to be competent. It is difficult to know what makes a competent supervisor when supervisors function in such diverse situations.

Supervisor Competence

Although minimal competence requirements for supervisors were suggested in the early 1970s (Schubert, 1974), the Communication Disorders profession continued to operate on the assumption that the skills needed by supervisors are the same as those needed by clinicians. In fact, a report on supervision from the Committee on Supervision of Speech Pathology and Audiology (ASHA, 1978) stated that after acquiring the Certificate of Clinical Competence (CCC), members "are assumed to be qualified not only as a clinician but as a supervisor. In other words, in the eyes of the Association, to be a qualified clinician is also to be a qualified supervisor" (p. 482). However, professionals who have been actively involved in supervision realize that clinical competence and supervision competence are not the same thing. Through diligent study, such professionals have begun to understand the complexities of the supervision process. One result has been a listing of qualifications and competencies for speech-language pathology and audiology supervisors.

A position statement on clinical supervision in speech-language pathology and audiology, the culmination of dedicated work by ASHA's Committee on Supervision in Speech-Language Pathology and Audiology and by the Council on Professional Standards, was published in the May 1985 issue of *Asha*. The document addressed three areas: tasks of supervision, competencies for effective supervision, and preparation of supervisors.

It is still generally accepted that demonstration of quality clinical skills is a prerequisite for supervisors. The committee (ASHA, 1985, p. 59) suggested that beyond clinical proficiency, supervisors could acquire the specific skills and competencies for supervision through special training including, but not limited to:

1. Specific curricular offerings from graduate programs; examples include doctoral programs emphasizing supervision, other postgraduate preparation, and specified graduate courses.
2. Continuing educational experiences specific to the supervisory process (e.g., conferences, workshops, self-study).
3. Research-directed activities that provide insight in the supervisory process.

The position statement lists 13 tasks and defines them more precisely through 81 associated competencies (see appendix A).

Although the tasks of supervision have been defined and the special skills and competencies needed to accomplish them have been identified, some elements of the total supervision process remain unclear.

The first problem relates to the concept of the supervisory competencies, or skills. A skill is a developed or acquired excellence in the performance of technical acts, as measured by some set of performance criteria. But experience has shown that supervision competence requires not only skills but the companion element of *dispositions*. Dispositions are the attributions, or internalized, integrated skills, that summarize the trends of a supervisor's actions in particular contexts; they are summaries of technical act frequencies. Dispositions indicate whether the supervisors actually employ, as a natural part of their professional services, the knowledge and skills that were developed in the training program. The following equation is used to describe supervision competence: Supervision Competence (SC) = Supervisory Skills (SS) + Supervisory Dispositions (SD).

A second concern with the committee's position statement is its limited focus on the *multiple roles* of supervisors; it emphasizes only the Educator role in the Pentagonal Model of Communication Disorders supervision. The document states that clinical supervision "refers to the tasks and skills of clinical teaching related to the interaction between a clinician and a client and the evaluation or management of communication skills" (p. 57). The committee's tasks and competencies, accordingly, address the other four domains of the Pentagonal Model only secondarily or not at all. Table 2–1 presents each of the 13 tasks relative to the five domains. This analysis shows that all of the tasks relate to the Educational domain but that only three tasks (11.0, 12.0, and 13.0) are germane to the Professional and Clinical domains. It is important for the development of Communication

TABLE 2-1 Relation of Communication Disorders supervision tasks to supervision roles

Task		P	R	Role E	A	C
1.0	Establishing and maintaining an effective relationship with the supervisee.		X	X	X	
2.0	Assisting the supervisee in developing clinical goals and objectives.			X		
3.0	Assisting the supervisee in developing and refining assessment skills.			X		
4.0	Assisting the supervisee in developing and refining clinical management skills.			X		
5.0	Demonstrating for and participating with the supervisee in the clinical process.		X	X	X	
6.0	Assisting the supervisee in observing and analyzing assessment and treatment sessions.		X	X	X	
7.0	Assisting the supervisee in the development and maintenance of clinical and supervisory records.			X	X	
8.0	Interacting with the supervisee in planning, executing, and analyzing supervisory conferences.		X	X	X	
9.0	Assisting the supervisee in evaluation of clinical performance.		X	X	X	
10.0	Assisting the supervisee in developing skills of verbal reporting, writing, and editing.		X	X	X	
11.0	Sharing information regarding ethical, legal, regulatory, and reimbursement aspects of professional practice.	X	X	X	X	X
12.0	Modeling and facilitating professional conduct.	X	X	X	X	X
13.0	Demonstrating research skills in the clinical or supervisory processes.	X	X	X	X	X
	Totals	3	9	13	10	3

Disorders supervisors that the basic 13 tasks and 81 competencies be supplemented, as the ASHA Committee on Supervision has suggested, to take into account the Professional, Research, Educational, Administrative, and Clinical domains.

A third issue is that the tasks and competencies tend to emphasize supervision in university settings and do not adequately address supervision in other worksites that serve unique populations (e.g., multiply- and severely-handicapped, linguistically different, or incarcerated persons). Obviously lacking is a focus on professional technology (primarily electronics) that is used in the five supervision domains.

A fourth limitation is that, while the position statement may imply that clinicians will be supervised from the time they enter the clinical process during the training program through most, if not all, of their professional careers, it does not make clear the status of the *long-term supervisee*. Supervisors need special competencies in order to supervise experienced, long-term supervisees (staff clinicians).

To summarize, supervision competence needs further consideration for at least four reasons: First, the clinical process requires that a clinician employ both skills and dispositions. Clinicians learn personal skills and dispositions through the clinical education provided by supervisors. Therefore, supervisors must know how to facilitate the development of both skills and dispositions. As more and more educational programs begin to educate and train Communication Disorders personnel in the supervision process, professionals must take care not to emphasize skill development to the exclusion of disposition development. Second, supervisors must be prepared to work in all five domains in order to meet the demands of many supervisory positions. Third, supervisors must be prepared to work in many different sites with different populations. Fourth, supervisors must be prepared to supervise both beginning student clinicians and long-term staff clinicians.

All four of the limitations mean that supervisor competence has been only partially defined. This fact reduces the potential for supervision to function adequately as a specialty area within the Communication Disorders profession. Because education and training in supervision appear to be the best ways to develop competent supervisors, it is critical that academic or continuing education programs address the 13 tasks and associated competencies *plus* the additional four issues presented here.

Education and Training in Supervision

The need to prepare for the process of supervision will be present always, either to update practicing supervisors or to educate and train new ones. The most common method of becoming a supervisor in an applied training field such as Speech-Language Pathology or Audiology has been by credentials (e.g., ASHA certification) and position (e.g., availability or length of employment). However, it is now being acknowledged that to be competent supervisors, speech-language pathologists or audiologists must have background knowledge and skills associated with the supervision process. Thus, they need education and training beyond what is necessary for the clinical process. In addition, the Committee on Supervision in Speech Pathology and Audiology (ASHA, 1978) recommended that the American Speech-Language-Hearing Association encourage the development of training programs in supervision, as well as continuing education programs. This suggestion is based on five concerns: (a) most of the personnel currently doing supervision have not been prepared to be supervisors, and they are the ones teaching supervision courses; (b) few Communication Disorders training programs have a supervision course (approximately 10 to 15% of the graduate programs), and many of those are taught only intermittently (Pickering, 1985); (c) it is unclear what content and experience should be included in supervision training (Anderson, 1980); (d) the quality of continuing education courses varies greatly; and (e) it has not been well documented that supervision preparation facilitates change in supervisors' behavior. Anderson (1974) argued that it is unwise to wait to develop training models until all relevant data become available. Instead, she suggested, supervision training programs should be established concurrently with research effort. The same principle has been applied to programs for educating and training in the clinical process; academicians have not waited for all the data about stuttering to come in before they educate and train clinicians to deliver services to individuals who stutter. We must simply acknowledge that methods of preparing supervisors are based on current knowledge and that our understanding of the process will change, requiring change in turn on the part of supervisors and supervisees.

Currently, the most likely source of supervision preparation information is continuing education offerings. Local, state, regional, and national workshops, colloquia, seminars, teleconferences, and meetings occur regularly, so that personnel can acquire supervision preparation experiences with some effort. Microcomputer technology has made possible national networking through the modem, and video technology allows us to share information for purposes of knowledge, skill development, and research. To insure that quality continuing education programs are developed, Oas (1987) suggested a six-stage program design process based on the work of Brinkerhoff (1987): (a) needs assessment, (b) design of a program, (c) operation, (d) assessment of learning, (e) implementation (retention and transfer), and (f) value.

Supervisor preparation has two components, education and training. The difference between them is represented in Figure 2-1. The figure places the two concepts on a preparation continuum based on the source of control (*external*, from the instructor; *internal*, from the learner) and the direction of the preparation (the instructor providing experience *to* the learner, in training, or experiences developing *with* the learner, in education). Teachers need to blend education and training by combining academic knowledge with supervision practicum experience. The concept of skills versus dispositions becomes relevant here also; skills result from training, whereas dispositions emerge from educational interactions with instructors who routinely model competence as part of their professional behavior. Research has shown that specific supervision skills such as critical observation (Farmer, 1984) and supervisor conference techniques (Dowling, 1983) can be trained. However, little information is available about whether the new behaviors are then implemented in supervision contexts.

In the past, the concern has been what topics, concepts, issues, and skills should be presented in supervisor preparation programs, whether they are part of a Communication Disorders curriculum or continuing education offerings. The literature identifies numerous items that are considered important in training supervisors. The information can be divided into two major areas, theoretical dimensions and human dimensions.

Theoretical Dimensions. Theoretical dimensions of Communication Disorders supervision training include such ideas and issues as systems theory, models, styles, forms and types of supervision, differential supervision, change, supervision in Speech-Language Pathology versus supervision in Audiology, and supervision as a specialty area in the Communication Disorders

FIGURE 2-1
Philosophical and psychological belief systems continuum

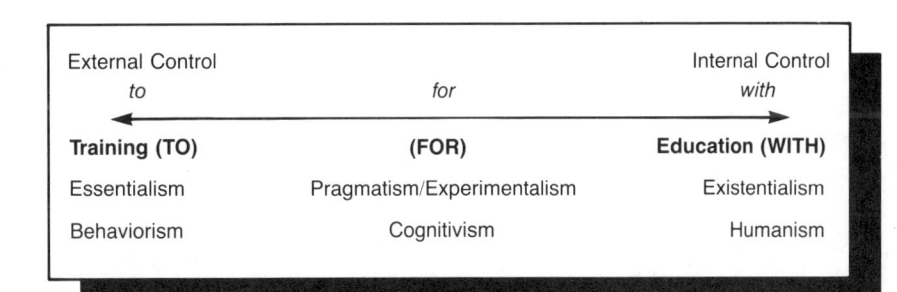

External Control		Internal Control
to	for	with
Training (TO)	**(FOR)**	**Education (WITH)**
Essentialism	Pragmatism/Experimentalism	Existentialism
Behaviorism	Cognitivism	Humanism

profession. Because the focus of this chapter is on the people involved in the process, chapter 3 will cover the theoretical dimensions of supervision. The remainder of this section on supervisors details the human dimensions of educating and training Communication Disorders supervisors and presents ideas about assessing and developing each dimension.

Human Dimensions. An initial step in supervision preparation is the supervisors' development of self-awareness about their own predispositions and characteristics. Specifically, these include their philosophical and psychological beliefs about the teaching-learning process, beliefs that are the foundation of the supervision process. Learning styles, personality types, cognitive styles, inquiry modes, communication styles, and leadership styles are also important areas for self-exploration.

Supervisors should develop self-knowledge for three purposes: (a) to assist both supervisors and supervisees to be better participants in the supervision process; (b) to help pre-service supervisees determine whether they might be effective supervisors sometime in their careers and, if so, to begin preparing them for that position; (c) to aid the professional development of present supervisors so that they become more proficient in the five supervision domains. Developing self-awareness and its complementary competencies will ultimately improve communication disorders supervision.

Philosophy of learning. Supervisors possess a philosophy of learning whether or not they are aware of it. Individuals' philosophies, personal values, and beliefs form the foundation of their choices or decisions throughout their lifetimes. Professionally, all supervisors apply more or less conscious principles for living, learning, and functioning as supervisors. In addition, how supervisors feel about themselves—their psychological postures or styles—influences what transpires in their everyday living, learning, and working in the Professional, Research, Educational, Administrative, and Clinical domains of supervision.

The various philosophies and psychologies of learning have been combined and then grouped into three camps by Dobson, Dobson, and Kessinger (1980; Dobson & Dobson, 1981). As applied to Communication Disorders supervision, the educational philosophies and psychological styles are grouped according to whether supervisors are primarily concerned with doing *to, for,* or *with* supervisees. The *philosophies* of learning are represented by essentialism, experimentalism, and existentialism.

According to Dobson and Dobson (1981), the *essentialist* learning philosophy mediates between the extremes of the realist and the idealist modes of inquiry. Essentialists believe that certain truths exist and that they must be at the core of all teaching-learning situations. Within this philosophy, supervisors are the dominant active agents and provide supervision *to* their supervisees. All supervisees learn the same clinical competencies in the same ways under maximum supervisor control.

Experimentalism (also called *pragmatism*) represents the second group of educational philosophies. Pragmatism emphasizes active learning rather than deductive reasoning. Experimentalism, a branch of pragmatism, stresses the scientific method of learning through experiences, the importance of individual differences and interests, and the presence of alternatives to prompt freedom of choice combined with personal responsibility. Supervisors who are guided by a pragmatic/experimental philosophy of learning stress the importance of "learning by doing." However, the supervisor still exerts some external control by helping supervisees determine what competencies are important. The supervisor will then create learning situations in which supervisees can develop the skills they and the supervisor have jointly deemed important. In other words, supervisors supervise *for* the good of their supervisees or *for* the good of the clients.

The third philosophical camp is represented

by *existentialism*, which holds that the ultimate questions of life cannot be answered with finality; trying to answer them by understanding oneself is what life and learning are all about. Supervisors who follow this philosophy of learning believe that knowledge is a lifelong process of developing oneself through experiential discovery. Therefore, supervisors and supervisees together create environments in which they can learn about themselves actively in their quest for professional knowledge. The need for specific competencies emerges uniquely from each context, and the competencies are developed from experiencing that situation personally. Existential supervisors supervise *with* their supervisees, developing themselves as their supervisees develop.

Supervisors' basic teaching-learning philosophies are strong determinants of how they will supervise. The second such influence is psychological styles.

Psychology of learning. The three psychological styles described by Dobson and Dobson (1981) are behaviorism, cognitivism, and humanism. *Behaviorism* limits psychological knowledge to objective, observable phenomena associated with learning. Objectives, stimuli, responses, criteria, and consequences are important to supervisors who espouse a behaviorist psychology of learning. Supervision is applied *to* supervisees through external control in the form of goals and objectives.

Cognitivism defines reality in subjective, perceptual terms rather than in objective, physical terms. The process of discovering and using information is important to supervisors who subscribe to cognitivism. Supervisors supervise *for* the development of the supervisee and/or the client.

The psychology of *humanism* states that all learning is motivated by striving to attain one's potential. Humanists believe that learning and improvement are internally reinforcing, that humans are guided by the desire to develop themselves, and that external reinforcement such as grades or specific competency levels is not needed.

Although perceptions expressed collectively as beliefs ultimately result in personal philosophies and psychological styles, it is important to remember that the above classification systems help individuals organize their perceptions and do not express absolute truths. Individuals or institutions usually do not reflect a particular educational philosophy or psychological style in pure form. Rather, they hold some attitudes derived from all three camps, falling somewhere on a continuum in their predominant approach to teaching-learning. Dobson, Dobson, and Kessinger (1980) developed two data gathering instruments, the *Educational Beliefs System Inventory* and the *Educational Practice Belief Inventory*, to help individuals identify personal beliefs about learning. Results of the inventories identify predominant belief patterns that fit on the continuum that was shown in Figure 2-1.

Table 2-2 presents characteristics of the three categories of educational philosophy, essentialism, experimentalism, and existentialism, and of the three categories of psychological styles, behaviorism, cognitivism, and humanism.

Supervisors and supervisees can assess their beliefs about teaching and learning by self-administering the *Educational Beliefs System Inventory* and the *Educational Practice Belief Inventory*. The importance of self-awareness for supervisors is to help them identify their personal profile, evaluate its advantages and disadvantages, and work toward complementing their predominant strategies with alternative patterns of interacting with others.

Supervisors and supervisees will act from a predominant philosophical and psychological base when participating in the supervision process. It is essential to recognize when the supervisor's and supervisee's orientations toward learning are compatible and when they are incongruent. Sometimes compatible orientations lead to productive supervision; at other times incongruent ones create a more dynamic super-

TABLE 2-2
Characteristics of educational philosophical and psychological belief systems

PHILOSOPHY

	Essentialism (Idealism + Realism)	Pragmatism/ Experimentalism	Existentialism
Theorists	Idealism: Plato, Johnson, Kant, Hegel, Berkeley. Realism: Aristotle, Locke, Russell, Whitehead. Essentialism: Kneller.	James/Dewey.	Kierkegaard.
Human Nature	Humans are potentially evil.	Humans are potentially both good and bad or blank slate.	Humans are potentially good.
Nature of Learning	Truth exists separate from the individual. There are basic facts that are necessary for all. Learning occurs by reaction.	Truth is relative and subject to the condition of the learner and the environment. Learning occurs by action.	Truth is an individual matter. Learning occurs when the information encountered takes on personal meaning for the learner. Learning occurs by transaction and interaction.
Nature of Knowledge	Logical structure. Information. Subject matter. Vertical relationship. Universal.	Psychological structure. Vertical and horizontal. Relationships and interrelationships.	Perceptual structure. Relationships and Interrelationships. Personal. Gestalt.
Nature of Society	Closed. Ordered. Institutionalized. Static Grouping. Control.	In flux. Democratic. Relative values. Experimentation.	Open. Self reviewing. Individual. Liberating. Distribution. Egalitarian.
Purpose of Education	To understand and apply knowledge. To control the environment. To learn absolute truth.	To learn prerequisite skills for survival. To learn conditional truths.	To live a full life. To experience the environment. To continue learning personal truth.

PSYCHOLOGY

	BEHAVIORISM	COGNITIVE	HUMANISM
Theorists	Watson, Thorndike, Skinner.	Lewin, Bruner, Piaget.	Maslow, Perls, May, Rogers.
Human Growth and Development	Growth is environment determined.	Growth is the realization of one's potential.	Growth is the experiencing of one's potential.

TABLE 2–2
continued

PSYCHOLOGY

	BEHAVIORISM	COGNITIVE	HUMANISM
Concept of Self	Determined by what others think. Focuses on personality deficiencies.	Determined by how the individual perceives the social environment (becoming-future orientation).	Determined and created by each individual (being-now orientation).
Human Emotions	Controlled. Closed. Unaware. Masked.	Circumstantial Objective. Based on position. Well-adjusted.	Free. Openness Spontaneity. Aware. Transparency. Experienced.
Interpersonal Interactions	Role Playing. Manipulative games. Defensive. Detached. Distrusting. Dependent.	Minimum risk. Selective. Objective. Exclusive. Encountering. Independent.	Sharing. Risking, Trusting.

OPERATIONAL

Instructional Behavior	Transmission of facts and content. Purposeful. Management is teacher directed.	Grouping for instructional convenience Inquiring. Discovering. Open questions with multiple answers. Teacher invitation.	Learner directed. Learner invitations. Teacher functions as source of safety and support.
Evaluation	Measurement of facts and content. Determined by authority Imposed. Product oriented.	Critical thinking. Problem solving. Tests higher cognitive skills. Focuses on what is learned.	Feedback by invitation. Cooperative pupil and teacher evaluation. Nondamaging comparison. Focuses on how one feels about what is learned as well as what is learned.

From *Staff Development: A Humanistic Approach* (pp. 56–58) by R. Dobson, J. Dobson, and J. Kessinger, 1980, Lanham, MD: University Press of America. Copyright 1980 by the University Press of America. Reprinted by permission.

vision environment. A supervisor should be able to mix and match teaching-learning approaches to create the most productive supervision experience possible.

Learning styles. It has been suggested that adults learn differently from children and therefore must be taught differently. Knowles (1970, 1973) compares *pedagogy* (how children learn) with *andragogy* (how adults learn).

A pedagogical mode of supervision is a process in which information is transmitted from the supervisor to the supervisee, with the supervisor assuming full responsibility for what, when,

TABLE 2-3
Employment aspects of Myers-Briggs preference-types

Introverts	Extroverts
Like quiet for concentration	Like variety and some distractions
Are more careful with details	Are faster, dislike complicated procedures
Have trouble remembering names and faces	Are good at greeting people
Don't mind working on one project for a long time uninterruptedly	Are impatient with long, slow jobs
Dislike telephone interruptions	Often enjoy telephoning
Like to think before they act	Usually act quickly, sometimes without thinking
Are interested in the idea behind their job	Are interested in how other people do the job
Work contentedly alone	Like to have people around
Have some problems communicating	Communicate freely

Intuitive Types	Sensing Types
Like solving new problems	Dislike problems unless there are standard ways to solve them
Dislike doing the same thing over and over again	Don't mind routine
Enjoy learning a new skill more than using it	Enjoy using skills already acquired
Work in bursts of energy powered by enthusiasm	Work more steadily; more realistic about how long it will take
Are patient with complicated situations	Are impatient when there are too many complicated details to remember
Are impatient with routine details	Are patient with routine details
Follow their inspirations, good or bad	Don't usually get inspired
Reach a conclusion quickly	Usually reach a conclusion step by step
Frequently make errors of fact	Seldom make errors of fact
Tend to be good at precise work	Dislike taking time for precision

how, and to whom the information is presented. Some pedagogical characteristics are that the supervisor decides content; supervisees use rote memory to learn new material because they are inexperienced in the topic areas; the supervisor dictates the need for learning and is the source of wisdom and information; the need for learning the material is delayed rather than immediate; lecture, demonstration, and practice are common instructional strategies; and the supervisor evaluates, doing so on the basis of "right" answers.

In an andragogical approach to supervision both the supervisee and the supervisor assume responsibility for what, when, how, and to whom information is presented. The supervisee accepts the content based on evidence, not blind faith; the supervisee brings past experiences to the learning situation and, therefore, has needs that must be addressed; the supervisee is active, rather than passive, in the learning process and often applies information immediately; discussion and experimentation are common teaching-learning strategies; and the supervisee participates in a contextually-based evaluation process, where "correctness" is relative to context.

Some supervisees seem to learn better from a pedagogical approach to teaching-learning; others develop better with an andragogical approach. A supervisor should be able to assess which style is appropriate with which supervisees and then to implement the appropriate strategies.

TABLE 2-3
continued

Feeling Types	Thinking Types
Are very aware of other people and their feelings	Are not very interested in people's feelings; relatively unemotional
Like to please people or help them	May hurt people's feelings without knowing it
Like harmony; efficiency may be badly disturbed by office feuds	Like analysis; enjoy putting things into logical order
Have decisions influenced by personal likes and wishes	Make decisions impersonally, sometimes ignoring people's wishes
Need occasional praise	Need to be treated fairly
Dislike telling people unpleasant things	Are able to reprimand people or fire them when necessary
More people-oriented—respond to people's values	More analytically oriented—respond to people's thoughts
Sympathetic	Firm-minded
Perceptive Types	**Judging Types**
Like to adapt to changing situations	Like to plan their work and be able to get it finished on schedule
Like to leave things free for alterations	Like to get things settled and wrapped up
May have trouble making decisions	May decide things too quickly
May start too many projects and finish too few	May not like to interrupt one project for a more urgent one
May postpone unpleasant jobs	May not notice new things which need to be done
Want to know all about new jobs	Want only the essentials needed to begin work
Tend to be curious	Tend to be satisfied once a judgment is made

Reproduced by special permission of the Publisher, Consulting Psychologists Press, Inc., Palo Alto, CA 94306, from *Manual: A Guide to the Development of the Myers-Briggs Type Indicator* by Isabel Briggs Myers and Mary McCaulley, © 1985. Further reproduction is prohibited without the Publisher's consent.

Personality types. Personality is defined as a characteristic and distinctive way of behaving. Myers and McCaulley (1985) have used the dimensions of Extraversion-Introversion, Sensing-Intuition, Feeling-Thinking, and Judging-Perceiving to create 16 categories of personality.

The *Myers-Briggs Type Indicator (MBTI)* (Myers & McCaulley, 1985) has been helpful in identifying and understanding differences in personnel in various work forces. Supervisors have found the tool useful in managing supervision staffs. Responses to the *MBTI,* which is based on the psychological constructs of Carl Jung, a 20th-century analytic psychologist, produce a profile of contrasting preferences in the areas of (a) focus of interest: *Extraversion* (E) versus *Introversion* (I); (b) information gathering: *Sensing* (S) of facts and data versus using *Intuition* (N) to reveal theory and meaning; (c) involvement with information: *Feeling* (F) with subjectivity versus *Thinking* (T) with objective analysis; (d) information use: *Judging* (J) for decision making versus *Perceiving* (P) for awareness. These eight dimensions can be combined to produce 16 possible *MBTI* personality types: ISTJ, ISFJ, INFJ, INTJ, ISTP, ISFP, INFP, INTP, ESTJ, ESFJ, ENFJ, ENTJ, ESTP, ESFP, ENFP, ENTP.

Aspects of employment relevant to the eight preference types are presented in Table 2-3.

Sleight and Craig (1987) studied personality types relative to Communication Disorders supervision and found that a greater proportion of supervisors in their subject pool had profiles representing the INTJ and ENTJ patterns than any of the other patterns. In other words, Communication Disorders supervisors tended to be intuitive, thinking, and judging (see Table 2-3 for characteristic work patterns associated with these preferences).

According to Sleight and Craig (1987),

> The key to using *MBTI*-type information in supervision is to understand that each type has strengths and weaknesses. For example, a "judging" type needs a perceiver to instill flexibility in plans. A "feeling" type needs a thinker to maintain standards. Each of the types depends upon the others. It is through understanding why each type behaves as it does that we will improve our supervision. A perceiving student who fails to meet deadlines may not realize why turning reports in on time contributes to professionalism. A supervisor who comprehends which personality factors influence behavior may be better able to modify student behavior when necessary or understand when, instead, it is the supervisor's viewpoint that needs modification. (p. 68)

Cognitive styles. Cognitive style refers to a person's preferences of sensory modality (hearing, sight, touch, taste, smell), context (e.g., alone, in a group), and environment (e.g., heat, light, noise) for obtaining information. The preferences indicate how and where learning takes place most effectively. Although numerous cognitive styles models exist, three representative examples follow.

Erhardt and Corvey (1980) discuss the *Modified Hill,* a modification of the *Hill Educational Cognitive Style* developed by Joseph E. Hill. The *Modified Hill* is a "map" that describes individual cognitive styles by relating score results on 28 items on the *Cognitive Style Mapping Instrument* (*CSMI*). The map reflects a preferred learning environment. Farmer (1986a) discusses the application of cognitive style measurement to Communication Disorders supervision conferences. After completing the *CSMI,* an individual can determine the major, minor, and negligible sub-areas of cognitive salience within four major categories: Theoretical, Qualitative, Cultural, and Modalities of Inference. The idea is to use the preferences to facilitate optimum learning. In Communication Disorders supervision, the supervisor can use a supervisee's cognitive style map to help the supervisee gain as much as possible from the supervision experience. If supervisors know their own maps, they will be aware of their preferences for instructing and can either use their preferred style to facilitate certain supervisees' learning, or modify their preferred style to meet the needs of other supervisees.

The second model of cognitive style is Kolb's model of experiential learning (1978). Kolb's model identifies four phases in the experiential learning cycle: (a) *Concrete Experience* (CE), where learning takes place by the learner's immediate, direct involvement in the active learning event; (b) *Reflective Observation* (RO), where the learner mentally associates data that have been gathered by the senses; (c) *Abstract Conceptualization* (AC), where the learner derives hypotheses about the nature of observations that have been made; and (d) *Active Experimentation* (AE), where the learner tests hypotheses that have been generated to explain relationships among observed phenomena.

The experiential learning cycle suggests two primary dimensions of the learning process. Concrete experience is the polar opposite of abstract conceptualization; reflective observation is the opposite of active experimentation, or hypothesis testing. Ideally, the learner should enjoy using all four modes of the experiential learning cycle. However, the methods an individual consistently chooses to accomplish particular learning tasks often indicate distinct preferences for specific modes. The Communication Disorders supervisor can use this cycle information in two ways: (a) to identify the preferred learning modes for supervisees and use them accordingly, or (b) to facilitate supervisees' development of all four modes to increase the efficacy of their learning.

The third model of cognitive styles identifies aptitudes for learning. Greene and Lewis (1983) described nine aptitude areas considered to be important in a variety of professions: perceptual processing (accuracy and speed), language, scientific thinking, creative thinking, formal reasoning, hand/eye coordination (accuracy and speed), artistry, writing, and socialness. Greene and Lewis rated the importance of each aptitude in over 150 professions and occupations. If those ratings are adapted to the roles of Communication Disorders supervision, all nine aptitudes appear to be most important in the Clinical domain, followed by the Educational and Research domains, and then the Administrative and Professional areas. The perceptual processing (accuracy), creative thinking, writing, and social aptitudes are the most salient across domains.

Any task that a Communication Disorders supervisor does in any of the five roles will require some of the nine aptitudes discussed by Greene and Lewis (1983). By completing the Greene and Lewis inventory, *Nine Mind Tests*, persons will discover which of their aptitudes are well developed and which ones could be enhanced. In discussing each of the nine aptitudes, the authors suggest how certain scores might affect job performance of specific tasks and what effect the aptitudes have on leisure activities.

The aforementioned human characteristics have been applied to arrive at employee management styles. The concept of *inquiry modes* allows us to categorize the ways of interacting with employees.

Inquiry modes. Inquiry modes synthesize various parameters of cognitive styles into descriptions of types of thinking, or of organizing world experiences and knowledge, which are then used in employment contexts. Inquiry modes, or styles of thinking, have a definite effect on supervision. Harrison and Bramson (1982) discuss five styles of thinking: Synthesist, Idealist, Pragmatist, Analyst, and Realist. Their research, which is qualitative in nature (i.e., made up of observation, behavior analysis, behavior categorization, and generalization of subject behavior *in context*) led them to develop the *InQ Questionnaire*, which provides the empirical data on which the descriptions of their five inquiry styles are based. The questionnaire and detailed discussions of each mode are found in the book *The Art of Thinking* (Harrison & Bramson, 1982). As the authors point out, the convenience and predictive value of any typology of human characteristics cloud the fact that humans are seldom "ideal types." Instead, they are unique blends of behavioral tendencies. The *InQ* styles are presented as separate entities. However, Communication Disorders supervisors are more likely to be blends of at least two of the styles (e.g., Idealist-Analyst, Analyst-Realist, or Synthesist-Idealist). A small percentage of people who have taken the *InQ* show up as "three-way" thinkers. A supervisor with a "flat" profile shows no strong stylistic preference. Characteristics of the five inquiry modes are presented in Table 2–4. A unique feature of the table is the "Extending and Augmenting" area, which suggests things to do to acquire the characteristics of each mode. Modifying personal modes for productive supervision is an important ability for supervisors. Supervision personnel can discover their thinking style preferences by self-administering the *InQ* and then can develop alternative thinking patterns by following the "Extending and Augmenting" suggestions.

Leadership styles. Leadership is coordinating the activities of members of an organization or group toward some end. Leadership styles, then, are behavioral characteristics directed toward accomplishing tasks and toward recognizing the needs and relationships of members of a group or organization. Although many leadership models exist, five examples are discussed here.

The basis for most leadership models is the four-cell matrix of high and low emphasis on task and relationship dimensions. Blake and Mouton (1964) developed a sophisticated 81-cell managerial grid to define five ideal-type modes of leadership. The two dimensions of "concern for production" and "concern for people" are rated on a 9-point scale (1 = low, 9 = high) in terms of relative emphasis for efficiency of operation. The five ideal type patterns are 1.9

TABLE 2-4
Characteristics of five inquiry modes

SYNTHESIST

General Characteristics
1. Integrative view.
2. Sees likeness in apparent unlikenesses.
3. Seeks conflict and synthesis.
4. Interested in change.
5. Speculative.
6. Data meaningless without interpretation.

Specific Behavioral Characteristics

Apt to appear: Challenging, skeptical, amused; or may appear tuned out, but alert when disagrees.
Apt to say: "On the other hand...." "No, that's not necessarily so...."
Apt to express: Concepts, opposite points of view; speculates, may identify absurdities.
Tone: Sardonic, probing, skeptical; may sound argumentative.
Enjoys: Speculative, philosophical, intellectual argument.
Apt to use: Parenthetical expressions, qualifying adjectives and phrases.
Dislikes: Talk that seems simplistic, superficially polite, fact-centered, repetitive, "mundane."
Under stress: Pokes fun.
Stereotype: "Troublemaker"

Operational Strategies

Grand Strategy: Dialectic
1. Open argument and confrontation.
2. Asks dumb-smart questions.
3. Participates from sidelines.
4. Suspends opposing ideas.
5. Speculates and fantasizes.
6. Proposes "far out" ideas.
7. Uses negative analysis.

Strengths
1. Focus on underlying assumptions.
2. Points out abstract conceptual aspects.
3. Good at preventing over-agreement.
4. Best in controversial, conflict-laden situations.
5. Provides debate and creativity.

Liabilities
1. May screen out agreement.
2. May seek conflict unnecessarily.
3. May try too hard for change and newness.
4. May theorize excessively.
5. Can appear uncommitted.

Extending and Augmenting
1. Practice listening for conflict and disagreement.
2. Ask dumb-smart questions.
3. Develop the third-party observer viewpoint.
4. Look for relationships between things that have no apparent likeness.
5. Practice improving your tolerance for eccentricity.
6. When someone seems to come out of left field, stop and listen carefully.
7. Practice negative analysis.

TABLE 2-4
continued

IDEALIST

General Characteristics

1. Assimilative or holistic view.
2. Broad range of views welcomed.
3. Seeks ideal solutions.
4. Interested in values.
5. Receptive.
6. Data and theory of equal value.

Specific Behavioral Characteristics

Apt to appear: Attentive, receptive; often supportive smile, head nodding, much verbal feedback.
Apt to say: "It seems to me. . . ." "Don't you think that. . .?"
Apt to express: Feelings, ideas about values, what's good for people, concerns about goals.
Tone: Inquiring, hopeful; may sound tentative or disappointed and resentful.
Enjoys: Feeling-level discussions about people and their problems.
Apt to use: Indirect questions, aids to gain agreement.
Dislikes: Talk that seems too data-bound, factual, "dehumanizing"; and openly conflictual argument unless about issues of caring or integrity.
Under stress: Looks hurt.
Stereotype: "Bleeding heart"

Operational Strategies

Grand Strategy: Assimilative thinking

1. Focus on the whole.
2. The long-range view.
3. Setting goals and standards.
4. Receptive listening.
5. Search for aids to agreement.
6. Humanizing the argument.

Strengths

1. Focus on process, relationships.
2. Points out values and aspirations.
3. Good at articulating goals.
4. Best in unstructured, value-laden situations.
5. Provides broad view, goals and standards.

Liabilities

1. May screen out "hard" data.
2. May delay from too many choices.
3. May try too hard for "perfect" solutions.
4. May overlook details.
5. Can appear overly sentimental.

Extending and Augmenting

1. Focus on the whole, not the "one best way."
2. Focus on the long range.
3. Think about high standards and superordinate goals.
4. Listen for value statements and aspirations.
5. Try to fit a number of differing ideas under a common framework.
6. Encourage others to express their aspirations.

TABLE 2-4
continued

PRAGMATIST

General Characteristics
1. Eclectic view.
2. "Whatever works."
3. Seeks shortest route to payoff.
4. Interested in innovation.
5. Adaptive.
6. Any data or theory that gets us there.

Specific Behavioral Characteristics
- Apt to appear: Open, sociable; often a good deal of humor, interplay, quick to agree.
- Apt to say: "I'll buy that. . . ." "That's sure one way to go. . . ."
- Apt to express: Non-complex ideas; may tell brief personal anecdotes to explain ideas.
- Tone: Enthusiastic, agreeable; may sound insincere.
- Enjoys: Brainstorming around tactical issues; lively give-and-take.
- Apt to use: Case examples, illustrations, popular opinions.
- Dislikes: Talk that seems dry, dull, humorless; or too conceptual, philosophical, analytical, "nitpicking."
- Under stress: Looks bored.
- Stereotype: "Politician"

Operational Strategies
Grand Strategy: The contingency approach

1. Moving one step at a time.
2. Experiment and innovation.
3. Looking for quick payoff.
4. Tactical thinking.
5. The marketing approach.
6. Contingency planning.

Strengths
1. Focus on payoff.
2. Points out tactics and strategies.
3. Good at identifying impacts.
4. Best in complex, incremental situations.
5. Provides experiment and innovation.

Liabilities
1. May screen out long-range aspects.
2. May rush too quickly to payoff.
3. May try too hard for expediency.
4. May rely too much on what "sells."
5. Can appear over-compromising.

Extending and Augmenting
1. Practice thinking incrementally.
2. Allow others to experiment, and try to join in.
3. Look for the short-range payoff.
4. Learn to think tactically.
5. Practice being "marketing."
6. Try being less tediously serious and more playful, especially with ideas and plans.

TABLE 2-4
continued

ANALYST

General Characteristics
1. Formal logic and deduction.
2. Seeks "one best way."
3. Seeks models and formulas.
4. Interested in "scientific" solutions.
5. Prescriptive.
6. Theory and method over data.

Specific Behavioral Characteristics
Apt to appear: Cool, studious, often hard to read; may be a lack of feedback, as if hearing you out.
Apt to say: "It stands to reason. . . ." "If you look at it logically. . . ."
Apt to express: General rules; describes things systematically, offers substantiating data.
Tone: Dry, disciplined, careful; may sound set, stubborn.
Enjoys: Structured, rational examination of substantive issues.
Apt to use: Long, discursive, well-formulated sentences.
Dislikes: Talk that seems irrational, aimless, or too speculative, "far out," and irrelevant humor.
Under stress: Withdraws.
Stereotype: "Great Stone Face"

Operational Strategies
Grand Strategy: Search for the one best way
1. Systematic analysis of alternatives.
2. The search for more data.
3. Conservative focusing.
4. Charting the situation.
5. Constructive nit-picking.
6. Deductive reasoning.

Strengths
1. Focus on method and plan.
2. Points out data and details.
3. Good at model-building and planning.
4. Best in structured, calculatable situations.
5. Provides stability and structure.

Liabilities
1. May screen out values and subjectives.
2. May over-plan, over-analyze.
3. May try too hard for predictability.
4. May be inflexible, overly cautious.
5. Can appear tunnel-visioned.

Extending and Augmenting
1. Study statistics or operations research.
2. Learn to gather more data before a decision.
3. Learn to make a flowchart.
4. Learn to tolerate quantification.
5. Pay greater attention to detail.
6. Focus on constraints.

TABLE 2-4
continued

REALIST

General Characteristics
1. Empirical view and induction.
2. Relies on "facts" and expert opinion.
3. Seeks solutions that meet current needs.
4. Interested in concrete results.
5. Corrective.
6. Data over theory.

Specific Behavioral Characteristics
Apt to appear: Direct, forceful; agreement and disagreement often quickly expressed nonverbally.
Apt to say: "It's obvious to me. . . ." "Everybody knows that. . . ."
Apt to express: Opinions; describes factually, may offer short, pointed anecdotes.
Tone: Forthright, positive, may sound dogmatic or domineering.
Enjoys: Short, direct, factual discussions of immediate matters.
Apt to use: Direct, pithy, descriptive statements.
Dislikes: Talk that seems too theoretical, sentimental, subjective, impractical, "long-winded."
Under stress: Gets agitated.
Stereotype: "Blockhead"

Operational Strategies
Grand Strategy: Empirical discovery
1. Setting hard objectives.
2. The resource inventory.
3. Getting to specifics.
4. Simplification.
5. Using expert opinion.
6. Incisive correction.

Strengths
1. Focus on facts and results.
2. Points out realities and resources.
3. Good at simplifying, "cutting through."
4. Best in well-defined, objective situations.
5. Provides drive and momentum.

Liabilities
1. May screen out disagreement.
2. May rush to over-simplified solutions.
3. May try too hard for consensus and immediate response.
4. May over-emphasize perceived "facts."
5. Can appear too results-oriented.

Extending and Augmenting
1. Focus on concrete results.
2. Focus on resources.
3. Practice getting to the point quickly.
4. Practice writing short, declarative sentences.
5. Learn to paraphrase for precision.
6. Practice incisiveness.

Source: From *The Art of Thinking* (pp. 196–197) by A. F. Harrison and R.M. Bramson, 1984, New York: Doubleday. Copyright 1984 by A.F. Harrison and R.M. Bramson. Reprinted by permission.

(low emphasis on production, high emphasis on people); 1.1 (low emphasis on both production and people); 9.1 (high emphasis on production, low emphasis on people); 9.9 (high emphasis on both production and people); and 5.5 (moderate emphasis on both production and people).

Reddin (1970) offered a contrast to Blake and Mouton's "ideal" pattern, positing a three-dimensional quadrant matrix that is contextually based. Reddin suggests that the effectiveness of any leadership style can be understood only in context. Four basic styles that reflect high and low *Task Orientation* (TO) and *Relations Orientation* (RO) are presented. The styles of "Related" (low TO, high RO), "Separated" (low TO, low RO), "Dedicated" (high TO, low RO), and "Integrated" (high TO, high RO) are effective or ineffective depending on the situation (context) in which they are used. For example, a "Related" style has two counterparts, the "Missionary" and the "Developer." In some situations, it may be perceived as the less effective "Missionary" style, where supervisors are seen as being interested primarily in harmony. In others, a style with the same configuration can be perceived as a "Developer" style in which the supervisor's primary emphasis is developing personnel as individuals and professionals.

DeVille (1984) presents a third model of leadership based on the two continua of self-control/self-expression and cooperation/competition. This model again allows for description of four types of leaders. The "self-reliant" leader (controlling pattern) is competitive and self-controlled; the "factual" leader (comprehending pattern) is self-controlled but cooperative; the "loyal" leader (supporting pattern) is cooperative and self-expressing; the "enthusiastic" leader (entertaining pattern) is self-expressing but competitive. Supervisors can self-administer the *Management Style Assessment* instrument described by DeVille.

The *Supervision Style Index* (Farmer, 1986b) is the last quadrant-form model to be discussed. The *Supervision Style Index* is a modification of a model of four leadership styles based on the concept of whole-brain thinking. The original assessment inventory, which identifies the styles of Analyzer-Controller, Permitter-Observer, Developer-Feeler, and Expresser-Communicator, is part of the book *Whole-Brain Thinking* by Wonder and Donovan (1984). In the *Supervision Style Index*, STYLE I corresponds with the Analyzer-Controller style, STYLE II corresponds with the Permitter-Observer, STYLE III with the Developer-Feeler, and STYLE IV with the Expresser-Comunicator. (See chapter 3 for an additional discussion of supervision STYLES.) Again, suggestions are provided as to how to develop behaviors in non-predominant styles.

Price (1984) uses a three-category (ABC) classification system rather than the quadrant grids. He suggests that personal characteristics are blended from major tendency groups: (A)nalytical, (B)old, and (C)aring. The three tendency groups, used separately and blended, form seven leadership styles: Analyst, Challenger, Motivator, Developer, Inspirer, Instructor, and Catalyst. Characteristics of the ABC leadership styles are presented in Table 2–5.

Leadership is one of the most critical characteristics of supervision. It is important, therefore, that supervisors have some knowledge of their predominant leadership style and can evaluate the effect of the style in the five domains of supervision.

Communication styles. Underlying all of these human dimensions of supervision is communication. A supervisor's communication style can be assessed formally by means of the *Communicator Style Measure* instrument (Norton, 1983). Respondents' answers categorize them into 10 subconstructs of communicator style: Dominant, Dramatic, Contentious, Animated, Impression Leaving, Relaxed, Attentive, Open, Friendly, and Communicator Image. The inventory does not place value judgments on the categories. Rather, it describes, for the purpose of heightening awareness, how the supervisor communicates.

Communication styles, including the four interpersonal communication styles described by

TABLE 2-5
Characteristics of the A B C leadership styles

STYLE A: Analyzer/Organizer

Descriptors:	Conscientious, economical, fair, methodical, orderly, practical, precise, sensitive, stable, systematic, tactful, thorough, thoughtful, traditional
Strengths:	Accurate, cautious, conserving, orderly, persevering, self-dependent
Possible Problems:	Overly sensitive, procrastination, won't delegate
Conflict: (When dealing with others, I should...)	Introduce change slowly, be sensitive to feelings, take organized and well-planned action, use logic, treat fairly, allow self-checking, use tact when criticizing
Discipline: (When dealing with others, I should...)	Take a logical approach, have them analyze the problem, use facts and logic, emphasize the "Big Picture," give them a chance to improve, be consistent with policy
Communication: (When communicating with others, I should...)	Minimize interruptions, giving advance notice for changes, be tactful, supply complete information, ask for their input and opinions, listen closely
Appreciation: (When showing appreciation, I should...)	Recognize quality of work, point out cost savings, compliment their organized approach, comment on their ability to persevere, reinforce a willingness to change, note ability to follow a procedure
Interesting Work: (To make jobs more interesting, I should...)	Assign specific and detailed tasks, establish and document procedure and instruction, ask for input on "doing it better," have them investigate a problem, consider training into a better-matched position, reinforce methods and results

STYLE B: Bold/Challenger

Descriptors:	Achiever, assertive, change-oriented, commanding, dominant, forceful, impatient, proud, risk taker
Strengths:	Ambitious, confident, decisive, innovative, persuasive
Possible Problems:	Acts too quickly, impatient, lacks caution, not sensitive
Discipline: (When dealing with others, I should...)	Speak directly, let them "ventilate," calm them down, defend self with facts, stay in control, ask questions, follow-up
Conflict: (When dealing with others, I should...)	Have them think it through again, be open to new ideas, use incentives and challenges, ask more questions, put them in charge of the problem, have them slow down, be more direct
Communication: (When communicating with others, I should...)	Be direct and to the point, show confidence, make sure they are listening, maintain control, create a relaxed environment, be alert for impulsive or unfounded statements, ask more questions
Appreciation: (When showing	Recognize accomplishment, encourage improvements and new ideas, comment on initiative and ability to take charge, reinforce an organized approach, compliment

TABLE 2-5
continued

appreciation, I should. . .)	thoroughness and caution, reinforce their being sensitive to others' work
Interesting Work: (To make jobs more interesting, I should. . .)	Have them consider new approaches, assign tasks requiring a decision or action, put them in charge of a small group or a committee, change environment and tasks as frequently as possible, add an element of risk or change, use incentive and rewards for accomplishment

STYLE C: Caring/Motivator

Descriptors:	Gregarious, idealist, optimistic, idealistic, people-oriented, talkative
Strengths:	Cooperative, flexible, helpful, motivating, supportive
Possible Problems:	Misallocate time, lack enough facts, compromise too often
Discipline: (When dealing with others, I should. . .)	Ask for input and suggestions; compliment where possible; make sure they're listening; state conclusions first; stress the effect on material, plant, and finances; use constructive criticism
Conflict: (When dealing with others, I should. . .)	Have them declare a course of action, keep them near people, make them aware of talking too much, request more facts, set schedules and deadlines (NOTE: Style C leaders have a natural tendency to avoid conflict)
Communication: (When communicating with others, I should. . .)	Ask specific questions, be alert, get their opinion first, make sure they stick to the subject, make sure they're listening, have them defend their statements
Appreciation: (When showing appreciation, I should. . .)	Comment on improving morale, encourage thoroughness and documentation, note their ability to get their point across, notice their willingness to help, reinforce efficiency and good use of time, recognize how flexibility helps
Interesting Work: (To make jobs more interesting, I should. . .)	Allow freedom and flexibility for results, assign tasks that require different viewpoints and multiple approaches, get input and improvements from them, give them an idea of cause to promote, keep them around other people, let them be helpful to others (orientation, training)

STYLE A + B: Developer

Descriptors: Creative, industrious, self-confident, well-disciplined

STYLE B + C: Inspirer

Descriptors: Confident, optimistic, persuasive, spirited

STYLE A + C: Instructor

Descriptors: Convincing, diplomatic, intuitive, open-minded

STYLE A + B + C: Catalyst

Descriptors: Balanced, cooperative, flexible, harmonious

Source: Reprinted by permission of John Price and SourceCom ™.

Knapp (1978) and the five conflict communication styles described by Kilmann and Thomas (1975), are important tools for supervisors. The interpersonal communication styles of Amiable, Analytical, Driver, and Expressive and the conflict communication styles of Accommodation, Avoiding, Competition, Collaboration, and Compromise not only constitute a supervisor's persona, they also elicit specific patterns of behavior from supervisees. Therefore, supervisors need to know about communication generally and their own communication specifically in order to use it to facilitate productive supervision experiences. Communication competence is such an important aspect of the Constituents component of the Trigonal Model of Communication Disorders supervision that the topic is covered in detail in chapter 5.

If supervisors assess themselves, then they can synthesize the results of their assessments on the Personal Supervision Characteristics Profile shown in Table 2–6. The profile will show patterns of behavior that can either facilitate or interfere with productive supervision. The profile provides data for use in supervisors' Professional Development Plans, discussed in chapter 11.

Although the Personal Supervision Characteristics Profile is described here in reference to supervisors, many of the same inventories and resultant profiles can be used by supervisees.

Human dimensions of supervision are applied to differential supervision in chapter 3, the chapter on concepts. Supervisors who are serious about a career of supervision in Communication Disorders should plan the course of personal assessment and development in their professional life.

Career Development

Supervision offers speech-language pathologists and audiologists opportunities for career development. Building on their basic role as clinicians, they can add competencies for any of the other four supervision domains and increase the flexibility of their professional careers.

A job description is an important part of a supervisor's career development plan for at least three reasons. First, it defines the domains in which the supervisor will have responsibilities. Some supervisory positions require work in all five domains; other positions emphasize one, two, three, or four domains. Employees can make an informed decision about whether to accept a given position based on the defined duties and responsibilities. Second, a job description will direct the supervisor toward areas of competence that need to be developed. For example, if a supervisory position requires activity in the research or classroom education domains and the supervisor does not have strong competencies in those areas, she or he can direct preparation efforts accordingly. Finally, a job description can protect the supervisor during performance evaluation periods; it ensures that an employee is evaluated only on the assigned responsibilities.

Unfortunately, not all supervisor positions have job descriptions, and the documents may not be well developed if they do exist. Good job descriptions should include (but not be restricted to) the following items:

1. Position title
2. Nature and purpose of the work
   a. Duties (listed with a percent of time devoted to each)
   b. Hierarchy of responsibility
3. Scope and effect of the work
4. Supervision and guidance to be received
5. Mental and physical demands
6. Personal qualifications
7. Salary and benefits
8. Career ladder options (e.g., tenure track)

Employers may not be aware of the multiple roles of Communication Disorders supervisors and, therefore, may neglect to assign rank in the personnel hierarchy: is the Communication Disorders supervisor to be considered part of the administration, faculty, or staff? Each position

THE TRIGONAL MODEL OF COMMUNICATION DISORDERS SUPERVISION: CONSTITUENTS 43

TABLE 2-6
Personal Communication Disorders Supervision Characteristics Profile

Instructions: Mark the appropriate results from your inventories. Discuss with a colleague how these results affect your supervision.

Educational Philosophy	Educational Psychology	Inquiry Modes	Cognitive Styles	Supervision Style Index
1. Essentialism	1. Behaviorism	1. Synthesist	1. 1.a-1	1. STYLE I
2. Experimentalism	2. Cognitive	2. Idealist	2. 1.a-2	2. STYLE II
3. Existentialism	3. Humanism	3. Pragmatist	3. 1.a-3	3. STYLE III
4. 1 & 2	4. 1 & 2	4. Analyst	4. 1.b-1	4. STYLE IV
5. 2 & 3	5. 2 & 3	5. Realist	5. 1.b-2	5. I & II
6. 1 & 3	6. 1 & 3	6. I-A	6. 1.b-3	6. II & III
7. 1 & 2 & 3	7. 1 & 2 & 3	7. A-R	7. 2-1	7. III & IV
		8. S-I	8. 2-2	8. IV & I
		9. I-R	9. 2-3	9. II & IV
		10. P-R	10. 3-1	10. I & III
		11. I-P	11. 3-2	11. I & II & III
		12. A-P	12. 3-3	12. II & III & IV
		13. A-S	13. 4-1	13. I & III & IV
		14. S-P	14. 4-2	14. I & II & IV
		15. S-R	15. 4-3	15. I & II & III & IV
		16. 3-way	16. 5-1	
		17. Flat	17. 5-2	

Cognitive Style Map			
	M	m	N
T(AL)	___	___	___
T(AQ)	___	___	___
T(VL)	___	___	___
T(VQ)	___	___	___
Q(A)	___	___	___
Q(O)	___	___	___
Q(S)	___	___	___
Q(T)	___	___	___
Q(V)	___	___	___
Q(P)	___	___	___
Q(CEM)	___	___	___
Q(CES)	___	___	___
Q(CET)	___	___	___
Q(CH)	___	___	___
Q(CK)	___	___	___
Q(CKH)	___	___	___
Q(CP)	___	___	___
Q(CS)	___	___	___
Q(CT)	___	___	___
Q(CTM)	___	___	___
A	___	___	___
F	___	___	___
I	___	___	___
M	___	___	___
D	___	___	___
R	___	___	___
L	___	___	___

Communicator Styles
1. Friendly
2. Impression Leaving
3. Relaxed
4. Contentious/Argumentative
5. Attentive
6. Precise
7. Animated/Expressive
8. Dramatic
9. Open
10. Dominant
11. Communicator Image

Interpersonal/Conflict Style
1. Driver "Dominator" — Competition
2. Analytical "Computer" — Avoiding
3. Amiable "Pleaser" — Accommodation
4. Expressive "Leveler" — Collaboration
5. _____ — Compromise

18. 5-3
19. 6.a-1
20. 6.a-2
21. 6.a-3
22. 6.b-1
23. 6.b-2
24. 6.b-3
25. 7-1
26. 7-2
27. 7-3
28. 8-1
29. 8-2
30. 8-3
31. 9-1
32. 9-2
33. 9-3
34. 9-4
35. 9-5
36. 9-6
37. 9-7
38. 9-8
39. 9-9

Myers-Briggs

ISTJ	ISFJ
INFJ	INTJ
ISTP	ISFP
INFP	INTP
ESTJ	ESFJ
ENFJ	ENTJ
ESTP	ESFP
ENFP	ENTP

ABC Leadership

A A + B
B B + C
C A + C
   A + B + C

TABLE 2-6A Key to individual protocols in Table 2-6

Item	Protocol and Reference
Educational Philosophy	Educational Beliefs System Inventory
Educational Psychology	Educational Practice Belief Inventory (Dobson, Dobson, & Kessinger, 1980)
Inquiry Modes	InQ (Harrison & Bramson, 1982)
Cognitive Styles	9 Mind Tests (Greene & Lewis, 1983)
Supervision Style Index	4 Management Styles (Wonder & Donovan, 1984)
Cognitive Style Map	Hill's Modified Cognitive Style Mapping Instrument (Mountain View College, 1980)
Communicator Styles	Communicator Style Measure (Norton, 1983)
Interpersonal Styles	Four Interpersonal Styles (Knapp, 1978)
Conflict Styles	Five Conflict Styles (Kilmann & Thomas, 1975)
Myers-Briggs	Myers-Briggs Type Indicator (Myers & McCaulley, 1985)
ABC Leadership Styles	Personal Inventory (Price, 1984)

has advantages and disadvantages for individual personnel. Salary, fringe benefits, status and power within the employment system, and performance evaluation may differ for each title. Until supervisors become more knowledgeable and secure in what it is they do and can do, they may not be able to bargain effectively with employers in matters of status.

The possibilities of career development have career conflicts associated with them (Gavett, 1985). Hall (1976) identified four stages of career growth: Stage I, Exploration and Trial (ages 15 to 25 years); Stage II, Establishment and Advancement (ages 25 to 45 years); Stage III, Mid-Career Growth, Maintenance, or Stagnation (ages 45 to 65 years); and Stage IV, Disengagement (after age 65). According to Gavett (1985), the path of Communication Disorders supervisors does not follow that model. Stage I appears to be an area of breakdown for at least two reasons. First, speech-language pathologists and audiologists do not begin supervision careers at the same age as peers begin their professions; Communication Disorders personnel tend to work clinically for a substantial time before moving into supervisory positions. In the past, supervision has not been emphasized as a career option in many Communication Disorders training programs. The emphasis has been on clinical employment. Consequently, the process of Exploration and Trial comes at a time when peers may be well into Stage II, Establishment and Advancement. Second, Communication Disorders supervisors tend to spend an inordinate amount of time in the Exploration and Trial stage, perhaps for two reasons: (a) they do not have a good sense of professional identity because of insufficient preparation in their clinical training or through continuing education programs, or (b) employers do not know how to make maximum use of the supervisors' preparation. As a consequence, much time is spent in Stage I trying to find the niche that will lead to Stage II. If supervision is presented as a viable career option in clinical training programs and if students receive preparation for supervision, then well-developed job descriptions can be of value for Communication Disorders supervisors in Stage I.

Problems at Stage II relate to the job description issue also. The descriptions must include the possibility for upward mobility with clear criterion statements at each rung of the career ladder. Because most Communication Disorders supervisors have not left Stages I and II, little is known about the career ladder for these people at Stages III and IV. The situation can change with increased efforts to prepare supervisors and employers for the roles of supervision.

Another issue in the career ladder dilemma is that of gender. Since a majority of Communication Disorders supervisors are female, when they accept a supervision position that includes multiple roles, they have had to compete in traditionally male-dominated administrative echelons. Even though female supervisors may function in a variety of capacities, due respect and compensation is rarely afforded them, especially in the form of career ladder options commensurate with those of male counterparts (Langellier & Natalle, 1987). (The concept of genderlect is discussed in greater detail in chapter 5.)

Stress and Burnout

A consequence of career ladder problems for some Communication Disorders supervisors is stress and, perhaps, burnout. Stress, defined as "a coordinated organismic response of all components, all systems of the organism—physical, emotional, cognitive, behavioral, interpersonal—to perceived threat or disequilibrium" (Block, 1980, p. 134), is generally considered to be a negative force in most lives, though stress in moderation can stimulate optimum performance in many individuals. Stress is considered to be cumulative both vertically (i.e., within one dimension of life, such as the professional or personal) and horizontally (i.e., across all dimensions of life). Supervisors without clear professional identity, job descriptions, or career development options are in disequilibrium and may perceive this situation as threatening to their professional and personal lives. According to Block (1980), stress and burnout are deleterious not only to the person who experiences the phenomena but to entire professions. Excellent employees may be lost to these areas because of what seem like untenable professional conditions.

Current thinking about stress considers it an ongoing, rather than episodic, aspect of living and working and argues that people should learn to *manage* (not eliminate) stress through active strategies. Stress management has three components: knowledge, skill, and resources. Awareness is the first level of knowledge; supervisors must have information about stress and burnout in general and know specifically what causes stress in their own lives. The knowledge about stress will include elements of attribution theory, which identifies the aspects of life over which individuals have control. Bourne and Ekstrand (1982) discuss the basic dimensions of attribution theory:

1. *Personal vs. universal* dimension. A personal attribution (something an individual has potential control over) will lead to more severe symptoms than a universal attribution (something that is totally out of the individual's control). For example, in the area of grantsmanship, if a supervisor is not a good grant writer (an ability that belongs to the Research and Administrative domains), then the organization may not receive adequate funding to support a strong supervisory staff. This is a personal attribute that can contribute strongly to stress. On the other hand, if the federal government has stopped all funding of grants to Communication Disorders programs, the supervisor has no control over this universal attribution and therefore perceives the lack of money from the federal source as a less stressful condition.
2. *Stable vs. unstable* dimension. Stable attributions (those not likely to change over time) produce more severe effects than unstable ones. A supervision position with no advancement possibilities (stable attribution) is a stronger contributor to stress than positions that offer opportunities for advancement.
3. *Global vs. specific* dimension. Global attributions (e.g., no supervisor has good working conditions) lead to more serious consequences than specific ones (e.g., one's personal situation is considered intolerable).

Supervisors are most likely to experience stress and burnout when they lack control of important dimensions of their lives and identify a *personal-stable-global* attribution pattern of why control is lacking.

Another aspect of awareness is knowledge of what strategies are available for managing stress. After effective management strategies are identified, skills can be developed for employing them as necessary. Although stress is a personal phenomenon (i.e., different things are stressful to different people; people have varying degrees of stress tolerance), some generic management strategies include: developing realistic, clearly stated personal and professional goals; developing a strong, distinctive guiding philosophy; taking time for periodic stress and burnout checkups; developing skills that are not strong to improve overall competence; arranging each day so that rewarding and unrewarding activities alternate; becoming knowledgeable about and skillful in creative problem management (see chapter 8) and conflict management (see chapter 5); and developing support groups and/or resource exchange networks. (If this final strategy is to involve using community resources, they must be available and readily accessible.)

In short, it is important that supervisors become prepared for the multifaceted work of Communication Disorders supervision. Self-assessment measures, career development, and stress management are ways for clinical personnel to develop into the specialty area of Communication Disorders supervision. Chapters 6 through 11 contain specific information about areas of professional competence that supervisors need in order to work effectively in the five domains of Communication Disorders supervision.

SUPERVISEES

The second group of people involved in Communication Disorders supervision, the supervisees, must also prepare for the supervision process.

Types

Many different people may be supervisees, including undergraduate and graduate student clinicians; graduate students doing clinical supervision practicum and being supervised by faculty/staff supervisors; peers; clinical fellows; paraprofessionals and aides; ancillary personnel; and clients' family members, primary caregivers, or significant others. These different types of supervisees have different supervision needs, different knowledge and skill levels, and different degrees of willingness to be supervised. Within the Communication Disorders profession itself, Dowling and Wittkopp have documented differential needs of supervisees (1982). Other studies have shown that different levels of supervisees ranked in different orders the importance of the 13 supervisor tasks developed by the ASHA Committee on Supervision (Hull & Kramer, 1985; Mornout, Siegle, & Solomon, 1985). As a group, the 83 respondents in the Mornout et al. study (representing six groups from beginning undergraduate clinicians to advanced graduate clinicians and supervisors) ranked the 13 tasks in this order of priority: 4.0, 1.0, 2.0, 3.0, 9.0, 6.0, 5.0, 12.0, 10.0, 8.0, 7.0, 11.0, 13.0 (see appendix A). However, each of the six groups ranked the tasks differently.

Levels

Most Communication Disorders training programs categorize supervisees into levels based on experience, such as the following example:

- *Level 0:* paraprofessionals and aides; parents, family members, and significant others; ancillary personnel.
- *Level I:* student clinicians who have completed 0–100 clock hours of clinical practicum.

- *Level II:* student clinicians who have completed 101–200 clinical clock hours; experienced paraprofessionals and aides.
- *Level III:* student clinicians who have completed 201–300+ clinical clock hours; ancillary personnel trained in teamwork.
- *Level IV:* professional peers; graduate students doing clinical supervision practicum; clinical fellows.

A categorical system such as this can be used for differential supervision.

Differential Supervision

Differential supervision allows the people who are involved in the supervision process to participate to the best of their abilities. If supervisees are differentiated by level of knowledge and willingness to participate, each of the levels requires a different supervisory tack. A supervisor must be able to match the needs of supervisees with appropriate modes of action. One way to attain participant congruence is for supervisors to find out as much as possible about the people with whom they will be interacting and adjust their own modes of action accordingly.

The *Educational Beliefs System Inventory* (Dobson et al., 1980), the *Cognitive Style Mapping Instrument* (Erhardt & Corvey, 1980), Kolb's (1978) *Model of Experiential Learning*, the *Nine Mind Tests* (Greene & Lewis, 1983), or the *Myers-Briggs Type Indicator* (Myers & McCaulley, 1985), all described earlier as tools to help supervisors develop self-awareness, may also prove beneficial to supervisees in identifying their learning strategies. Supervisees then can work with supervisors to create preferred learning conditions.

Hersey and Blanchard (1982) have written about the *readiness states* of individuals, using the parameters of ability (the necessary knowledge, experience, and skill) and willingness (the necessary confidence, commitment, and motivation). The concept of readiness states (RS) is applicable to Communication Disorders supervisees: RS1 = unable and unwilling or insecure; RS2 = unable but willing or confident; RS3 = able but unwilling or insecure; and RS4 = able and willing or confident. Once a supervisor has identified a supervisee's readiness state, supervision can be transacted in the most appropriate manner.

In the clinical process, learning occurs most readily when the clinician's modes of interaction are congruent with those of the client (Weiss, 1983). A parallel assumption can be made about the supervisor-supervisee relationship during supervision (Farmer, 1984). The process of matching the cognitive, linguistic, and social components of communication is called *Interpersonal Communication Pacing* and is described in detail in chapter 5.

Brasseur (1987) offers another view of supervisee preparation. She suggests preparing supervisees by informing them of the components of the supervision process, discussing their perceptions about supervision, setting goals and objectives for supervision, exploring supervisees' prior experiences in supervision, identifying their style preferences, exploring their anxieties, and establishing their baseline needs and competencies.

It is useful for supervisees at any level to prepare to be active participants in supervision. To accomplish this goal for all supervisees, some form of differential preparation is necessary.

OTHERS

Clients/Patients

Differential supervisee preparation can, in turn, maximize the quality of service provided to clients or patients. Too often clients are overlooked as an integral part of the constituent paradigm. However, in some situations it is appropriate to involve them heavily in the supervision process, from the beginning (setting client and clinician goals and objectives) to the end (evaluation of client progress and clinician effectiveness). This client involvement is the essence of Wholistic Supervision (Farmer, 1986c). No matter how actively clients are involved in the supervision process, they must always be considered a part of the constituency.

Other Constituents

Occasionally other individuals may be included in the Constituents component of the Trigonal Model. For example, the ancillary personnel on multi-, inter-, or transdisciplinary teams may participate in the supervision process, not necessarily as supervisees. Family members, primary caregivers, and significant others of the client or patient may fall into this same category of participants but not supervisees. No matter to what degree a person participates in the supervision process, it is wise to prepare him or her to take part productively.

SUMMARY

Four groups of people make up the Constituents component of the Trigonal Model of Communication Disorders supervision: supervisors, supervisees, clients/patients, and others. All four groups of people need some preparation for the supervisory process. The most extensive preparation is done by supervisors, who prepare by gaining knowledge (through self-awareness assessment, academics, training, and continuing education) and competencies to operate in the five supervision roles (Professional, Researcher, Educator, Administrator, and Clinician). Supervisors are classified as clinical or staff, primary or secondary, generic or categorical, on-site or field.

All Constituents need some type of preparation to participate productively in the supervision process. The differences in this preparation are an integral part of differential supervision. Differential supervision, which means adapting supervision efforts to the ability and willingness of the participants, is one way to enhance supervision. It contributes to the process of developing and maintaining competent speech-language pathologists and audiologists, and it also improves the quality of services to consumers.

With education and training in supervision, supervisors gain career development opportunities that other speech-language pathologists and audiologists do not have.

APPLICATIONS

Discussion Topics

1. Discuss the five roles, or domains, of Communication Disorders supervision. What kind of preparation is needed for each?
2. Discuss the differences between generic and categorical supervisors.
3. Discuss the four problems identified in this chapter that are associated with the 13 tasks and 81 competencies developed by the ASHA Committee on Supervision.
4. Discuss the levels of supervisees and their differential preparation needs.

5. Discuss the advantages and disadvantages for supervisors of being ranked as administration, as faculty, and as staff in college and university settings.

Laboratory Experiences

1. Design a continuing education workshop to teach about the Administrator role of supervisors.
2. Develop procedures to prepare supervisors and supervisees for supervising beginning students, peers/colleagues, parents or significant others, graduate students, CFY supervision (as supervisee and supervisor); and paraprofessionals or aides.
3. Complete a Personal Communication Disorders Supervision Characteristics Profile (see Table 2-6).
4. Develop three job descriptions to represent these combinations of roles:
   a. P + R + E + A + C
   b. E + A + C
   c. P + R + E
5. Develop and implement a stress reduction program for the supervisors in your worksite.

Research Projects

1. Design and conduct a study to explore stress and burnout in Communication Disorders supervisors.
2. Design and conduct a study to validate the concept of differential supervision.
3. Design and conduct a study using the five inquiry modes.
4. Design and conduct a study using one of the models of cognitive styles.
5. Design and conduct a study using one of the models of leadership styles.

REFERENCES

American Speech and Hearing Association. (1976). *Comprehensive Assessment and Service Evaluation (CASE) Information System*. Rockville, MD: Author.

American Speech and Hearing Association. (1978). Current status of supervision of speech-language pathology and audiology. Committee on Supervision in Speech Pathology and Audiology. *Asha, 20,* 478–486.

American Speech-Language-Hearing Association. (1982). *Child Services Review System*. Rockville, MD: Author.

American Speech-Language-Hearing Association Committee on Supervision in Speech-Language Pathology and Audiology. (1985). Clinical supervision in speech-language pathology and audiology (position statement). *Asha, 7,* 57–60.

Anderson, J. (1974). Supervision of school speech, hearing, and language programs: An emerging role. *Asha, 16,* 7–10.

Anderson, J. (Ed.). (1980). *Proceedings of the conference on training in the supervisory process in speech-language pathology and audiology.* Bloomington: Indiana University.

Anderson, J. (1988). *The supervisory process in speech-language pathology and audiology.* Boston: Little, Brown/College-Hill Press.

Barnes, K., & Pines, D. (1982). Assessing and improving services to the handicapped. *Asha, 24,* 555–559.

Blake, R., & Mouton, J. (1964). *The managerial grid.* Houston: Gulf.

Block, J. (1980). Stress and burnout in supervisors. In J. L. Anderson (Ed.), *Proceedings of the conference on training in the supervisory process in speech-language pathology and audiology* (pp. 128–161). Bloomington: Indiana University.

Bourne, L., & Ekstrand, B. (1982). *Psychology: Its principles and meanings.* New York: Holt, Rinehart & Winston.

Brasseur, J. (1987). Preparation of supervisees for the supervisory process. In S. Farmer (Ed.), *Clinical supervision: A coming of age. Proceedings of a national conference on supervision.* Las Cruces: New Mexico State University.

Brinkerhoff, R. (1987). *Achieving results from training.* San Francisco: Jossey-Bass.

Council of University Supervisors of Practicum in Speech-Language Pathology and Audiology. (1982). Constitution of the Council of University Supervisors of Practicum in Speech-Language Pathology and Audiology. *SUPERvision, 6* (1), 8–10.

deVille, J. (1984). *The psychology of leadership.* New York: New American Library (Mentor).

Dobson, R., & Dobson, J. (1981). *The language of schooling.* Lanham, MD: University Press of America.

Dobson, R., Dobson, J., & Kessinger, J. (1980). *Staff development: A humanistic approach.* Lanham, MD: University Press of America.

Dowling, S. (1983, November). *The impact of training in supervision upon conference talk behaviors.* Paper presented at the annual convention of the American Speech-Language-Hearing Association, Cincinnati, OH.

Dowling, S., & Wittkopp, J. (1982). Students' perceived supervisory needs. *Journal of Communication Disorders, 15,* 319–328.

Dublinske, S., & Grimes, J. (1971). *Program Planning Evaluation.* Unpublished workshop materials available from the authors, ASHA, Rockville, MD.

Erhardt, H., & Corvey, S. (1980). *Cognitive style: In search of buried treasure.* Dallas, TX: Mountain View College.

Farmer, S. (1984). Supervisory conferences in communicative disorders: Verbal and nonverbal interpersonal communication pacing. *Dissertation Abstracts International, 44,* 2715 B. (University Microfilms No. 84-00, 891)

Farmer, S. (1985, November). *Supervision in communicative disorders: Metalinguistic analysis of assumptions and predictions. Phase I.* Paper presented at the annual convention of the American Speech-Language-Hearing Association, Washington, DC.

Farmer, S. (1986a). Relationship development in supervisory conferences: A tripartite view of the process. *The Clinical Supervisor, 3*(4), 5–21.

Farmer, S. (1986b). *Supervision Style Index*. Unpublished inventory. New Mexico State University, Las Cruces, NM.

Farmer, S. (1986c). *Wholistic supervision*. Unpublished manuscript, New Mexico State University, Las Cruces.

Gavett, E. (1985). Clinical supervision in a university setting. In J. Bernthal (Ed.), *Proceedings: Sixth Annual Conference on Graduate Education* (pp. 20–25). Lincoln: University of Nebraska, Department of Special Education and Communication Disorders.

Greene, J., & Lewis, D. (1983). *Know your own mind*. New York: Rawson Associates.

Hall, D. (1976). *Careers in organization*. Goodyear Publishing.

Harrison, A., & Bramson, R. (1984). *The art of thinking*. New York: Doubleday.

Hersey, P., & Blanchard, K. (1982). *Management of organizational behavior: Utilizing human resources* (4th ed.). Englewood Cliffs, NJ: Prentice-Hall.

Hull, R., & Kramer, W. (1985, November). *Graduate and undergraduate ratings of thirteen ASHA approved supervision competences*. Paper presented at the annual convention of the American Speech-Language-Hearing Association, Washington, DC.

Kilmann, R., & Thomas, K. (1975). Interpersonal conflict: Handling behavior as reflections of Jungian personality dimensions. *Psychological Reports, 37,* 971–980.

Knapp, M. (1978). *Social intercourse: From greeting to goodbye*. Boston: Allyn & Bacon.

Knowles, M. (1970). *The modern practice of adult education: Andragogy versus pedagogy*. New York: Association Press.

Knowles, M. (1973). *The adult learner: A neglected species*. Houston: Gulf.

Kolb, D. (1978). *Learning style inventory: Technical manual* (rev. ed.). Boston: William McBee.

Langellier, K., & Natalle, E. (1987). Communication, gender perspectives, and the clinical supervisor. In S. Farmer (Ed.), *Clinical supervision: A coming of age. Proceedings of a national conference on supervision* (pp. 14–38). Las Cruces: New Mexico State University.

Mornout, C., Siegle, D., & Solomon, B. (1985, November). *Which competencies are important for clinical supervision?* Paper presented at the annual convention of the American Speech-Language-Hearing Association, Washington, DC.

Mountain View College. (1980). *Hill's Modified Cognitive Style Mapping Instrument*. Dallas, TX: Author.

Myers, I., & McCaulley, M. (1985). *Manual: A guide to the development of the Myers-Briggs Type Indicator*. Palo Alto, CA: Consulting Psychologists Press.

Norton, R. (1983). *Communicator style: Theory, applications, and measures*. Beverly Hills, CA: Sage.

Oas, D. (1987). Establishing and maintaining an effective working relationship with the supervisee. In S. Farmer (Ed.), *Clinical supervision: A coming of age. Proceedings of a national conference on supervision* (pp. 45–49). Las Cruces: New Mexico State University.

Pickering, M. (1985). Clinical supervision in a university setting. In J. Bernthal (Ed.), *Proceedings: Sixth Annual Conference on Graduate Education* (pp. 15–19).

Lincoln: University of Nebraska, Department of Special Education and Communication Disorders.

Price, J. (1984). *Personal Inventory: Planning For On-The-Job Growth.* Assessment materials, Keye Productivity Center, Shawnee Mission, KS.

Rassi, J. (1987). The questions of self-evaluation. *SUPERvision, 10*(4), 2–3.

Reddin, W. (1970). *Managerial effectiveness.* New York: McGraw-Hill.

Schubert, G. (1974). Suggested minimum requirements for clinical supervisors. *Asha, 16,* 10.

Shewan, C. (1988). ASHA members at work. *Asha, 30,* 49.

Sleight, C., & Craig, C. (1987). Personality types and supervision. In S. Farmer (Ed.), *Clinical supervision: A coming of age. Proceedings of a national conference on supervision* (pp. 66–72). Las Cruces: New Mexico State University.

Ulrich, S. (1987). Supervision: A developing specialty. In M. Crago & M. Pickering (Eds.), *Supervision in human communication disorders: Perspectives on a process* (pp. 3–29). Boston: Little, Brown/College-Hill Press.

Weiss, R. (1983). *INREAL Training Evaluation Model (ITEM)* (revised). Unpublished interaction analysis system used in INREAL Training.

Wonder, J., & Donovan, P. (1984). *Whole-brain thinking.* New York: Random House (Ballantine).

3
The Trigonal Model of Communication Disorders Supervision: Concepts

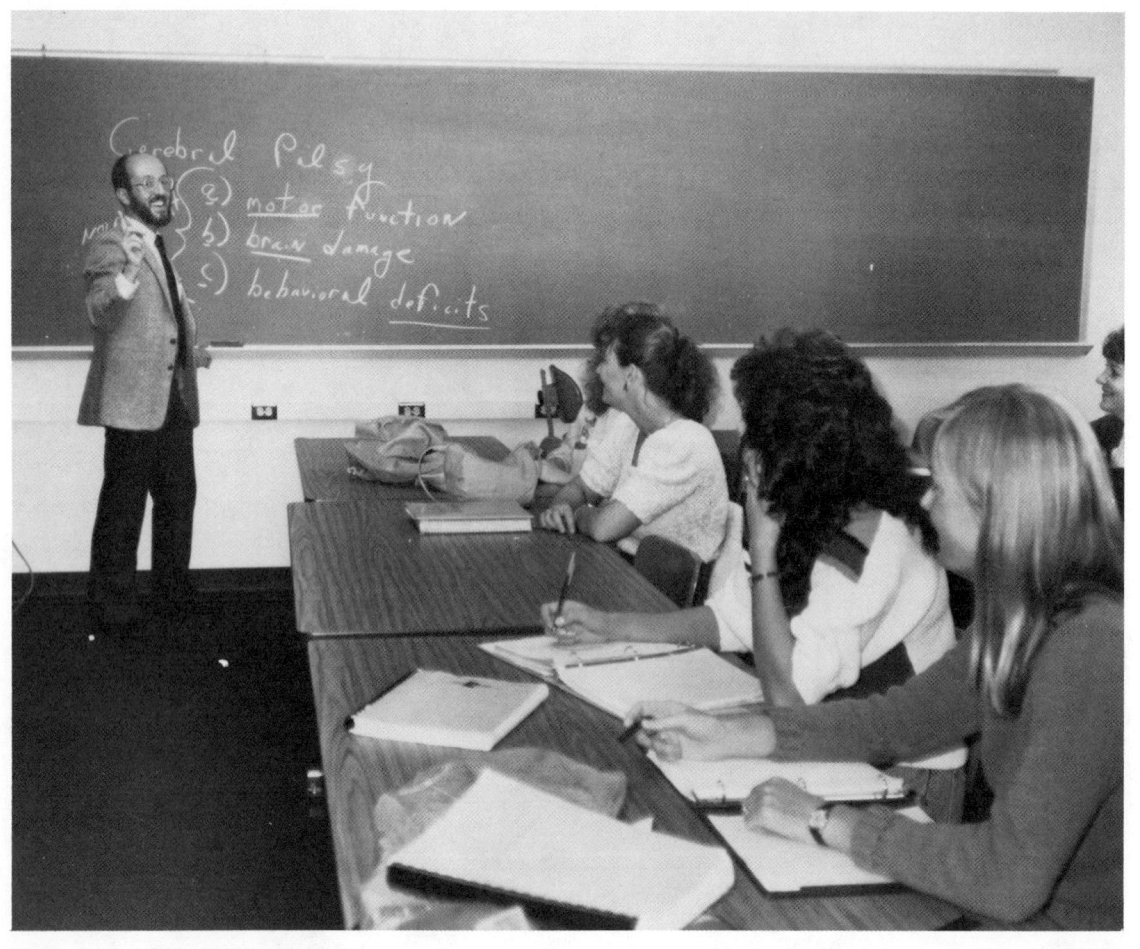

CRITICAL CONCEPTS

- *The model of supervision as a process evolved from general systems theory.*
- *Four STYLES combined with two forms make eight types of communication disorders supervision.*
- *Differential supervision involves preparing constituents to participate in the supervision process.*
- *Supervision involves change.*
- *Supervision in Speech-Language Pathology and Supervision in Audiology have commonalities.*
- *Supervision is a specialty area of Communication Disorders.*

OUTLINE

INTRODUCTION

IDEAS AND ISSUES
  Systems
  Theories of Supervision
  Styles of Supervision
  STYLES of Communication Disorders Supervision
  Forms of Supervision
  Types (STYLES + Forms) of Communication Disorders Supervision
  Differential Supervision
  Change
  Supervision in Speech-Language Pathology versus Supervision in Audiology
  Supervision as a Specialty Area in Communication Disorders

SUMMARY

APPLICATIONS

INTRODUCTION

The Concepts component of the Trigonal Model of Communication Disorders supervision includes ideas and issues studied and written about in the general body of supervision literature, as well as work specific to Communication Disorders supervision. The Concepts component may be the most complex of the three. Material in this chapter blends old with new, familiar with unfamiliar, strong data-based information with hypotheses and theories. Readers who are experienced in supervision will be familiar with, or will readily apply, many of the concepts. However, they will find others that will trigger fruitful future study to expand their knowledge. Beginning students of supervision will be exposed to some of the basic thoughts about the topic and can also gain a sense of its complexity.

IDEAS AND ISSUES

The Concepts component of the Trigonal Model of Communication Disorders supervision has four major subdivisions: (a) theories and models used to discuss the supervision process, (b) differential supervision, (c) supervision in Speech-Language Pathology versus supervision in Audiology, and (d) supervision as a specialty area

---

This chapter was contributed by Stephen S. Farmer, New Mexico State University.

in Communication Disorders. All four issues affect all domains of the Pentagonal Model of Communication Disorders supervision.

Systems

To understand the process of supervision in Communication Disorders, it is important to review the concept of *systems*. In General Systems Theory (GST) a system is defined as a group of entities and the relations among them as they function as a whole or a unit (Bertalanffy, 1968). The components of Communication Disorders supervision are not static entities, but dynamic processes, or systems, having form and movement; they must be conceptualized as such for future productive study. Hall and Fagin (1956) and Watzlawick, Beavin, and Jackson (1967) have developed principles of systems that are germane to supervision:

1. Systems can be *closed or open*; supervision interactions should be open systems.
2. Systems exhibit *wholeness*; all parts of the systems are related, and change in one part causes change in others.
3. Systems exhibit *equifinality*; similar initial conditions can yield different outcomes and similar outcomes can result from different initial conditions.
4. A *morphostatic process* is feedback that maintains a system.
5. A *morphogenic process* is a mechanism of change in a system (Hall & Fagin, 1956).
6. The constant stream of events is divided, or *punctuated*, into sequences of cause and effect, determined by human initiations or responses (Watzlawick et al., 1967)

The concepts of systems are complex and difficult to comprehend. However, general systems thinking appears to be a beneficial tool for studying the Communication Disorders supervision process.

General systems thinking (also called dialectical or postformal thinking) is a specialized area of cognitive psychology. Its paradigms include the notion that forms or systems undergo transformations, moving in the direction of greater differentiation of parts, greater integration of those parts, and greater inclusiveness with other seemingly unrelated forms or systems. Ultimately all systems are unitary. Their progress to this end is moved by interactions within the boundaries of any system, between a system and others within its contextual location, and between systems interacting among themselves within that space. All interactions affect the given system. Growth toward general systems thinking involves understanding four basic components of systems: movement, form, relationship and value, and metaformal issues (Coulter, 1986).

In short, supervision can be thought of as a system composed of forms that interact through movement toward some goal. The systems theory of supervision has evolved from a series of other theories of supervision.

Theories of Supervision

Theories of supervision are built out of the philosophical and psychological ideas about learning, personality type, cognitive style, inquiry mode, and leadership style discussed in chapter 2. Theories form the framework of supervision; classifications, competencies, styles, forms, and types of supervision make up the patterns of the different theories.

Historically, supervision has progressed through a series of four theoretical models: (a) Scientific Management, (b) Human Relations Supervision, (c) Neoscientific Management, and (d) Human Resources Supervision (Sergiovanni & Starratt, 1979). The four models are differentiated as follows:

1. *Scientific Management* represents the classical autocratic philosophy of supervision in which supervisees are viewed as extensions of administration and as such are expected to carry out prespecified duties according to the

administration's wishes. The method emphasizes control, accountability, and efficiency in a closed, inflexible system of boss-subordinate relationships. In Scientific Management, supervisees are managed extensively and dictatorially in an effort to ensure (for administrators, supervisors, and the public) that good professional service is provided. In practice, supervisees were not satisfied with such a task-oriented approach to supervision. The pendulum then swung to the opposite end of the task oriented-relation oriented continuum, that is, to individuals and their relationships.

2. *Human Relations Supervision* had its beginning in the democratic movement of the 1930s. Supervisees were viewed as complete individuals rather than as packages of needed energy, skills, and aptitudes to be used by administrators and supervisors. Supervisee participation was to be a method of making them feel useful and important. This participation was to create a feeling of satisfaction among the personnel; it was assumed that a satisfied workforce would work harder and would be easier to work with, to lead, and to control. "Feelings" and "meaningful relationships" were the watchwords of human relations supervision. However, even though supervisees were feeling good about themselves and their relationships, some were not being effective, efficient employees. This led supervision back toward a task product orientation.

3. *Neoscientific Management* developed as a reaction to Human Relations Supervision and shares with traditional Scientific Management an emphasis on control, accountability, and efficiency. Its methods include competencies, performance objectives, and cost-benefit analysis. In Neoscientific Management, impersonal, technical, or rational control mechanisms substitute for face-to-face close supervision. It is assumed that if supervisors can set visible standards of performance, list objectives, or identify competencies, then they can control supervisees by holding them accountable for these standards, thereby ensuring excellent work for administrators and for the consumer. But even though supervisors shared decision making responsibility, they overemphasized the technical aspects of external control (goals and objectives) and underemphasized personal contact between supervisor and supervisee. This need led to the fourth, and current, theoretical phase of supervision.

4. *Human Resources Supervision* combines aspects of both the Scientific Management and the Human Relations methodologies; it is the approach that receives most support in Communication Disorders supervision. Whereas shared decision making in Human Relations Supervision is designed to increase supervisee satisfaction in order to increase work effectiveness, the emphasis is reversed in Human Resources Supervision: the purpose of the shared decision making is to increase work effectiveness, which in turn increases supervisee satisfaction. According to this view, satisfaction results from the successful accomplishment of important and meaningful objectives, and this accomplishment is the key to effectiveness. The human resources view appears to provide the necessary integration between person and organization, personality and accomplishment, relationships and tasks. Specific models of Human Resources Supervision include Clinical Supervision, or Colleagueship (Cogan, 1973; Goldhammer, 1969), Humanistic Supervision (Abrell, 1974), the Molar Model (Oratio, 1977), the Clinical Theory of Instruction (Hunter, 1978), ASSIST-M (Crago, 1983), Diagnostic Supervision (Duffy, 1984), the Integrative Task-Maturity Model of Supervision (ITMMS) (Mawdsley, 1985), and Collaborative Consultation (Idol, Paolucci-Whitcomb, & Nevin, 1986).

The *Colleagueship* model is presented as a cycle of eight phases in which quality of work depends on the relationship of the supervisor and supervisee. *Humanistic Supervision* attempts to create an environment that encourages human growth and fulfillment of goals among supervisees and supervisors through constructive, other-centered action that leads to the growth of others, to the improvement of the teaching-learning process, and to self-development. This model is based on the educational psychology theory of humanism and the concept of andragogical, or adult, learning style (Knowles, 1970, 1973). The *Molar Model* was proposed by Oratio as a transactive model that integrated the cognitive, emotional, and experiential elements of the supervision process. Oratio, like Crago and other Human Resources theorists, stressed the importance of self-exploration as facilitating self-supervision. The *Clinical Theory of Instruction* emerged from educational research in human learning. Hunter analyzed the instructional decisions and actions that teachers make either consciously or by default. Instruction—a teacher's deliberate action to increase the probability of learning—provides the theoretical and clinical framework to guide the substance, not the form, of those decisions and actions so that they promote intended learning more effectively. This model of supervision incorporates a process for identifying potentially effective management solutions to instructional problems regardless of goals. *ASSIST-M* is an interactional, self-exploratory approach to supervisee training. *Diagnostic Supervision* is a mutual process of recognizing needs, defining problems, and agreeing on objectives so as to increase the professional effectiveness of both supervisor and supervisee. The supervisee completes a Diagnostic Conference Planning Questionnaire that is used by the supervisor during the diagnostic conference. The *Integrative Task-Maturity Model of Supervision* (ITMMS) was developed by Mawdsley (1985) to help users arrive at an appropriate supervisor-supervisee match for supervision style (direct or indirect) and the accompanying specific techniques. The *ITMMS* is a composite of the Situational Leadership Model of Hersey and Blanchard (1982), the *Wisconsin Procedure for Appraisal of Clinical Competence* (W-PACC) (Shriberg, Filley, Hayes, Kwiatkowski, Schatz, Simmons, & Smith, 1975), Cogan's (1973) phases of colleagueship, and techniques from Acheson and Gall (1980), Boone and Prescott (1972), and Ingrisano, Hebalk, and Rathmel (1979). *Collaborative Consultation* is an interactive process that enables professionals from different disciplines to collaborate in solving mutually defined problems so as to reach outcomes that are enhanced or different from the solution that any individual would produce independently.

Theories of supervision are often associated with styles of supervision.

Styles of Supervision

Historically, two problems have been associated with the study of supervision styles. First, styles have been imagined as falling along unidimensional continua, or strands (e.g., direct-indirect, unilateral-bilateral). Such models are limited and simplistic. Second, styles have been represented as holding a single position along one of the strands (e.g., a "direct" style on the direct-indirect continuum). This approach is not flexible enough to convey the complexity of supervision styles. The result of these two problems is a fractured, static picture of solitary concepts, rather than a wholistic view of dynamic systems of behavior. A more complete method of describing supervision styles (Farmer & Farmer, 1986) is to synthesize single-point styles data into models of *composite actions,* or Communication Disorders supervision STYLES. The single-point concept of styles (lowercase) and the concept of STYLES (uppercase) as composite actions will be differentiated by upper and lowercase print throughout the text.

A review of the information available about supervision styles shows that they can be categorized as focusing on (a) people and their relationships; (b) tasks and their products; or (c) supervision as a process. Examples of representative styles follow:

1. A *unilateral-bilateral* style targets the respective *amounts* of input the supervisor and the supervisee(s) have into the process. Supervisors who follow unilateral practices establish goals and objectives and hold the supervisee accountable to those standards. In bilateral styles, supervisor and supervisee set goals and objectives jointly and determine jointly whether or not those standards were met. "Pure" forms rarely occur, and supervisor and supervisee input should be viewed on a continuum from unilateral to bilateral (Flower, 1984).
2. *Direct-indirect* supervision, though similar to the unilateral-bilateral orientation, focuses on the *quality* of communication in addition to the amount of talk. For example, indirect supervisors encourage more supervisee talk, use supervisees' ideas, ask the supervisees for opinions and suggestions, make no direct criticism, and try to reflect and extend supervisees' ideas. Direct supervision shows opposite patterns (Blumberg, 1974; Flanders, 1960; Oratio, 1977).
3. *Supervisee-oriented* supervision has as its focus the development of supervisees into competent professionals. This approach may emphasize the acquisition of skills, dispositions, or professional competence, as jointly determined by the supervisor and supervisee (Ward & Webster, 1965a, 1965b).
4. *Supervisor-oriented* supervision has the supervisor (rather than supervisees, clients/patients, the organization, etc.) as its focus. All phases of supervision revolve around the supervisor. This approach may emphasize supervisees' acquisition of skills, dispositions, or professional competence, as determined by the supervisor (Sergiovanni & Starratt, 1979).
5. *Client-oriented* supervision focuses on the communication needs of clients. The development of supervisees' professional competence is secondary to their meeting the needs of clients/patients (Prather, 1967; Starkweather, 1974).
6. *Clinical skill-interpersonal skill* supervision focuses on the skill development of supervisees (Farmer & Farmer, 1986).
7. *Clinical disposition-interpersonal disposition* supervision focuses on the dispositions development of supervisees (Farmer & Farmer, 1986).
8. *Professional competence* supervision focuses on a blend of supervisees' acquisition of skills and of dispositions (Farmer & Farmer, 1986).
9. *Task-oriented-relations-oriented* supervision focuses either on the development of supervisees' clinical skills (task-oriented), on the change in a client's communication behavior (client-oriented), or on the interpersonal skills of the supervisee (relations-oriented) (Sergiovanni & Elliot, 1975).
10. *Product concern-people concern* supervision focuses either on the clinical process (product) or on the client-clinician relationship (people). Another application is the focus on development of supervisees' skills (product) or on the development of supervisees as total professionals (people) (Blake & Mouton, 1964).
11. *Instructive-communicative* supervision focuses on the *intent* of the supervision process. If the supervisor's intent is to teach *to* the supervisee, then the style is instructive; if the intent is that learning occur through communication *interactions,* then the style is communicative. These styles can include orientations toward skills, dispositions, competence, the supervisee, the supervisor, client, tasks, relations, products, people, or goals (Farmer & Farmer, 1986).
12. *Goal-oriented* supervision focuses on the goals and objectives of the supervisor, supervisee, client, or organization. The goals, not the people involved in the process, are what is important (Sergiovanni & Starratt, 1979).

13. *Goal-directed* supervision uses goals to help direct the development of the supervisor, supervisee, client, or organization. The goals are a means to an end, not the end (Sergiovanni & Starratt, 1979).
14. *Self-directed* supervision is characterized by the supervisee's use of self-exploration strategies (Crago, 1983).
15. *Mutually-directed* supervision is similar to indirect supervision (Crago, 1983).

Each of the 15 items has in the past been thought of as a specific style. However, because supervision is now being understood as a multidimensional process, the concept of STYLES is more often used so as to represent the multidimensional and movement aspects of supervision systems. The following discussion presents this perspective.

STYLES of Communication Disorders Supervision

The concept of STYLES is unique to Communication Disorders supervision. It synthesizes information from sources in other professions (e.g., medicine, business, education, management, psychology) in order to define specific modes of action in the supervision process. An operational definition of Communication Disorders supervision STYLES follows:

> Supervision STYLES are distinctive, characteristic, identifiable *aggregates of behavior* that form *modes of action* focused on people and their relationships, on tasks and their products, and on the process of supervision.

The General Systems Theory helps us understand the evolution of the concept of STYLES. The evolutionary process and associated descriptions are illustrated in Figures 3-1 through 3-5.

STYLES of Communication Disorders supervision can be viewed as continua or as matrices. The concept of the continuum allows us to consider movement from point to point along one plane, shifting degrees of focus from one pole to another. Three examples of single strand continua, such as direct/indirect, are shown in Figure 3-1.

The historical concept of styles typically used one continuum. However, the combination of continua allows for creating double-strand or multiple-strand STYLES. The double- and multiple-strand concept is presented in Figure 3-2.

Each supervision styles strand can also be conceptualized in more than one plane, or as a matrix with a horizontal (abscissa, or X) axis and a vertical (ordinate, or Y) axis. To form a style matrix, a strand is divided in the middle; low and high degrees of each dimension are marked. The strand is rotated to form a 90° angle and then the defined square is divided into quadrants, each of which represents a high or low degree of each of the two dimensions of the strand. The continuum-to-matrix transposition and three examples of single-strand matrices are shown in Figure 3-3.

FIGURE 3-1 Single-strand continua

Unilateral ——————————— Bilateral

Clinical Skills ··············· Interpersonal Skills

Clinical Dispositions — — — — Interpersonal Dispositions

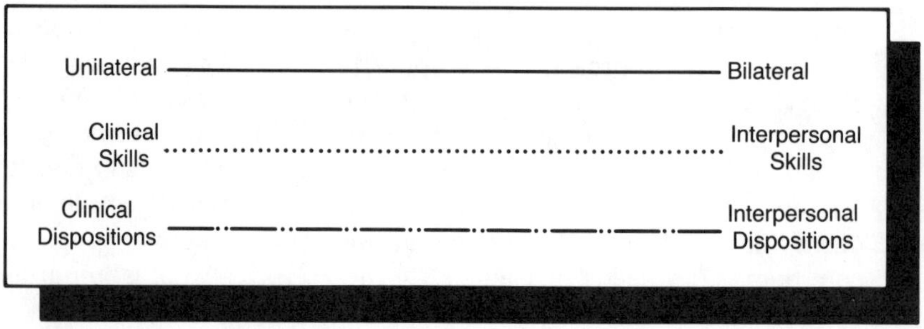

THE TRIGONAL MODEL OF COMMUNICATION DISORDERS SUPERVISION: CONCEPTS   61

FIGURE 3-2
Double- and multiple-strand continua

DOUBLE-STRAND CONTINUA

Unilateral ——————————— Bilateral
Clinical Skills ················· Interpersonal Skills

Unilateral ——————————— Bilateral
Clinical Dispositions —··—··—··— Interpersonal Dispositions

Clinical Dispositions ——————— Interpersonal Dispositions
Clinical Skills ················· Interpersonal Skills

MULTIPLE-STRAND CONTINUA

Unilateral ——————————— Bilateral
Clinical Skills ················· Interpersonal Skills
Clinical Dispositions —··—··—··— Interpersonal Dispositions

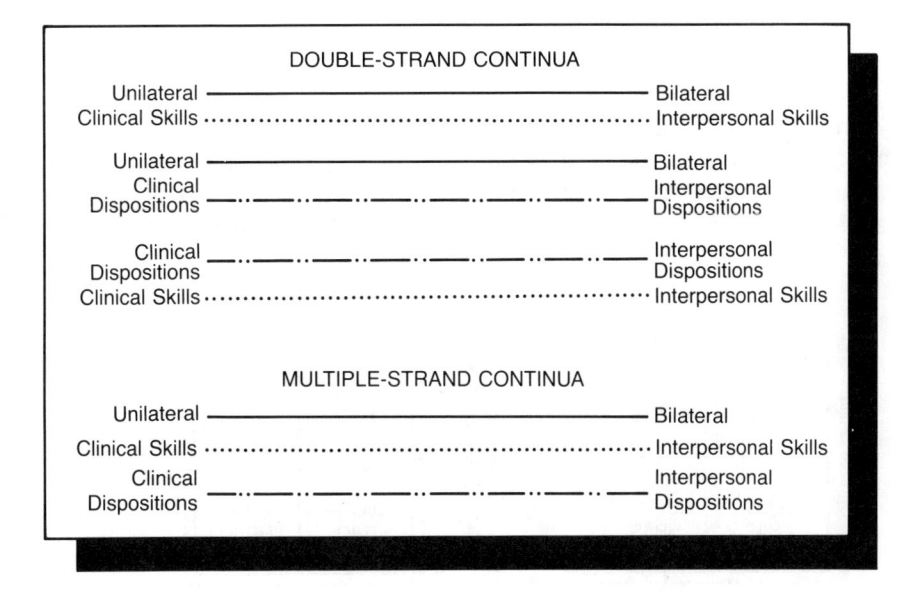

FIGURE 3-3
Continuum-to-matrix transposition

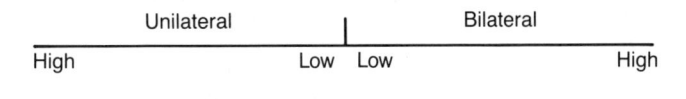

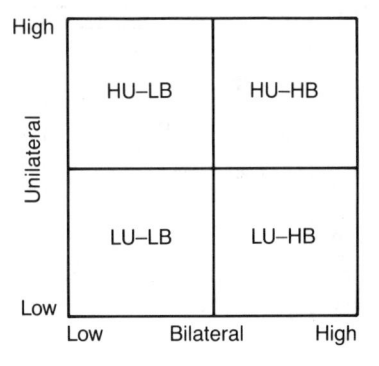

Unilateral | Bilateral
High   Low Low   High

	High	
Unilateral	HU–LB	HU–HB
	LU–LB	LU–HB
	Low	
	Low Bilateral High	

SINGLE-STRAND MATRICES

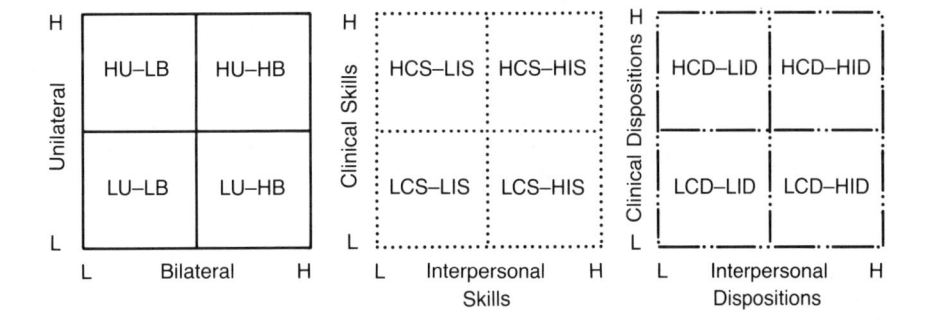

Unilateral	HU–LB	HU–HB
	LU–LB	LU–HB
L	Bilateral	H

Clinical Skills	HCS–LIS	HCS–HIS
	LCS–LIS	LCS–HIS
L	Interpersonal Skills	H

Clinical Dispositions	HCD–LID	HCD–HID
	LCD–LID	LCD–HID
L	Interpersonal Dispositions	H

Multiple-strand matrices combine many dimensions of Communication Disorders supervision into a format that clearly illustrates the complexity of the supervision process. The combinatorial effect of the double- and multiple-strand matrices is demonstrated in Figure 3-4.

The supervision concepts from different perspectives can be combined into a four-cell matrix, as shown in Figure 3-5.

Each quadrant is considered a specific S̄TYLE. Each STYLE is distinctive, is characteristic, and has identifiable *modes of action*. The modes are composed of aggregates of behavior used to manage people and their relationships, tasks and

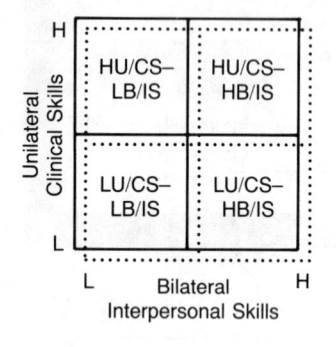

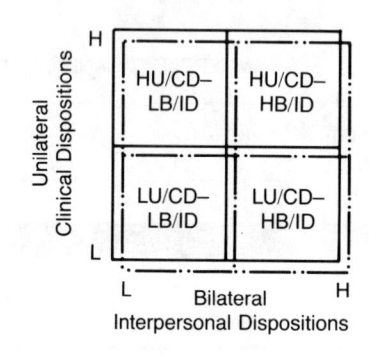

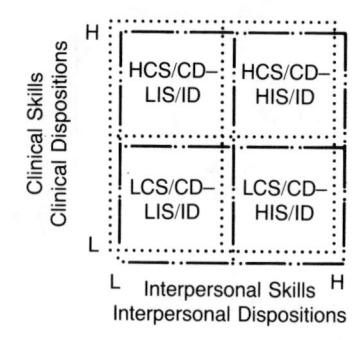

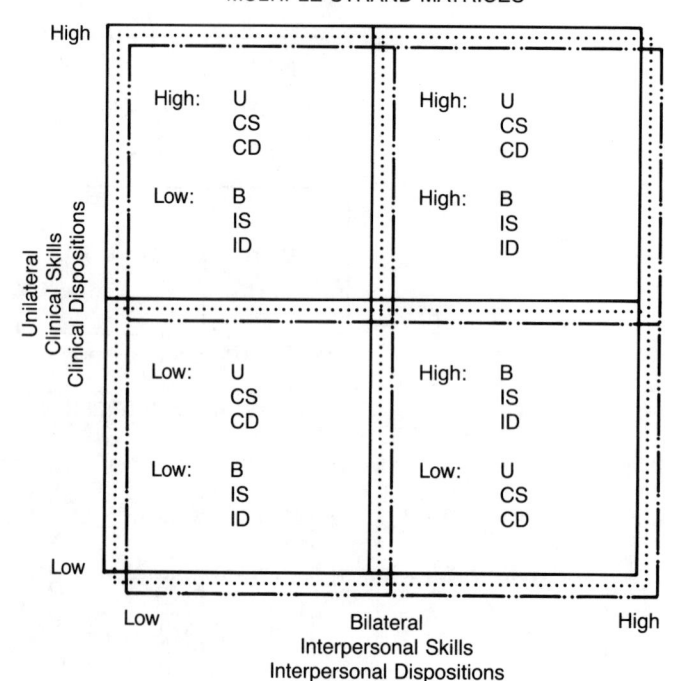

DOUBLE-STRAND MATRICES

MULTIPLE-STRAND MATRICES

FIGURE 3-4
Double- and multiple-strand matrices

FIGURE 3-5 Multiple-strand Communication Disorders supervision STYLES matrix

STYLE I	STYLE IV
Key Descriptor: Training Purpose: To teach cognitive development (skill and information) Philosophical Orientation: Essentialism Psychological Orientation: Behaviorism Inquiry Mode: Realist Interpersonal Commun. Style: Driver Conflict Commun. Style: Competitive Decision Style: Supervisor decisions Leadership Style: Directive Examples of Single Strands: 1. High unilateral–low bilateral 2. High CS–low IS 3. High CD–low ID 4. High direct–low indirect (Style B) 5. High TO–low RO 6. High instructive–low communicative	Key Descriptor: Transacting Purpose: To facilitate affective and cognitive development (professional competence) through genuine communication Philosophical Orientation: Experimentalism Psychological Orientation: Cognitivism Inquiry Mode: Synthesist and pragmatist Interpersonal Commun. Style: Expressive Conflict Commun. Style: Collaboration Decision Style: Mutually negotiated decisions between supervisor and supervisee Leadership Style: Collaborative Examples of Single Strands: 1. High unilateral–high bilateral 2. High CS–high IS 3. High CD–high ID 4. High direct–high indirect (Style A) 5. High TO–high RO 6. High instructive–high communicative
STYLE II	**STYLE III**
Key Descriptor: Monitoring Purpose: To teach cognitive development with some attention to affective development Philosophical Orientation: Essentialism Psychological Orientation: Behaviorism Inquiry Mode: Analyst Interpersonal Commun. Style: Analytical Conflict Commun. Style: Avoiding Decision Style: Supervisor decisions Leadership Style: Administrative Examples of Single Strands: 1. Low unilateral–low bilateral 2. Low CS–low IS 3. Low CD–low ID 4. Low direct–low indirect (Style D) 5. Low TO–low RO 6. Low instructive–low communicative	Key Descriptor: Advising Purpose: To facilitate affective development (relationships and dispositions) through genuine communication Philosophical Orientation: Existentialism Psychological Orientation: Humanism Inquiry Mode: Idealist Interpersonal Commun. Style: Amiable Conflict Commun. Style: Accommodation Decision Style: Supervisor & supervisee decisions or supervisee decision with supervisor encouragement Leadership Style: Consultive Examples of Single Strands: 1. Low unilateral–high bilateral 2. Low CS–high IS 3. Low CD–high ID 4. Low direct–high indirect (Style C) 5. Low TO–high RO 6. Low instructive–high communicative

FIGURE 3-5
continued

Strand	Theorist
1. Unilateral-bilateral (Interactant participation in the supervision process)	Flower (1984)
2. Clinical skill-interpersonal skill	Farmer & Farmer (1986)
3. Clinical disposition-interpersonal disposition	Farmer & Farmer (1986) Katz & Raths (1985)
4. Interactive supervision styles (direct and indirect)	Blumberg (1974)
5. Reddin's 3-D theory of leadership (task-oriented–relations oriented)	Reddin (1970)
6. Instructive-communicative supervision (intent of communication during supervision process)	Farmer & Farmer (1986)

their products, and the process of supervision in Communication Disorders. Characteristics of each STYLE are described in detail in appendix B.

The strength of the concept of supervision STYLES lies in the theory that the whole is greater than the sum of its parts. Therefore, the validity of this model comes from the combined force of the validity of each of the styles presented in Figure 3-5.

A companion issue to *how* supervision is done (i.e., STYLE) is the question *with whom* it is done. Supervision is done with individuals or with groups, and this dimension of the process is referred to as *form*.

Forms of Supervision

Supervision in Communication Disorders can take two *forms*, dyadic or group. In dyadic supervision, a supervisor and a supervisee join together to accomplish goals through communication. Dyads occur in supervision conferences, interviews, and counseling. Group supervision, on the other hand, involves at least one supervisor and two or more supervisees or others (e.g., a client, family or significant others, or other professionals) who join together to accomplish goals through communication. Group supervision occurs in staff meetings, lectures, inservice programs, and committees. Both dyadic and group forms of supervision have advantages and disadvantages. The forms are compared in Table 3-1.

Seven examples of group Communication Disorders supervision have been discussed in the literature. Some of the models have received intensive scrutiny through research (e.g., Teaching Clinic, Microteaching) and others, although grounded in strong pragmatic theory, are without detailed study to document their efficacy (e.g., In Absentia Supervision). All seven are presented here to encourage future use of and research in group supervision.

Teaching Clinic (Dowling, 1979; Olsen, Barbour, & Michalak, 1971) is a group format developed by Olsen et al. and adapted for Communication Disorders supervision by Dowling. The Teaching Clinic is a voluntary form of peer group supervision. In it, individuals can develop clinical competence by analyzing behavior and interacting with each other. Each teaching clinic meets weekly for approximately 1 1/2 hours and follows six sequential steps that parallel Cogan's (1973) cycle of colleagueship supervision:

1. Review of the previous Teaching Clinic
2. Planning session
3. Observation session
4. Critique preparation session
5. Critique and strategy development session
6. Clinic review

The content of the meetings comes from a videotaped therapy session presented by one of the team members for group observation and analysis. Team members of the Teaching Clinic fulfill various rotating roles: (a) *clinic leader,* the

TABLE 3-1
Comparison of dyadic and group supervision

Dyadic	Group
1. Attends to specific needs of individual supervisees and/or clients	1. Attends to needs of majority of group members
2. May be better for marginal supervisees	2. May be too confusing for marginal supervisees
3. May be difficult to schedule meetings with 25 separate supervisees	3. May be easier to schedule one meeting with 25 supervisees in a group
4. May facilitate supervisor-supervisee relationship	4. May facilitate supervisee-supervisee relationships
5. Does not facilitate supervisor-supervisor relationship	5. May facilitate supervisor-supervisor relationship
6. Does not facilitate teamwork	6. May facilitate teamwork
7. Does facilitate development of supervisee's professional competence (skills and dispositions)	7. Does facilitate development of supervisee's professional competence (skills and dispositions)
8. May be a source of interpersonal conflict between supervisor and supervisee	8. Is less likely to be a source of interpersonal conflict between supervisor and supervisee
9. Is less likely to be a source of interpersonal conflict between supervisees	9. May be a source of interpersonal conflict between supervisees
10. May facilitate intrapersonal competition	10. May create interpersonal competition
11. May be used for evaluation and appraisal	11. Is less likely to be used for evaluation and appraisal
12. May be threatening to some supervisees	12. May be threatening to some supervisees
13. Is less likely to be threatening to supervisors	13. Is more likely to be threatening to some supervisors
14. May be time efficient	14. Is generally considered to be time efficient
15. May be cost efficient	15. May be cost efficient
16. Limits exposure to variety of ideas, methods, materials	16. Expands exposure to variety of ideas, methods, materials
17. Disseminates information slowly to one supervisee at a time	17. Disseminates information quickly to all supervisees at once
18. Increases possibility of lack of information, misinformation, or misunderstanding	18. Decreases possibility of lack of information, misinformation, or misunderstanding
19. Does not develop networking or linkages	19. Does develop networking and linkages
20. Unlikely to lead to groupthink	20. May lead to groupthink
21. Process is generally more predictable	21. Process may be less predictable
22. May be less motivating to supervisee and supervisor	22. May be more motivating to supervisee and supervisor
23. May not facilitate morale of supervisees or supervisors	23. May facilitate morale of supervisees or supervisors
24. Supervisee may develop dependence on supervisor	24. Supervisee less likely to develop dependence on supervisor
25. Impossible to do In Absentia Supervision	25. Possible to do In Absentia Supervision
26. May not facilitate a sensitivity to others	26. Does facilitate a sensitivity to others
27. Supervisors (and maybe supervisees) may need special training in dyadic dynamics and processes	27. Supervisors (and maybe supervisees) may need special training in group dynamics and processes

TABLE 3-1
continued

Dyadic	Group
28. Takes up less physical space	28. Takes up more physical space
29. May require more supervisors	29. May require fewer supervisors
30. May increase or decrease supervisee talk time	30. May increase or decrease supervisee talk time
31. Interaction analysis is relatively uncomplicated	31. Interaction analysis is relatively complicated
32. Record keeping is relatively easy	32. Record keeping may be difficult
33. Developing goals and objectives for clients and supervisees is relatively easy	33. Developing goals and objectives for clients and supervisees may be difficult
34. Wholistic Supervision is impossible	34. Only way Wholistic Supervision can be done
35. Teaching Clinic and Case Staffings models of supervision are impossible	35. Teaching Clinic and Case Staffings models of supervision are inherent

Groups Can Be Formed by:

Discipline (all audiology personnel; all speech-language pathology personnel)

Experience (beginning vs. advanced)

Topics (writing goals/objectives; report writing; IEP writing; new audiogram format; new testing format; etc.)

Specific techniques (masking; Air Flow technique; etc.)

Worksite (all supervisees who work in schools; hospitals; hearing aid centers; etc.)

Age (all supervisees who work with preschoolers; schoolage children; the elderly; etc.)

Disorder (all supervisees who work with articulation; fluency; aural rehabilitation; tinnitus; etc.)

Medical condition (all supervisees who work with laryngectomy; mental retardation; language/learning disability; central auditory processing; etc.)

Heterogeneous mixture (of any of the above categories)

Wholistic mixture (including supervisor, supervisee, client, parent or significant other, other professional, etc.)

supervisor who guides discussion and stimulates interaction among team members; (b) *demonstration clinician,* the supervisee being observed; (c) *peers,* supervisee observers who assist in analyzing, discussing, and supporting the demonstration clinician; (d) *group monitor,* a supervisee who monitors the group process to see that ground rules are followed. The Teaching Clinic is considered by many to be an efficient, effective group process for developing supervisees' self-supervisory skills. It can be used with supervisees from pre-service through service levels. It can also be applied to pre-clinical academic education, where videotapes of a variety of clients might be shown to students who could learn to collect and analyze data and make inferences from those data.

Case Staffings (Farmer, 1980) are formal presentations about particular clients and are prepared by a clinical team (senior clinician, junior clinician, clinical supervisor). Case Staffings share many of the elements of the Teaching Clinic. The team makes a 1-hour presentation before all clinical colleagues involved in practicum. Staffings follow this format: (a) a statement of case staffing objectives; (b) a summary of pertinent case history information; (c) a summary of pertinent diagnostic communication evaluation results; (d) semester goals for the client; (e) semester goals for the clinicians; (f) sample lesson plans typifying therapy tasks; (g) examples of data/record keeping; (h) a videotape, audiotape, or live sample of the client; (i) discussion; (j) a critique of the Case Staffing by observer colleagues; (k) a conference and critique review by presenter colleagues. The Case Staffing process includes:

1. Selection. At the beginning of the term, clients to be used for Case Staffings are selected. Staffers select clients who are of interest because of disorder type, management procedures, or other unique factors.
2. Preparation. Clinical teams prepare for the staffing by deciding as a group what information to present and by developing appropriate objectives. Preparation may include doing research on specific diseases, syndromes, medications, or treatment procedures; contacting other professionals who also may be working with the client; and arranging a videotaping schedule.
3. Presentation. During the presentation, the observer colleagues are instructed to record data or make some type of objective notation about client and/or clinician behavior. In addition, at the end of the staffing, each observer colleague lists three positive aspects of the management program set up and executed by the team, and three suggestions for improving the program. Because observers critique the management program, and because the staffers work as a team, there is less chance of discussing the personalities of the team members. Working as a junior clinician on a team is a good way for a beginning clinician to ease into the colleagueship process.
4. Review. After the Case Staffing, the presenter colleagues meet as a group to discuss the critiques of the observer colleagues. Each clinician has individual conferences with clinical supervisors throughout the semester.

Microteaching is a group supervision approach used by Irwin (1971) to train speech-language pathologists. The first step of microteaching is a supervisor-supervisee preconference. The supervisee then conducts a 5-minute therapy session during which a specific technique, strategy, or principle is stressed. A second conference is held to discuss the short segment of therapy. The supervisee makes appropriate modifications and re-presents the segment. A final conference is held for closure on that specific topic. In microteaching, group members can assist in the planning as well as in evaluation.

Quality Circles is a management technique that originated in Japan in 1962 and has been modified to serve Communication Disorders supervision (Buckberry & White, 1987). A Quality Circle is a group of supervisors and supervisees who meet to manage work-related problems. The unmodified Quality Circle concept is a participative management approach that accepts supervisees as experts at their own jobs. The point is to develop cooperation between supervisors and supervisees, with a joint dedication to doing a better job.

The objectives of a Quality Circle program can be as varied as the problems managed by the circles, but improvement can come in three general areas: quality, productivity, and the working environment. Quality of service delivery is the most common concern for circle supervision. A Quality Circle also can be concerned with problems of productivity, which is generally defined in terms of the number of units produced but may also be related to increases and decreases in employee or client absenteeism, or to employee productivity. Quality Circles often center on improving the working contexts, including safety, personnel relations, contextual ecology, and so forth.

The Quality Circle approach provides a formal means for developing and sustaining worker input into production and service management. Circle members receive training in problem management and hold regular meetings to work on the problems they face. Supervisees make presentations to supervisors who are committed to supporting the circle's problem-managing activities. The changes that supervisees see themselves making in their work can lead to overall improvements in quality, quantity, pride, and morale. The Quality Circle concept succeeds where a reciprocal, cooperative relationship between supervisors and supervisees exists (Dewar, 1980).

Wholistic Supervision (Farmer, 1986a) is an interreactive, collaborative process that allows people with diverse perspectives in a teaching-learning context to contribute creative ideas to the development of the personnel and the educational process within that context. Wholistic Supervision addresses the whole individual within a whole teaching-learning (or habilitation-rehabilitation) context. The results are enhanced or different from those that any one person would produce independently. Wholistic Supervision is grounded in the premise that all the people within a given clinical or supervision context are educators as well as learners and have the right and the responsibility to contribute to the teaching-learning process.

The concept of Wholistic Supervision aligns with that of INter-REActive Learning (INREAL) (INREAL Staff, 1983), which takes place when interactants work in a partnership based on genuine communication and when all interactants learn (i.e., achieve new successes in performance and interpersonal relations). Wholistic Supervision, which utilizes General Systems Theory, places the responsibility for education not solely on supervisees nor supervisors but also on the supervisees' colleagues, the clients, and the parents or primary caregivers of the clients. All of these participants also are responsible for evaluating the amount and quality of learning that transpires.

Philosophically, Wholistic Supervision is based on reverence for the individual person. Wholistic Supervision uses many of the basic tenets of humanistic supervision (Abrell, 1974), but adds group supervision methods to the more traditional forms of dyadic supervision. By including all the interactants who have responsibility for education in the supervision process, this model departs drastically from the traditional supervisor-supervisee model and will require participants to move through the stages of change: (a) awareness, (b) understanding, (c) commitment, (d) change or exchange.

In Absentia Supervision is a group form used by Farmer (1986b). Advanced supervisees meet as a group using an agenda developed by the supervisees, by the supervisor, or by both. The supervisor is not present during the supervision meeting, but the group is videotaped. If uncertainties or problems arise that the group members cannot manage to their satisfaction, they direct their questions to the camera to solicit input from the supervisor, who views the videotape at a later time. The supervisor can then meet with the group of supervisees to discuss their self-supervision process in general and to address the questions.

Multi-, inter-, and transdisciplinary teams provide opportunities for generic or categorical supervision for both supervisors and supervisees. McCormick and Goldman (1979) summarize the three kinds of teams as follows. In the *multidisciplinary* model, professionals from each discipline evaluate a client but do not communicate or coordinate across disciplines. Evaluation results may be collected and collated by some person (e.g., a supervisor) who interprets them according to personal discipline biases, or, more typically, may be presented at a staffing. There is no formal attempt to allocate resources by prioritizing clients' needs or by considering the disciplines' overlap of services, nor is there any arrangement for feedback and revision of original findings.

The *interdisciplinary* approach resembles the multidisciplinary in most respects but advocates establishing formal communication channels and assigning a case manager (e.g., the Communication Disorders supervisor) so as to avoid compartmentalization and fragmentation of services. The case manager does not provide or monitor services, but simply directs the flow of information. Theoretically the method fosters group decision making, development of a unified service plan, and multiple opportunities for interaction among discipline representatives. In practice, however, the responsibility is often diffused, in a way that precludes recycling data, revising program recommendations, or implementing new methods.

In the *transdisciplinary* model, the discipline representatives are responsible (as in the other two models) for initial assessments in their respective fields. In addition, they are expected to collaborate in developing a comprehensive individualized treatment program. The three models differ at the point of program implementation. In the transdisciplinary approach, responsibility for client behavior change falls on one team member called the *primary therapist* rather than being divided among the disciplines according to specialty. The other team members are available on a continuing basis for consultation and direct assistance. This approach requires that transdisciplinary participants (including Communication Disorders supervisors) become multidiscipline professionals, at the same time releasing some of their primary discipline role to other team members. The phase of *role release* includes (a) providing general information about one's discipline to team members from other disciplines, (b) teaching information skills to others for one's discipline, (c) training others in performance competencies for one's discipline, and (d) following up to ensure appropriate application.

Table 3–2 outlines advantages and disadvantages of each of the seven models of group supervision discussed in this section.

Types (STYLES + Forms) of Communication Disorders Supervision

By combining the four STYLES of supervision with the two forms, we can examine, discuss, and use eight *types* of supervision: Type 1 = STYLE I/dyadic; Type 2 = STYLE I/group; Type 3 = STYLE II/dyadic; Type 4 = STYLE II/group; Type 5 = STYLE III/dyadic; Type 6 = STYLE III/group; Type 7 = STYLE IV/dyadic; Type 8 = STYLE IV/group. The concept of supervision types grows out of the ideas that different kinds of information (content) need to be imparted in different ways; that supervisees (constituents) have different needs and supervisors (constituents) have different personal and professional strengths and weaknesses; that worksites (contexts) are not uniform; and that all these differences require different STYLES and forms of supervision. No single "right" or "best" way of supervising has been discovered in the Communication Disorders profession. Instead, appropriate modes of supervision must arise from the interaction of the Constituents, Concepts, and Contexts. To select these appropriate supervision techniques, supervisors need academic knowledge about the concepts of systems, philosophical and psychological orientations to teaching and learning, inquiry modes, cognitive styles, leadership styles, theoretical models, professional competence, classifications, and the STYLES, forms and types of Communication Disorders supervision; they also need the professional competence (skills and dispositions) to utilize that knowledge. When a supervisor is knowledgeable about and skillful in using the various types of supervision, differential preparation of supervisees can occur.

Differential Supervision

The concept of differential supervision was introduced in chapter 2. There it was suggested that supervisees have varying degrees of knowledge, skill, experience, and interest in the process of supervision and that in order to receive the most productive learning experiences for each supervisee, supervisees need to be prepared for supervision and the process must be individualized. The information from the previous Concepts sections contributes to a theoretical model of differential supervision. Table 3–3 shows the five supervisee levels and their associated knowledge and skills. The combination of supervisees' levels and their Readiness States (RS) leads to the suggested type(s)

TABLE 3-2
Comparison of models of group Communication Disorders supervision

Model	Advantages	Disadvantages
Teaching Clinic (Dowling, 1979)	increases staff morale and results in better social and personal relationships develops leadership skills stimulates better planning broadens scope of knowledge allows participants to try new ideas with colleague feedback allows individuals with expertise to share it with others learning occurs as a result of interaction may be a source of security	deprives individuals of guidance from one-to-one relationships may emphasize group harmony rather than individual learning; may increase interpersonal tension may emphasize conflict resolution rather than conflict management and innovative solutions some people can't function in a group group may be a source of anxiety
Case Staffings (Farmer, 1980)	develops teamwork supervisees function in different roles develops oral communication competence develops presentation skills develops affective as well as observational skills develops a video bank develops a sample lesson plan bank allows peers to observe peers provides samples of different diagnostic and treatment methods and materials provides samples of different recording and data keeping procedures provides examples of case management develops criteria for judging effectiveness of diagnostic and treatment programs introduces and develops use of professional terminology develops self-knowledge develops ability to accept and grow from constructive critiques	requires coordination of time among team members requires knowledge of videotaping and perhaps editing requires equipment and facilities participants need training in visual literacy in order to comment objectively on a videotaped session
Microteaching (Irwin, 1971)	follows colleagueship format uses short 5-minute segments and one target area includes follow-up	may be difficult to develop disposition—uses primarily skill-based instruction may be difficult to synthesize and integrate short segments of target behaviors

TABLE 3-2
continued

Model	Advantages	Disadvantages
Quality Circles (Dewar, 1980; Buckberry & White, 1987)	uses upward and downward (vertical) communication requires supervisor to accept ideas of supervisees	requires time from job to meet as a group requires a formal proposal for suggested changes
Wholistic Supervision (Farmer, 1986a)	emphasizes team effort for diagnosis and treatment brings together *all* members of clinical team (clients, supervisor, ancillary personnel, etc.) for more complete evaluation of supervisee competence and of effectiveness of intervention program requires cooperation in developing goals and objectives—cannot be developed just by clinician and/or supervisor	requires training of supervisee to accept evaluation from others requires preparation of others (client, parents, etc.) to evaluate effectiveness of intervention program requires different criteria for evaluation
In Absentia Supervision (Farmer, 1986b)	emphasizes self-supervision because of absence of supervisor from group and because of delayed supervisor feedback emphasizes team/peer supervision allows flexible scheduling for supervisor allows multiple replay of videotapes for detailed analysis; good for research	supervisees may be anxious about being videotaped; may require period of desensitization delayed feedback may be deleterious to case management video equipment is expensive
Multi-, Inter-, and Transdisciplinary Supervision (McCormick & Goldman, 1979)	may result in better management for client extends knowledge across disciplines	may be no one responsible for management (multi- or inter-) may be difficult to accept generic supervision may be difficult to develop team unity requires training in group process

TABLE 3-3
Preparation of five levels of supervisees for the Communication Disorders supervision process

Level 0 Supervisees (Paraprofessionals, Aides, Parents, Family, Significant Others, Ancillary Personnel)	Level II Supervisees (101–200 clinical hours)	Level IV Supervisees (Professionals; peers)
NEEDS	**NEEDS**	**NEEDS**
Knowledge	*Knowledge*	*Knowledge*
1. Mindset of selves as a resource	1. Secondary knowledge of the clinical process	Level III knowledge, plus:
2. An attitude of partnership with the client and supervisor	2. Secondary knowledge of the supervision process	1. Continuing education in the clinical process
3. Self-knowledge (strengths and weaknesses)	a. Level II Clinician responsibilities	2. Continuing education in the supervision process
4. Basic information about communication	b. Types (STYLES + forms) of supervision	3. Career ladder options
5. Basic information about communication disorders	*Skills*	*Skills*
6. Information about client(s)	1. Level I Supervisee skills, plus:	Level III skills, plus:
7. Information about expectations of client, clinician, self, supervisor	a. Primary formal interactional analysis: clinical	1. Advanced professional competence (skills + dispositions)
Skills	b. Primary conflict management strategies	2. Continuing education in clinical skills and dispositions
1. Ability to share information	2. Primary organizational communication strategies	3. Continuing education in the supervision process (prepare for supervision position)
2. Ability to establish goals and objectives	3. Primary planning and problem management strategies	a. Strengthen professional networks
3. Ability to assist in planning and problem management	4. Secondary microcomputer use	b. Active involvement in researcher role
4. Communication competence		c. Active involvement in educator role
5. Ability to observe (watch what clients do, listen to what clients say, read what clients write, see what clients draw)		d. Active involvement in administrator role
		4. Develop a career ladder

Level I Supervisees (0–100 clinical hours)	Level III Supervisees (201–300 + clinical hours; Clinical Fellows)	Readiness States (Hersey & Blanchard, 1982)	Appropriate Types of Supervision
NEEDS	**NEEDS**	RS1 = Unable and unwilling or insecure	Type 1 (STYLE I/Dyadic)
Knowledge	*Knowledge*		Type 2 (STYLE I/ Group)
Primary (overview) knowedge of:	1. Tertiary knowledge of the clinical process	RS2 = Unable but willing or confident	Type 1 (STYLE I/Dyadic)
1. ASHA clinical requirements	a. Skills + dispositions = professional competence		Type 2 (STYLE I/ Group)
2. Program clinical requirements	2. Tertiary knowledge of the supervision process		Type 3 (STYLE II/Dyadic)
3. Disorder types	a. Level III Clinician responsibilities	RS3 = Able but unwilling or	Type 4 (STYLE II/Group)
4. Worksites (contexts)	b. Supervision roles		Type 5 (STYLE III/Dyadic)
5. The clinical process	1) Professional		
a. Diagnosis	2) Researcher		
b. Treatment	3) Educator		
c. Case management	4) Administrator		
d. Counseling	5) Clinician		
e. Reporting			
1) Oral			
2) Written			

6. The supervision process
   a. A theoretical model of human resources (e.g., colleagueship)
   b. Constituents
      1) Supervisors
      2) Supervisees
      3) Clients/patients
   c. Content
      1) Level I Clinician responsibilities
      2) Personal goals and objectives
      3) Scheduling
      4) STYLES of supervision
      5) Forms of supervision
         a) Dyadic: conferences
         b) Group: clinical team meetings; clinical staff meetings
      6) Supervisor observations
         a) Live: participant and non-participant
         b) Closed-circuit
         c) Videotape
         d) Audiotape
         e) Lesson plans
      7) Evaluation and grading
         a) Supervisor evaluation and grading of supervisee
         b) Supervisee evaluation of supervisor
   c. ASHA Supervision Tasks and Competencies
   d. Systems theory
   e. Philosophical orientations
      1) Essentialism
      2) Experimentalism
      3) Existentialism
   f. Psychological orientations
      1) Behaviorism
      2) Cognitivism
      3) Humanism
   g. Inquiry modes
      1) Synthesist
      2) Idealist
      3) Pragmatist
      4) Analyst
      5) Realist
   h. Cognitive styles (learning aptitudes)
      1) Perceptual processing
      2) Language
      3) Scientific thinking
      4) Creative thinking
      5) Formal reasoning
      6) Hand/eye coordination
      7) Artistry
      8) Writing
      9) Socialness
   i. Leadership styles
   j. Decision making
   k. Change theory
   l. Secondary knowledge of contexts
   m. Research

Skills

Primary (basic) skills in:
1. Visual literacy
   a. Observation
   b. Reporting (oral and written)
   c. Interpersonal communication
   d. Self-confrontation from videotape
   e. Videotape equipment use
2. Microcomputer use
   a. Word processing
   b. Data bases

Level II Supervisee skills, plus:
1. Personal Supervision Profile
2. Primary Professional role activity (beginning professional networking)
3. Primary supervision research activity
4. Primary educator role activity
   1) Demonstration clinician role
   2) Cosupervision practicum
   3) Evaluation/grading
5. Primary administrator role
6. Tertiary clinical skills and dispositions
   a) Administration practicum
7. Tertiary microcomputer use

RS4 = Able and willing or confident ... insecure

Level	RS	Type
0	RS1	1
		2
	RS2	3
		4
	RS3	5
		6
	RS4	7
		8
I	RS1	1
		2
	RS2	3
		4
II	RS1	1
	RS2	2
III	RS3	3
	RS4	4
		5
		6
		7
		8
IV	RS3	5
	RS4	6
		7
		8

Type 6 (STYLE III/Group)
Type 7 (STYLE IV/Dyadic)
Type 8 (STYLE IV/Group)

of supervision to be utilized. For example, Level I supervisees will have minimal information about the supervision process, and thus their readiness for supervision is RS1 or RS2. The difference between RS1 and RS2 depends on the willingness, security, or confidence of the supervisees. As shown in Table 3-3, supervision types 1 through 4 would be appropriate approaches for a supervisor to try with Level I supervisees.

Preparation Level III includes clinical fellows. Clinical fellows are those speech-language pathologists and audiologists with master's degrees who are working to attain the ASHA Certificate of Clinical Competence (CCC-SLP or CCC-A). They work as interns under the supervision of ASHA certified professionals during the Clinical Fellowship Year (CFY). Clinical fellows span the gap between preservice and service level personnel. Supervision strategies seem to be more determinate for novices and for professional personnel than for clinical fellows as emerging professionals.

A conference was held in 1964 to establish guidelines for the CFY, including the requirements for supervision and supervisors (Kleffner, 1964). Changes have occurred over the years, and current requirements are presented in the *Membership and Certification Handbook* (ASHA, 1985). A proposal to abolish the CFY has been debated by various ASHA committees (ASHA, 1987). Some of the reasons supporting abolition relate to supervision issues: difficulty finding supervisors who can meet the CFY supervision requirements, especially in rural areas; untrained supervisors; lack of knowledge about effective strategies to use with developmental clinical fellows; lack of evidence of the efficacy of CFY supervision.

Minimal research has been done on the CFY. Schubert and Lyngby (1977), Fein (1983), Crichton and Oratio (1984), and Hyman (1986) have studied various aspects of the internship period. Three conclusions emerge from those studies: (a) the internship year would have been as beneficial without the required supervision; (b) quality interpersonal communication is a critical supervisor competence; and (c) differential supervision is a necessity.

Differential supervision requires supervisor education and training, which in turn results in change—a sequence that may be at the heart of how the specialty area of Communication Disorders supervision develops in the future. Because change is such an important concept in the development of the supervision process, it will be discussed in detail in the next section.

Change

To implement into the Communication Disorders supervision process any of the Concepts described in this chapter, change must occur at various levels of the process: ASHA, CUSPSPA, colleges and universities, supervisors, supervisees, employers, and worksites. Change is often traumatic and unsuccessful in improving the status quo. Loucks, Newlove, and Hall (1975) suggest that the failure to incite successful change is due to a lack of knowledge and attention to the process of change and to what constitutes successful change.

Watzlawick, Weakland, and Fisch (1974) discuss two types of change. *First-order* change (from the theory of groups) is defined as change that occurs within the members of a system while the system itself remains invariant. *Second-order* change, based on the theory of logical types, involves altering the system itself by changing the body of rules governing the system's structure or internal order. Productive supervision requires both first- and second-order change. Both supervisees and supervisors change by developing new skills (first-order change). The rules of supervisory interaction must then change to accommodate the new skills (second-order change). If second-order change does not occur, professional dispositions do not develop and professional competence remains only at a skill level.

From extensive research on adopting program innovations, Hall and Loucks (1978) report six assumptions that provide insight into the complexity of the change process:

1. Change is a *process*, not a single event or decision point; it is ongoing, not episodic.
2. *Individuals* must be the primary targets of interventions designed to facilitate change.
3. Change is a highly *personal* experience.
4. Individuals involved in the change process go through *stages* in their perceptions and feelings about the innovation, as well as in their skill, sophistication, and disposition in using the innovation.
5. Change can best be facilitated by using a *client-centered diagnostic/prescriptive model* rather than in-service training.
6. Change facilitators need to work in *adaptive, systematic* ways. They must stay in contact with the progress of (first-order) change in individuals who operate within the larger context of the total organization supporting the change (e.g., ASHA, CUSPSPA, a university, a clinic, or a public school). They must be able to examine and reexamine the change process and be able to modify interventions to accommodate the latest assessment data. At the same time, they should look for the "ripple effect" that first-order change may have on other parts of the system, which is a sign of second-order change.

Implementing supervision innovations requires second-order, or whole-system, change. To accomplish whole-system change, supervisors need a conceptual model of the change process that provides practical reference points on a constantly changing array of events. The *Stages of Concern* (*SoC*) (Hall, George, & Rutherford, 1974) and *Levels of Use* (*LoU*) (Loucks et al., 1975) segments of the *Concerns-Based Adoption Model* (*C-BAM*) (Hall & Loucks, 1978) provide a structure that can be used to implement innovations in the communication disorders supervision process. The *C-BAM* instrument can help supervisors diagnose, plan, deliver, and assess the effects of supervision innovations.

Research has verified six stages of concern that people appear to move through as innovations occur: awareness, informational, personal, management, consequence, collaboration, and refocusing. The *SoC* instrument can be a key diagnostic tool for determining the content and delivery of Communication Disorders supervision preparation programs. A companion tool, the *LoU* scale, can be used to assess how supervision innovations are being integrated into a system (by checking the implementation of professional skills and dispositions). The levels on the scale include non-use, orientation, preparation, mechanical use, routine, refinement, integration, and renewal.

The psychological theory of cognitive dissonance (Myers & Myers, 1973) is relevant to the phenomenon of change. Festinger (1957) states that the existence of dissonance (inconsistency among values, beliefs, attitudes, or knowledge) will motivate people (a) to attempt to reduce it so as to reestablish consonance (consistency), and (b) actively to avoid situations or information likely to increase it. This principle is important at two levels of Communication Disorders supervision: for the supervisor trainee and for the clinical supervisee. Supervisors must address three considerations when planning for change: (a) students (either supervisor trainees or clinical supervisees) must have a recognized or felt gap (dissonance) between the knowledge (concepts) and abilities they have in a given area and the knowledge and abilities they need to develop; (b) the program personnel must judge how wide the preparation gap is and provide learning experiences for the students at a level that will encourage them to move toward consonance; and (c) the students will not move on to new material until they reach some degree of consonance or equilibrium in the area(s) they are working on. This theory of cognitive dissonance coincides with the *SoC* and *LoU* segments of the *C-BAM*. Unless supervisors identify levels of cognitive dissonance and arrange learning experiences accordingly, they may not succeed in training speech-language pathologists and audiologists to become competent clinicians or supervisors.

Even with appropriate attitudes and desires, goals and objectives, cognitive dissonance, and a supportive environment, some individuals will still be unable to make the desired second-order changes in clinical or supervision behaviors. The Protective Motivation Theory (PMT)(Rogers, 1983) helps explain why some students do not incorporate new behaviors into existing patterns. This theory suggests that in feared situations (e.g., extreme cognitive dissonance), four mediators influence the decision to change or not change behavior: (a) the noxiousness of the feared outcome (the more personally disturbing, uncomfortable, or serious the outcome, the more likely it is that the behavior will change; (b) the perceived probability of the outcome's occurrence (the more likely it is that there will be a personally disturbing, uncomfortable, or serious outcome if the behavior is not changed, the more likely it is that the behavior will change); (c) the judged efficacy of the coping responses designed to prevent the behavior change (the less effective these responses are, the more likely it is that the behavior will change); and (d) the personal beliefs related to one's capacity for making the recommended change (the more strongly one believes that personal change is possible, the more likely it is that behavior will change).

The Protective Motivation Theory can be applied to Communication Disorders. Some individuals may not make changes in behavior if they:

1. Are not threatened by what might occur if they do not change their behavior. For some supervisors the threat of loss of employment if they don't receive training in supervision is not feared because they know that they can find employment elsewhere that doesn't require training. For supervisees, a failing grade if they don't improve their clinical work may not be feared. In both examples the personnel are not motivated to protect themselves by changing their behavior, because the result of not changing behavior is not personally disturbing.
2. Believe there is a low probability that the outcome will occur. If supervisors know that no supervisor has ever lost a job because of not receiving supervisory training, then they will consider that outcome unlikely. If supervisees know that no clinician has ever failed clinical practicum at their institution, they will not be afraid of receiving a failing grade.
3. Perceive that even their changing the behavior will not prevent the outcome from occurring. If supervisors believe that seniority has more weight in decisions about continued employment than competence, then they may not be sufficiently motivated to receive supervisory training. If supervisees think that even by improving clinical work they will still fail clinical practicum because of some other factor such as personality differences with supervisors, they may not be as motivated to improve their clinical competence.
4. Do not believe they are capable of becoming better supervisors or clinicians.

These mediators, individually or in combination, may explain why some personnel do not change behavior. It is important, therefore, to determine which mediator(s) is (are) the strongest deterrent(s) to the desired behavior, because each pattern must be approached differently. Two profiles are presented in Table 3–4 to illustrate this point.

Pattern A (5-4-1-3) indicates that the outcome for not changing the target behavior is very disturbing (5), the probability of the outcome occurring is perceived as high (4), the likelihood of the outcome occurring even with the behavior change is perceived as low (1), and the perceived ability to change is moderate (3). Pattern A represents strong motivation for changing behavior to protect oneself from an outcome. Pattern B (1-1-4-5), on the other hand, shows that the outcome is considered not to be disturbing (1), the probability of the outcome occurring is perceived as low (1), the perception is

TABLE 3-4
Protective motivation profiles

Mediators	Strength of Motivation

Profile A: Highly Motivated to Protect Self from Outcome (5-4-1-3 pattern)

1. How personally disturbing, uncomfortable, or serious the outcome (i.e., of not changing the behavior) is considered to be.
   1   2   3   4   **(5)**
   not very disturbing   very disturbing

2. Perceived probability of the outcome occurring.
   1   2   3   **(4)**   5
   not very probable   very probable

3. Perceived likelihood of the outcome occurring even if behavior is changed.
   (1)   2   3   4   5
   not very likely   very likely

4. Perceived ability to change behavior.
   1   2   **(3)**   4   5
   low ability   high ability

Profile B: Highly Unmotivated to Protect Self from Outcome (1-1-4-5 pattern)

1. How personally disturbing, uncomfortable, or serious the outcome (i.e., of not changing the behavior) is considered to be.
   (1)   2   3   4   5
   not very disturbing   very disturbing

2. Perceived probability of the outcome occurring.
   (1)   2   3   4   5
   not very probable   very probable

3. Perceived likelihood of the outcome occurring even if behavior is changed.
   1   2   3   **(4)**   5
   not very likely   very likely

4. Perceived ability to change behavior.
   1   2   3   4   **(5)**
   low ability   high ability

that if the outcome does occur it will do so whether or not the behavior is changed (4), and the ability to learn is considered strong (5). Pattern B represents low motivation to change behavior to protect oneself from an outcome, despite the high rating on the fourth mediator. Personnel who exhibit these and other patterns need differential learning experiences in order to change their behavior. Education and training must be designed to provide the strongest motivations to change behavior.

To summarize, the following conditions will maximize the probability for behavior change: (a) an outcome (of not changing the behavior) that is personally disturbing or uncomfortable must exist, (b) individuals must perceive a high probability that the feared outcome of not changing the behavior will occur, (c) individuals must perceive that if the change in behavior does occur the outcome will definitely not occur, and (d) individuals must believe that they are capable of changing the behavior.

It is possible for supervisors to assess students (both supervisor trainees and clinical supervisees) to determine their stages of concern and levels of use, cognitive dissonance, and protective motivation about innovations in Communication Disorders supervision. This procedure will allow them to select appropriate intervention strategies to help supervisees, supervisors, and others learn to use innovative supervision tactics with a minimum of trauma.

Supervision in Speech-Language Pathology versus Supervision in Audiology

Rassi (1978) has argued that supervision in Audiology is sufficiently different from supervision in Speech-Language Pathology to warrant serious attention to the differences. However, another view is that there is very little difference in the supervision process itself, especially considering that supervision operates in different domains and, therefore, that supervisors function in multiple roles. The differences appear to be in the knowledge base and specific clinical procedures of each discipline, not in the process of supervision. Rassi, in her landmark text, *Supervision in Audiology* (1978), offers two premises to support the notion that Speech-Language Pathology requires a different supervision tack from Audiology. Both premises are grounded in the supposition that supervision is only clinical education. First, ongoing therapy sessions often follow a speech-language diagnostic workup, so that the clinician is likely to see a given client repeatedly. Second, although speech-language services frequently use test equipment, it is relatively uncomplicated and limited in variety. In other words, audiologists tend to spend more time in evaluation and diagnosis using highly technical equipment, while speech-language pathologists spend more time therapeutically using minimal and perhaps less sophisticated equipment. This distinction becomes the basis for arguing that speech-language pathologists and audiologists should be trained differently. However, because speech-language pathologists and audiologists engage in the same kinds of activities (diagnosis and treatment using equipment developed in their fields), a supervisor needs the knowledge and skill to supervise the similar diagnostic or therapeutic activities superimposed on the clinical knowledge base of either field. The amount of time devoted to diagnosis or treatment becomes irrelevant. This opposing viewpoint is important to consider when developing training programs in supervision: Is it necessary to develop separate courses and continuing education workshops in supervision for speech-language pathologists that are significantly different from those for audiologists? Or is it possible to offer education and training in the multirole process of supervision in Communication Disorders that can be combined with specialized work in either area of the profession? The view in this text is that it *is* possible to prepare Speech-Language Pathology and Audiology supervisors together, with the added benefit that each specialist will become more aware and appreciative of the expertise of others with a different specialization but within the same profession. As more and more training institutions and organizations develop coursework and workshops on supervision, separate training is an issue that must be considered.

As the importance of supervision in both speech-language pathology and audiology has been recognized and acknowledged, the issue of supervision as a specialty area in Communication Disorders has emerged.

Supervision as a Specialty Area in Communication Disorders

The Committee on Supervision of Speech Pathology and Audiology (ASHA, 1978) recommended that the American Speech-Language-Hearing Association establish a certification level for supervisors beyond the Certificate of Clinical Competence. A certificate of supervision competence would clarify the distinction between clinical and supervision roles and abilities and would identify those who had met certain supervision preparation standards. ASHA could also establish certification for subspecialties of supervision, such as certification by disorder type, by age group, by supervisee level, by context, or by differentiated domain emphasis. The supervision certification would provide another career development option for speech-language pathologists and audiologists.

SUMMARY

The Concepts component is important in the Trigonal Model of Communication Disorders supervision. Consistent and directed supervision depends on having theories and models for understanding differential supervision, supervision in speech-language pathology versus supervision in audiology, and supervision as a specialty area. These theories and models help define supervision as it is today and prepare the way for future development. The concept of change helps us understand how Constituents interact with Concepts in the process of introducing innovations into supervisory practice.

APPLICATIONS

Discussion Topics
1. Discuss the concept of styles versus that of STYLES.
2. Discuss the advantages and disadvantages of both dyadic and group supervision.
3. Discuss the various models of group supervision.
4. Discuss how General Systems Theory applies to the supervision process.
5. Discuss the concept of change as it applies to supervision and to training in supervision.

Laboratory Experiences
1. Observe a Speech-Language Pathology supervisor for a week and an Audiology supervisor for a week. Document their activities and roles. Are these different?
2. Choose a behavior that you have tried unsuccessfully to change. Complete a protective motivation profile to determine which mediator(s) is (are) keeping you from making the changes you desire.
3. Practice the behavior associated with each of the four STYLES of Communication Disorders supervision.
4. Participate in In Absentia supervision. Afterwards respond in writing to the advantages and disadvantages of this approach.
5. Use the *SoC* to identify the concerns of your colleagues about implementing an innovation in your existing supervision process.

Research Projects

1. Conduct a survey to find out the numbers of generic and categorical Communication Disorders supervisors in a given area or region.
2. Develop a research design to explore the relationship between the five inquiry modes and the five Communication Disorders supervision roles.
3. Develop a research design to explore the relationship between the nine aptitudes (cognitive styles) and the five Communication Disorders supervision roles.
4. Develop, implement, and evaluate a program for developing clinical and interpersonal dispositions in Communication Disorders supervisors.
5. Make a demonstration videotape showing 5-minute segments of the eight types of Communication Disorders supervision.

REFERENCES

Abrell, R. (1974, December). The humanistic supervisor enhances growth and improves instruction. *Educational Leadership, 32,* 212–216.

Acheson, K., & Gall, M. (1980). *Techniques in the clinical supervision of teachers.* New York: Longman.

American Speech and Hearing Association. (1978). Current status of supervision of speech-language pathology and audiology. Report of Committee on Supervision of Speech Pathology and Audiology. *Asha, 20,* 478–486.

American Speech-Language-Hearing Association. (1985). *ASHA membership and certification handbook.* Rockville, MD: Author.

American Speech-Language-Hearing Association. (1987). Legislative Council report. *Asha, 29,* 38.

Bertalanffy, L. von. (1968). *General systems theory: Foundations, development, application.* New York: Braziller.

Blake, R., & Mouton, J. (1964). *The managerial grid.* Houston: Gulf.

Blumberg, A. (1974). *Supervisors and teachers: A private cold war.* Berkeley, CA: McCutchan.

Boone, D., & Prescott, T. (1972). Content and sequence analysis of speech and hearing therapy. *Asha, 14,* 58–62.

Buckberry, E., & White, H. (1987). Use of quality circles in clinical supervision. In S. Farmer (Ed.), *Clinical supervision: A coming of age. Proceedings of a national conference on supervision* (pp. 204–207). Las Cruces: New Mexico State University.

Cogan, M. (1973). *Clinical supervision.* Boston: Houghton Mifflin.

Coulter, D. (1986). *General systems thinking.* Unpublished materials from 1986 INREAL Trainers Institute, Boulder, CO.

Crago, M. (1983, November). *A Student-Supervisor Interactional Self-Exploratory Training Model (ASSIST-M).* A short course presented at the annual convention of the American Speech-Language-Hearing Association, Cincinnati, OH.

Crichton, L., & Oratio, A. (1984). Retrospective study: Speech-language pathologists' clinical fellowship training. *Asha, 26,* 39–43.

Dewar, D. (1980). *The quality circle handbook.* Red Bluff, CA: Quality Circle Institute.

Dowling, S. (1979). The teaching clinic: A supervisory alternative. *Asha, 21,* 646–649.

Duffy, F. (1984). Diagnostic supervision. *Perspectives, 3*(2), 7–9.

Farmer, S. (1980). Case staffings: A way of developing the colleagueship supervisory process. *SUPERvision, 4*(4), 5–7.

Farmer, S. (1986a). *Wholistic supervision.* Unpublished manuscript, New Mexico State University, Las Cruces.

Farmer, S. (1986b). *In absentia supervision.* Unpublished manuscript, New Mexico State University, Las Cruces.

Farmer, S., & Farmer, J. (1986, November). Unilateral and bilateral styles of dyadic and group clinical education/supervision. Short course presented at the annual convention of the American Speech-Language-Hearing Association, Detroit, MI.

Fein, D. (1983). Survey report: 1982 ASHA Omnibus. *Asha, 25,* 53–57.

Festinger, L. (1957). *A theory of cognitive dissonance.* Evanston, IL: Row, Peterson.

Flanders, N. (1960). *Teacher influence–pupil attitudes and achievement* (U.S. Office of Education, Cooperative Reseach Project 397, final report). Washington, DC: U.S. Government Printing Office.

Flower, R. (1984). *Delivery of speech-language pathology and audiology services.* Baltimore, MD: Williams & Wilkins.

Goldhammer, R. (1969). *Clinical supervision.* New York: Holt, Rinehart & Winston.

Hall, A., & Fagin, R. (1956). Definition of *system. General Systems, 1,* 18–28.

Hall, G., George, A., & Rutherford, W. (1974). *Measuring stages of concern about the innovation: A manual for use of the SoC questionnaire.* Austin, TX: Research and Development Center for Teacher Education.

Hall, G., & Loucks, S. (1978). Teacher concerns as a basis for facilitating and personalizing staff development. *Teachers College Record, 80*(1), 36–53.

Hersey, P., & Blanchard, K. (1982). *Management of organizational behavior: Utilizing human resources* (4th ed.). Englewood Cliffs, NJ: Prentice-Hall.

Hunter, M. (1978). *A clinical theory of instruction.* El Segundo, CA: TIP.

Hyman, C. (1986). The 1986 Omnibus Survey: Implications for strategic planning. *Asha, 28,* 19–24.

Idol, L., Paolucci-Whitcomb, P., & Nevin, A. (1986). *Collaborative consultation.* Gaithersburg, MD: Aspen.

Ingrisano, D., Hebalk, B., & Rathmel, B. (1979, November). *From observation to management: Clarifying university training objectives.* Paper presented at the annual convention of the American Speech-Language-Hearing Association, Atlanta, GA.

INREAL Staff. (1983). *Training materials.* Unpublished materials used in INREAL Specialist and Trainer training program. University of Colorado.

Irwin, R. (1971, November). *Microsupervision: A study of the behaviors of supervisors of speech clinicians.* Paper presented at the annual convention of the American Speech and Hearing Association.

Katz, L., & Raths, J. (1985, March). *Teachers' dispositions as goals for teacher education.* Paper presented at the annual meeting of the American Educational Research Association, Chicago.

Kleffner, F. (Ed.). (1964). *Seminar on guidelines for the internship year.* Washington, DC: American Speech and Hearing Association.

Knowles, M. (1970). *The modern practice of adult education: Andragogy versus pedagogy.* New York: Association Press.

Knowles, M. (1973). *The adult learner: A neglected species.* Houston: Gulf.

Loucks, S., Newlove, B., & Hall, G. (1975). *Measuring levels of use of the innovation: A manual for trainers, interviewers, and raters.* Procedures for adopting Educational Innovations Project/C-BAM. Austin, TX: Research and Development Center for Teacher Education.

Mawdsley, B. (1985, November). *The Integrative Task-Maturity Model of Supervision (ITMMS).* A paper presented at the annual convention of the American Speech-Language-Hearing Association, Washington, DC.

McCormick, L., & Goldman, R. (1979). The transdisciplinary model: Implications for service delivery and personnel preparation for the severely and profoundly handicapped. *AAESPH Review, 4*(2), 152–161.

Myers, G., & Myers, M. (1973). *The dynamics of human communication.* New York: McGraw-Hill.

Olsen, H., Barbour, C., & Michalak, D. (1971). *The teaching clinic.* Washington, DC: National Education Associates.

Oratio, A. (1977). *Supervision in speech pathology: A handbook for supervisors and clinicians.* Baltimore, MD: University Park Press.

Prather, E. (1967). An approach to clinical supervision. *Asha, 9,* 472–473.

Rassi, J. (1978). *Supervision in audiology.* Baltimore, MD: University Park Press.

Reddin, W. (1970). *Managerial effectiveness.* New York: McGraw-Hill.

Rogers, R. (1983). Cognitive and physiological processes in fear appeals and attitude change: A revised theory of protection motivation. In J. Cacioppo & R. Petty (Eds.), *Social psychophysiology* (pp. 153–174). New York: Guilford Press.

Schubert, G., & Lyngby, A. (1977). The clinical fellowship year (CFY). *Journal of National Student Speech and Hearing Association, 5,* 22–29.

Sergiovanni, T., & Elliot, E. (1975). *Educational and organizational leadership in elementary schools.* Englewood Cliffs, NJ: Prentice-Hall.

Sergiovanni, T., & Starratt, R. (1979). *Supervision: Human perspectives.* New York: McGraw-Hill.

Shriberg, L., Filley, F., Hayes, D., Kwiatkowski, J., Schatz, J., Simmons, K., & Smith, J. (1975). The Wisconsin Procedure for Appraisal of Clinical Competence (W-PACC): Model and data. *Asha, 17,* 158–165.

Starkweather, C. (1974). Behavior modification in training speech clinicians: Procedures and implications. *Asha, 16,* 607–611.

Ward, L., & Webster, E. (1965a). The training of clinical personnel: I. Issues in conceptualization. *Asha, 7,* 38–40.

Ward, L., & Webster, E. (1965b). The training of clinical personnel: II. A concept of clinical preparation. *Asha, 7,* 103–106.

Watzlawick, P., Beavin, J., & Jackson, D. (1967). *Pragmatics of human communication.* New York: Norton.

Watzlawick, P., Weakland, J., & Fisch, R. (1974). *Change: Principles of problem formation and problem resolution.* New York: Norton.

4
The Trigonal Model of Communication Disorders Supervision: Contexts

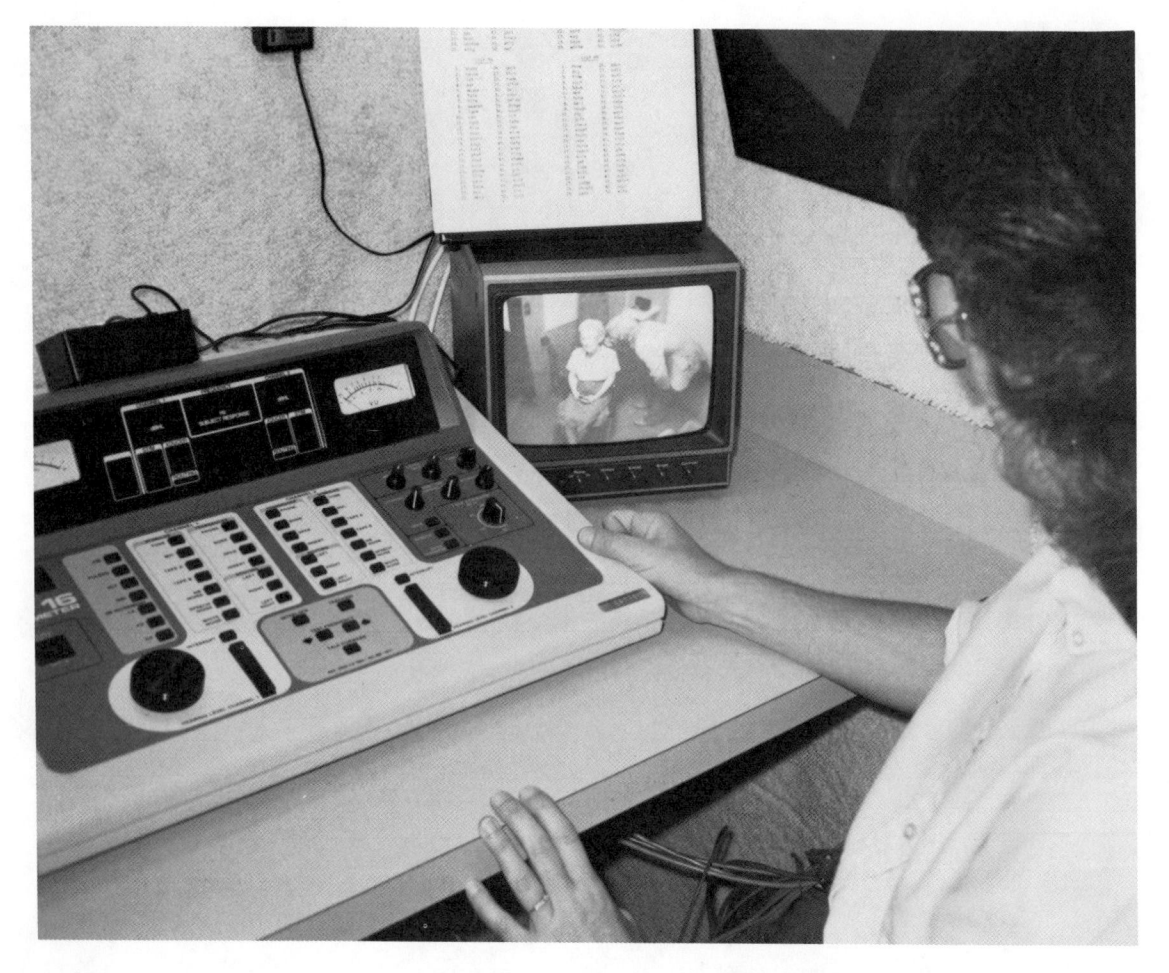

CRITICAL CONCEPTS

☐ *Communication Disorders supervisors work in five kinds of worksites.*
☐ *Three profiles characterize the distribution of work among supervision domains in every category of worksite.*
☐ *The 13 tasks of supervision have different relative importance in different worksites.*

OUTLINE

INTRODUCTION
WORKSITE PROFILES
   College and University Training Programs
   Schools
   Medical Settings
   Community Speech-Language and Hearing Centers
   Businesses
SUPERVISION TASKS RELATIVE TO WORKSITES
SUMMARY
APPLICATIONS

INTRODUCTION

Chapters 2 and 3 presented the Constituents and Concepts components of the Trigonal Model of Communication Disorders supervision. The third component of the model is Contexts: the worksites where supervisors are employed. Communication Disorders supervisors are typically employed in five general categories of contexts: college and university clinics, schools, medical settings, community speech-language and hearing centers, and businesses. Each worksite demands a somewhat different protocol for supervision, but the five contexts share three basic profiles of Communication Disorders supervisors. Table 4-1 presents the theoretical relative role emphasis for each of the three within each supervision context. Although these are the most typical profiles of Communication Disorders supervisors in the five contexts, they are by no means the only ones. Therefore, all organizations need to have well-developed job descriptions for supervisory personnel, for two reasons: (a) to use the supervisory personnel as effectively as possible by engaging their skills in all five roles, perhaps reducing the need for additional personnel in the organization; (b) to clarify for supervision personnel what is expected of them so that they can agree to those expectations and be compensated as multirole supervisors.

WORKSITE PROFILES

College and University Training Programs

Many supervisors work in clinics and ancillary and satellite facilities that are associated with college and university Communication Disorders training programs. These supervisors may be classified as primary (full-time in clinical/aca-

This chapter was contributed by Stephen S. Farmer, New Mexico State University.

TABLE 4-1
Communication disorders supervision roles relative to contexts

Context		Description	P	R	E	A	C
University clinics	A	Primary responsibility is education	2	2	3	1	2
	B	Equal distribution of roles	2	2	2	2	2
	C	Primary responsibilities are education and administration	2	2	3	3	2
		Subtotals	6	6	8	6	6
Schools	A	Primary responsibility is program management	2	1	2	3	1
	B	Primary responsibilities are program management and clinical service delivery	2	1	2	3	3
	C	Primary responsibilities are clinical service delivery, field clinical education for university, optional program management	2	1	3	1, 2, 3	3
		Subtotals	6	3	7	7, 8, 9	7
Medical settings	A	Primary responsibility is program management	2	1	2	3	1
	B	Primary responsibilities are program management and clinical service delivery	2	1	2	3	3
	C	Primary responsibilities are clinical service delivery, field clinical education for university, optional program management	2	1	3	1, 2, 3	3
		Subtotals	6	3	7	7, 8, 9	7

demic education) or secondary (part-time in clinical/academic education, part-time in other roles); faculty, staff, or adjunct; tenure track or non-tenure track; on-site or field supervisors; speech-language pathologists or audiologists. The classifications give little indication of what the supervisors do. However, because the primary mission of Communication Disorders training programs is to implement research-based methodologies for educating and training speech-language pathologists and audiologists to become competent professionals, it seems clear that supervisors affiliated with Communication Disorders training programs are responsible mainly for education, both clinical and academic, and for research. It is evident from Table 4-1 that the Educator role dominates all three profiles. The other roles are equally distributed across the college and university context. Profile A typifies the primary supervisor, for whom clinical education responsibilities predominate. The University-A supervisor's roles of Professional and Clinician will have subordinate emphasis; the role of Administrator is a tertiary function. A second category of university supervisors, University-B, shows an equal emphasis on all five roles. The third profile, University-C, emphasizes the Educator and Administrator

TABLE 4-1
continued

Context		Description	P	R	E	A	C
Community speech-language and hearing centers	A	Primary responsibility is program management	2	1	2	3	1
	B	Primary responsibilities are program management and clinical service delivery	2	1	2	3	3
	C	Primary responsibilities are clinical service delivery, field clinical education for university, optional program management	2	1	3	1, 2, 3	3
		Subtotals	6	3	7	7, 8, 9	7
Businesses	A	Primary responsibility is program management	1	1	1	3	1
	B	Primary responsibilities are program management and clinical service delivery	1	1	1	3	3
	C	Primary responsibilities are program management and clinical service delivery; field clinical education for university	1	1	2	3	3
		Subtotals	3	3	4	9	7

Code:
3 = Role has major emphasis in the context.
2 = Role has moderate emphasis in the context.
1 = Role has minor emphasis in the context.

Totals:
Professional: 27
Researcher: 18
Educator: 33
Administrator: 36-42
Clinician: 34

roles; the Professional, Researcher, and Clinician roles are subordinate. University B and C profiles are characteristic of Communication Disorders supervisors with titles like Clinic Coordinator or Clinic Director. Job descriptions for university-affiliated supervisors will be dictated by the institution's ranking guidelines for faculty and staff.

Schools

School contexts employ the most Communication Disorders supervisors. These contexts include urban, suburban, rural, preschool, elementary, and secondary institutions, and schools for exceptional learners, including handicapped, gifted, and incarcerated individuals. Rural schools sometimes present major problems for supervisors who must travel long distances to reach them. This problem might be alleviated with the development of alternatives to on-site supervision. Schools in rural areas need speech-language and hearing services but may have difficulty procuring them because of state or national supervision requirements. ASHA requires a minimum of ¼-time direct observation of all therapy and ½-time direct observation of all diagnostic work at the preservice level. Colleges and universities do not typically place student clinicians far away because the supervisor travel is not cost effective. Clinical fellows rarely choose rural sites because ASHA requires a minimum of 18 on-site visits by the Clinical Fellowship Year (CFY) supervisor (ASHA, 1985a). The advent of telecommunication through microcomputers and videotapes may guide researchers in the search for alternative supervision formats (see chapter 10). To work in schools for exceptional learners, supervisors may require additional preparation. University training programs may not give them adequate background and experience in (a) operating within the educational service delivery model, or (b) serving exceptional populations such as the multiple handicapped, the severely or profoundly handicapped, the gifted, or the incarcerated. However, supervisors should require no additional preparation for the other school contexts.

The first profile of supervisors in school contexts, School-A, describes supervisors who operate primarily as administrators. If the school has a large enough Communication Disorders staff, one person (typically a speech-language pathologist rather than an audiologist) will serve as a categorical supervisor of all the Communication Disorders personnel. If the staff is not large, it may be grouped with other rehabilitation and special education personnel such as physical therapists, occupational therapists, educational diagnosticians, counselors, social workers, and clinical psychologists. A Communication Disorders supervisor may function as a generic supervisor in that situation. The duties of the School-A supervisor revolve around program management. The Educator and Professional roles are secondary, and the Researcher and Clinician roles are tertiary. The School-B profile represents those whose responsibilities include part-time administrative and part-time clinical work. The Administrator and Clinician roles are of primary importance for them, the Educator and Professional are secondary, and the Researcher role receives minor attention. The third common profile of school supervisors, School-C, describes those who work as field supervisors for college or university training programs or who do CFY supervision. School-C supervisors place primary emphasis on the Educator and Clinician roles, some emphasis on the Professional, minor emphasis on Researcher, and variable emphasis on Administrator depending on how the roles are weighted on their job descriptions. The job description for a school supervisor will reflect the school's guidelines and, for a School-C supervisor, those of the college or university training program. As Table 4-1 shows, the Educator, Administrator, and Clinician roles are dominant in school contexts; the Professional and Research domains may not be emphasized in these settings.

Medical Settings

Communication Disorders supervisors may work in various medical settings, including hospitals, rehabilitation centers, extended care facilities, and nursing homes. In these facilities they may provide in- or out-patient, team, or one-on-one service. Supervision may be categorical or generic. Supervisors may need additional preparation in order to learn the medical model of service delivery and teamwork (multi-, inter-, or transdisciplinary). The Medical-A supervisor's profile parallels the School-A supervisor's: the dominant role is Administrator. The Medical-B supervisor profile, like the School-B, distributes the major emphasis between the Administrator and Clinician roles. The Medical-C profile, like the School-C, describes a field supervisor affiliated with a college or university training program. Table 4-1 shows identical patterns for the medical settings supervisors and the school supervisors.

Community Speech-Language and Hearing Centers

The role priority profiles for supervisors in community speech-language and hearing centers again follow the pattern described for supervisors in schools and medical settings. In other words, in the A profile for this context, major emphasis is placed on the Administrator role, a secondary emphasis on the Professional and Educator roles, and minor emphasis on the Researcher and Clinician roles. The B and C supervisor profiles are identical, respectively, to the School-B and Medical-B (which emphasize the Administrator and Clinician roles) and to the School-C and Medical-C (whose target is the Educational and Clinical domains, with flexibility in the Administrator role). Table 4-1 shows that the patterns for community speech-language and hearing center supervisors follow those of the previous two contexts. Job descriptions vary in accordance with the mission of each community speech-language and hearing center.

Businesses

Supervision in businesses includes private practices, hearing aid centers, group practices (e.g., with otolaryngologists, pediatricians, etc.), and corporations. The supervision is different in these situations because the focus is on the business aspects of service delivery and on peer rather than intern supervision. Medical and educational settings commonly have supervised services provided by interns, externs, or practicum students; business settings may not. Some clients purposefully choose practices that do not have preservice personnel. However, for businesses that do support intern training, supervision is an important facet of operations. Business-A and Business-B supervisors have role distributions similar to those of the other context A and B supervisors. The Business-C supervisor, however, is not as flexible as other context C supervisors, essentially because of the fee-for-service element of the business. Although other worksites often operate on a fee-for-service basis, the monetary aspect of administration is not always a top priority. Table 4-1 shows the importance of the Administrator and Clinician roles in most business enterprises.

The totals for each role in Table 4-1 show that the Administrator role receives the greatest emphasis across contexts, followed by the Clinician and Educator and then the Professional and Researcher roles.

SUPERVISION TASKS RELATIVE TO WORKSITES

The 13 tasks and 81 competencies defined by the ASHA Committee on Supervision (ASHA, 1985b) also have varying importance for different supervision roles in different worksites. Table 4-2 shows the theoretical relative importance of each task to each role within each worksite.

All 13 tasks are very important for supervisors in university clinics. The tasks vary in importance to the roles of Communication Disorders supervisors in the other four contexts (see p. 90). They are most important to the Educator role, with decreasing importance to the Clinician, Administrator, Professional, and Researcher roles, respectively.

In short, Communication Disorders supervisors who work in contexts where Speech-Language Pathology and Audiology services are provided under supervision align with one of three supervisor profiles that indicate the degree of emphasis on each of the five supervision roles. In addition, the ASHA tasks of supervision can be ranked in importance for each of the roles in each of the five Communication Disorders supervision contexts.

TABLE 4-2
ASHA supervision tasks relative to five Communication Disorders supervision roles within five contexts

Task*	University Clinics	Schools	Medical Settings	Community Speech and Hearing Centers	Businesses
1	REA 333	REA 133	REA 133	REA 133	REA 133
2	E 3	E 2	E 2	E 2	E 2
3	E 3	E 3	E 3	E 3	E 3
4	E 3	E 3	E 3	E 3	E 3
5	REA 333	REA 132	REA 132	REA 132	REA 132
6	REA 333	REA 132	REA 132	REA 132	REA 132
7	EA 33	EA 33	EA 33	EA 33	EA 33
8	REA 333	REA 131	REA 131	REA 132	REA 132
9	REA 333	REA 131	REA 131	REA 131	REA 131
10	REA 333	REA 133	REA 133	REA 133	REA 133
11	PREAC 33333	PREAC 21333	PREAC 21333	PREAC 21333	PREAC 21333
12	PREAC 33333	PREAC 33333	PREAC 33333	PREAC 33333	PREAC 33333
13	PREAC 33333	PREAC 13312	PREAC 13312	PREAC 13312	PREAC 13312

CODE:

3 = Supervision task is of major importance to the role within the context.
2 = Supervision task is of moderate importance to the role within the context.
1 = Supervision task is of minor importance to the role within the context.

SUMMARY:

	Pts./No.	Mean
Professional	33 /15	2.2
Researcher	79 /45	1.8
Educator	191 /65	2.9
Administrator	120 /50	2.4
Clinician	41 /15	2.7

*See appendix A for list of supervision tasks.

SUMMARY

The Trigonal Model of Communication Disorders supervision is made up of Constituents, Concepts, and Contexts. The Contexts component describes the locations where supervisors work. Supervisors are employed in five common worksites: college and university clinics, schools, medical settings, community speech-language and hearing centers, and businesses. Three supervision profiles characterize the work of supervision in each worksite. The interaction of Constituents, Concepts, and Contexts within the five supervision domains creates the modes of action that are the Communication Disorders supervision system.

APPLICATIONS

Discussion Topics

1. Discuss the three profiles of supervision in college and university speech-language and hearing centers. What other profiles are familiar to you?
2. Discuss the three profiles of supervision in school settings. What other profiles are familiar to you?
3. Discuss the three profiles of supervision in businesses. Should clients/patients pay the same amount for service to a business that uses interns who are being supervised?
4. Discuss the relative importance of the 13 supervision tasks to each worksite. Do you agree with the values given in Table 4–2?
5. Discuss the idea of differential preparation for supervision in specific worksites. Is it necessary to train personnel differently to supervise in medical settings? In businesses, schools, community centers, or college and university sites?

Laboratory Experiences

1. Write a job description and set up a career ladder for supervisors in each of the five worksites.
2. Design a continuing education workshop to teach about supervision in the five different worksites.
3. Develop laboratory experiences to prepare supervisor trainees for the five different worksites.
4. Develop a client/clinician schedule for each worksite.
5. Draw a visual representation of the Trigonal Model of Communication Disorders supervision for each of the five worksites. Are the triangles all equilateral?

Research Projects

1. Conduct a survey to find out what percentage of time is devoted to each role in each worksite within a given area or region of the country.
2. Develop a research design to explore the validity of the three work profiles.
3. Develop a research design to explore the relative ratings of importance of the 13 supervision tasks to the five worksites.

4. Develop, implement, and evaluate a training program for developing supervision skills and dispositions to work in the five worksites.

5. Make a videotape of 5-minute segments that demonstrate supervisor profiles in all five worksites.

REFERENCES

American Speech-Language-Hearing Association, Committee on Supervision in Speech-Language Pathology and Audiology. (1985a). *ASHA membership and certification handbook.* Rockville, MD: Author.

American Speech-Language-Hearing Association. (1985b). Clinical supervision in speech-language pathology and audiology (position statement). *Asha, 7,* 57–60.

PART THREE
Supervisor Development

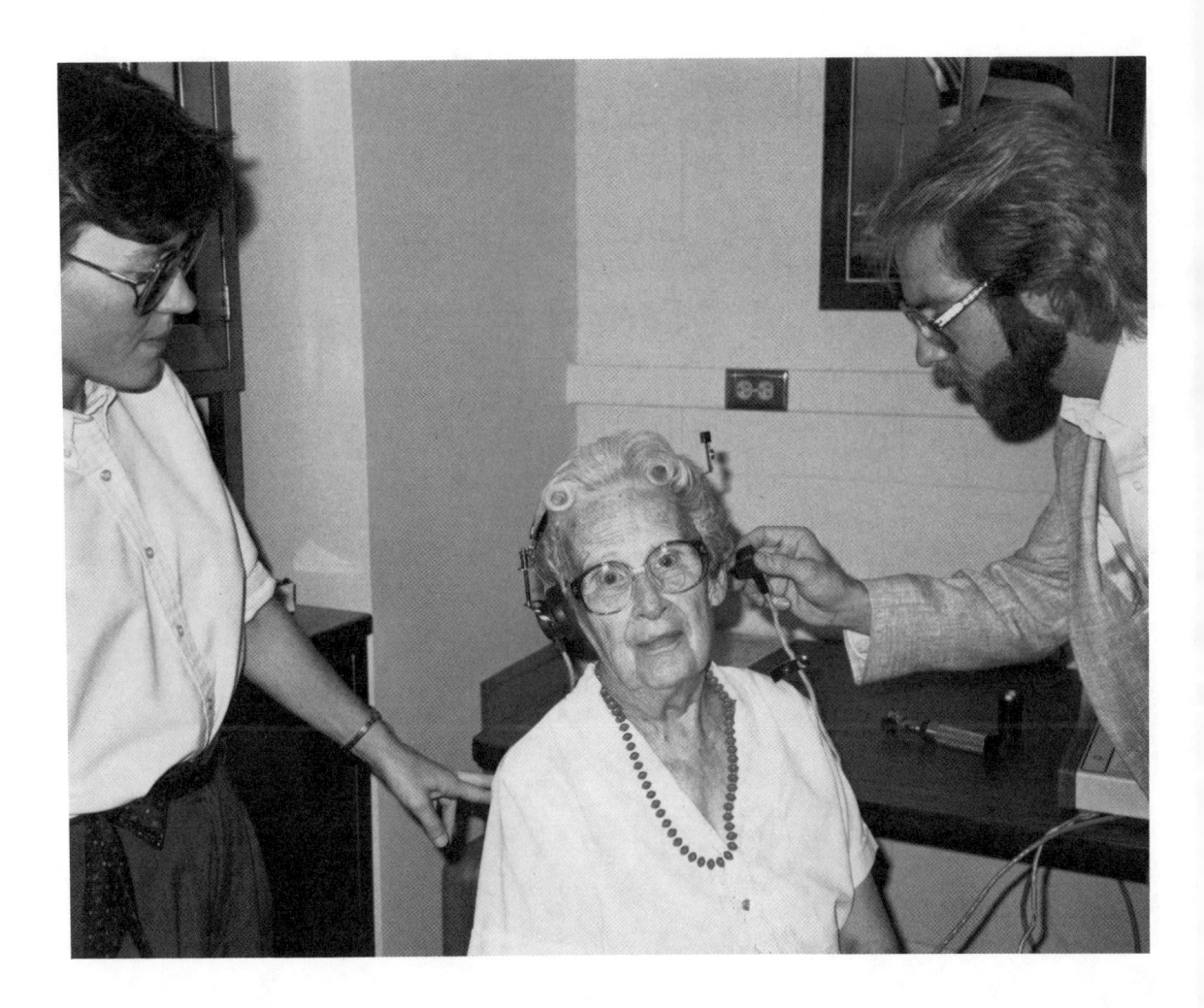

5
Communication Competence

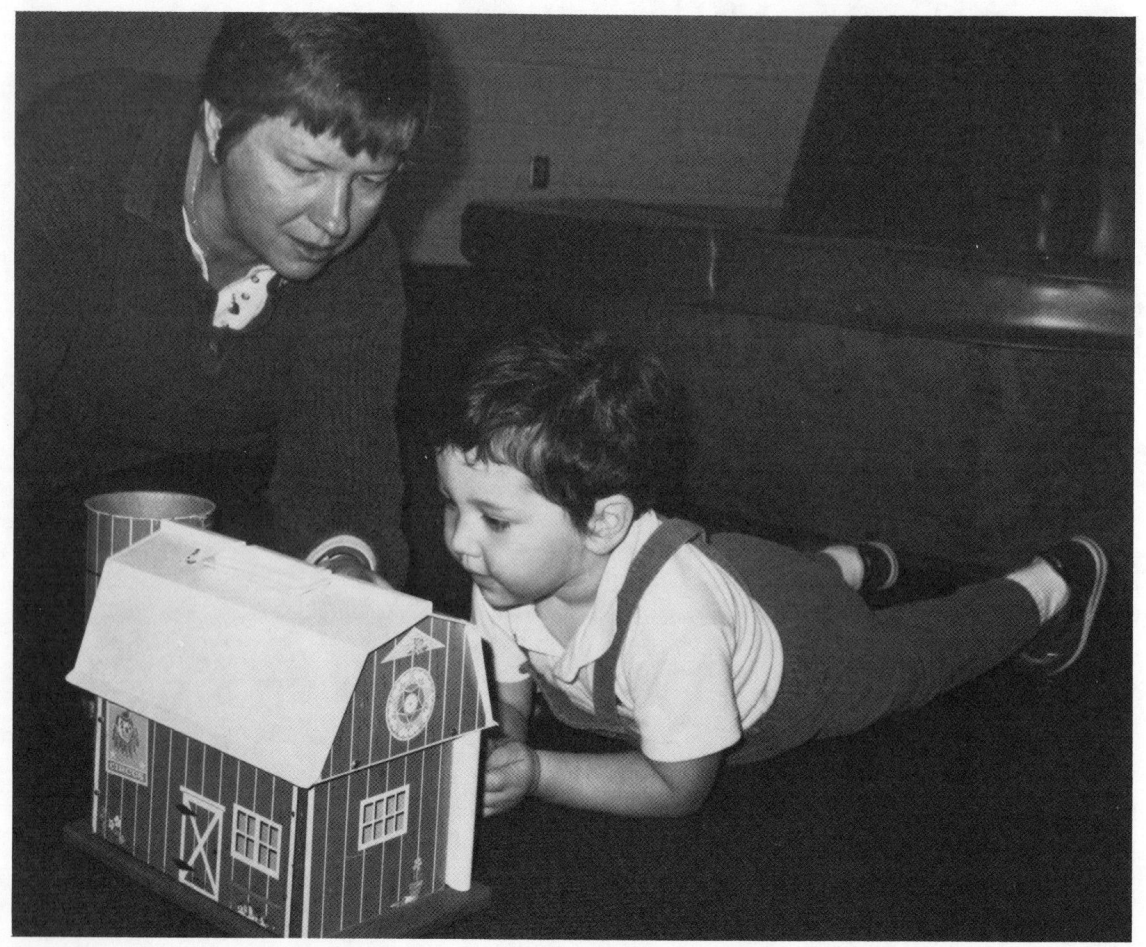

CRITICAL CONCEPTS

- *Communication is the cohesive agent in the Trigonal and Pentagonal Models of Communication Disorders supervision.*
- *Supervisors should know and be able to use 19 communication concepts.*
- *Supervisors can apply the 19 concepts in nine communication categories.*
- *Communication analysis is the first step toward developing communication competence.*

OUTLINE

INTRODUCTION

COMMUNICATION CONCEPTS
- Communication
- Language
- Axioms
- Metacommunication
- Listening
- Silence
- Channels
- Functions
- Intent/Force
- Communication Systems
- Registers/Codes
- Pragmatics
- Communication Style
- Rhetorical Sensitivity and Cognitive Complexity
- Life Scripts
- Conversational Competence
- Genderlect
- Question Types
- Humor

COMMUNICATION CATEGORIES
- Intrapersonal Communication
- Interpersonal Communication
- Small-Group Communication
- Organizational Communication
- Professional Communication
- Interviewing
- Supervision Conferences
- Nontraditional Communication
- Conflict Communication

COMMUNICATION ANALYSIS
- Personal Analysis
- Interaction Analysis (IA)
- Organizational Communication Audit
- Interview Analysis

COMMUNICATION COMPETENCE AND INCOMPETENCE

DEVELOPMENT OF COMMUNICATION COMPETENCE

SUMMARY

APPLICATIONS

This chapter was contributed by Stephen S. Farmer, New Mexico State University.

INTRODUCTION

Human relationships develop and are maintained through communication, the process of interaction between at least two people whose goal is the exchange of messages. Communication Disorders supervision is based on human relationships. This chapter presents general concepts associated with communication and argues that a supervisor's communication competence is a critical factor in supervision. Communication is the adhesive that conjoins the Constituents, Concepts, and Contexts and the five supervision roles into the Trigonal and Pentagonal Models of Communication Disorders supervision. Although competent communication is important in all human interactions, this chapter presents two perspectives on communication as a cohesive agent. First, communication competence emerges through an ongoing process of acquiring knowledge about the complexities of communication and acquiring skills and dispositions to use the knowledge. Supervisors need to be able to metacommunicate, that is, to communicate about communication. Although many professions depend on competent communication, not all of them demand the added step of analyzing and talking about the phenomenon. Second, supervisors, when fulfilling their five roles (Professional, Researcher, Educator, Administrator, Clinician), must communicate competently with many different communication partners (colleagues, parents, clients, ancillary personnel, etc.). Communication competence requires broad knowledge, skills, and dispositions that can be developed through academic and continuing education preparation programs. This competence forms the essential substructure for the Trigonal and Pentagonal Models of Communication Disorders supervision. Chapter 5 presents communication concepts (knowledge) as well as information about developing communication skills and dispositions.

COMMUNICATION CONCEPTS

Supervisors have the task of interacting with supervisees in such a way as to provide opportunities of genuine communication and, hence, learning for all the interactants. To do this, supervisors must be able to metacommunicate, to communicate about communication, from different perspectives: to discuss the communication of others (clients, clinicians, colleagues, etc.) and their own. To understand the vital importance of communication in supervision, and to develop metacommunication ability, it is necessary to understand the following 19 concepts.

Communication

Communication is a set of options used by speakers and listeners to negotiate the meanings of messages (Halliday, 1973). It can be viewed as a process composed of three single-strand continua: discrete-continuous; discursive-nondiscursive; and linear-intuitive (Hubbell, 1981). For example, a written memo from a supervisor to a supervisee is discrete, discursive, and linear. A conference between a supervisor and a partner may be discrete in the words used but continuous in tone of voice, posture, and facial expression; both verbal and nonverbal aspects of the message are fairly discursive. At the same time, the meaning of the conference in the relationship between the supervisor and the partner may have both linear and intuitive elements. *Genuine* communication is defined as a phenomenon that meets the sincerity and meaningfulness tests within the intentionality condition of Searle's speech act theory (Searle, Kiefer, & Bierwisch, 1980). Communication hinges on a symbol system for encoding and decoding messages.

Language

Language is the symbol system, a tool the supervisor or supervisee uses to send messages to the receiver; language is also a source of information used by the receiver to comprehend a message. Language has both nonverbal (including vocal and nonvocal) and verbal (oral, written, and sign) dimensions.

Nonverbal language falls into seven categories: (a) the symbols related to *time* (e.g., timing of discrete acts, *chronemics* (the use of time), and *silence*); (b) *kinesics* (e.g., body movements such as *emblems,* acts that have direct verbal translations or dictionary definitions, such as the "A-OK" or "peace" signs; *illustrators,* acts directly tied to or accompanying speech and serving to illustrate what is being said verbally; *regulators,* acts that maintain and regulate the back-and-forth nature of speaking and listening between two or more interactants; and *adaptors,* acts that are efforts to satisfy needs, perform actions, manage emotions, develop social contacts, or perform a host of other functions); (c) *proxemics,* such as body orientation and positioning; (d) *physical characteristics* (e.g., facial expressions; *oculesics,* such as winks, stares; personal accouterments, such as jewelry, a pipe; *organismics,* such as eye and skin color, body dimensions, prostheses); (e) *touch*; (f) *paralanguage,* such as *characterizers* (moan, laugh, cry, whisper, yell), *qualifiers* (intensity, pitch, quality of vocalizations), or *segregates* (nonfluencies, like *uh, ah, um*); and (g) the *environment* (e.g., furniture, temperature, light). Nonverbal language is often considered to be continuous, nondiscursive, and intuitive. Although communication is most often equated with verbal language, it has been estimated that between 65% and 80% of a message is coded on the nonverbal band (Knapp, 1978a). Nonverbal communication can repeat, contradict, substitute for, complement, accent, or regulate verbal behavior. A number of studies have dealt with the role of nonverbal communication in the clinical process; few studies have explored this aspect of the supervision process.

Verbal forms of language are the words used and their meanings (semantics), the grammar, the inflectional markers (morphology), and the order of the words used (syntax). Verbal language is most often thought of as oral. However, non-oral communication, such as a sign language or an augmentative communication system, may be classified either as verbal (because it involves semantics and syntax) or nonverbal. Writing is clearly verbal but non-oral. Thus, supervisors often encounter both oral and non-oral verbal communication situations.

Within the past decade, professionals have been reporting how verbal and nonverbal symbols work together in the communication process. Scherer (1980) states that future research will need to move from the dominant single-channel analysis to multichannel assessment of communication behavior. Theoretically, few pure verbal or nonverbal events occur in communication. Therefore, any methods that view the communication process from just one vantage point must, in Kendon's words, be thought of as "*special* language theories. *General* language theories must await the systematic development of a study of communicative behaviours which shows how all the different strands of behaviour function together" (Kendon & Ferber, 1973, p. 26). (Observation of verbal and nonverbal dimensions of communication is discussed in chapter 6.)

Based on what is known about verbal and nonverbal communication, theorists have proposed five universal principles or axioms.

Axioms

The axioms of communication describe how communication works in relationships. Wood (1981) summarizes these universal principles:

1. It is impossible to *not* communicate. All behavior, both verbal and nonverbal, is a form of language that is used in communication.
2. Messages have content and relationship components.
3. Communication exchanges are "punctuated," that is, feelings are attributed to the behavior of others.
4. Communication is digital and analogic. Digital communication uses verbal language; analogic communication includes the nonverbal channels of the message. Although digital language may be clear and precise in conveying a message, it is often unable to express the warmth of supervisor-supervisee relation-

ships. On the other hand, analogic communication is good for expressing feelings of affection or hostility, but the interpretation of an analogic message is not always clear and precise.

5. Relationships and messages can be symmetrical, complementary, or parallel. Historically supervisors have been afforded a higher status in the supervision process than supervisees (a complementary relationship). Currently other models equalize the status (symmetrical) or allow it to fluctuate (parallel) depending on the situation. Relationships can change every second or remain relatively constant. It is important to know that neither the symmetrical, the complementary, nor the parrallel pattern is best. Healthy supervisor-supervisee relationships flow back and forth among different roles and patterns.

Parks (1980) summarized research about symmetrical and complementary messages (as opposed to relationships). Symmetrical messages are equivalent messages (e.g., referential statement/referential statement; agreeing/agreeing; giving instructions/countering with instructions) while complementary messages are maximally dissimilar (e.g., giving/taking instructions; asking/answering; asserting/agreeing). Parks's synthesis showed that the greater the *symmetry,* the greater the frequency of unilateral action in a relationship, the lower the probability of relationship termination, and the greater the frequency of open conflict (which can be viewed as productive if the supervisor is skilled in conflict communication strategies). Further, the greater the *complementarity,* the less empathy and the greater the frequency of disconfirming messages.

Metacommunication

An important element of oral or written communication is the ability to use language to analyze communication. The process of appreciating and reflecting on communication is referred to as metacommunication and includes the ability to recognize and use component sounds, syllables, and words; grammatic and semantic rules; language as an interactive tool; and language as a tool for learning. Metacommunication requires a supervisor to shift focus to alternative uses, alternative meanings, or to the grammatical construction of verbal and nonverbal communication. To develop metacommunication ability, supervisors must have listening ability.

Listening

Listening, defined as the process by which the human organism selects, processes, and stores aural input data, is a major component of communication. Whitman and Boase (1983) found that adults spend an average of 70% of their waking hours communicating and that the time is divided as follows: writing, 9%; reading, 16%; talking, 30%; and listening, 45%. However, it is estimated that when people listen, they miss about half of what the speaker says; 2 months later, they will remember only one-fourth of what was said. In fact, people tend to forget within 8 hours one-third to one-half of what they hear (Myers & Myers, 1973). Lack of competence in this area is primarily responsible for many of the problems between supervisors and their communication partners. Listening is not an involuntary, automatic, or passive phenomenon; it requires active participation. Listening entails isolating the message, being ready to respond, decoding and assigning meaning, and forecasting, or predicting what is to come (Goss, 1983). Faulty listening affects not only the communication in progress but also future communication. Reasons for poor listening fall into three major categories: (a) *distraction,* the physical (external) and psychological (internal) "noise" that makes it difficult to concentrate on a speaker; (b) *disorientation,* when one is confused, bored, or critical of what the speaker is saying because of a dissonance between it and one's own background knowledge or interest; and (c) *defensiveness,* when one is threatened by the speaker, the message, or the situation (Goss, 1983).

Active, reflective, or responsive listening are antidotes to listening breakdowns. Consequences of active, reflective listening and responding as described by Long (1978) and applied to supervision include the following:

1. The partner communicates more thoroughly.
2. The partner is unthreatened because judgmental statements are not used.
3. Ideas become more clear and less biased by supervisor perception.
4. A conversational flow, rather than a clash of colliding statements, is established.
5. The partner's self-disclosure ability is enhanced.
6. The partner's feelings can be addressed.

A supervisor can either learn to be a poor listener and not operate to capacity or learn to be a good listener and come close to optimal performance. Good listening is both responsive and critical. Responsive listening is empathetic and other-oriented. Critical listening requires assessing the accuracy, acceptability (how reasonable the information is), facts, and inferences of messages. Specific strategies that have been shown to improve responsive and critical listening for Communication Disorders supervisors include the following:

1. S.O.U.L. (Silence, Observation, Understanding, Listening), an INter-REActive Learning (INREAL) strategy (Farmer, 1984b). Using this strategy, the supervisor can learn about a supervisee's world, understand that person's perceptions better, and thereby establish a relationship based on transactional mutuality. The supervisee begins the interaction so that the supervisor can then react to his or her present state of being. Meaning is negotiated from accurate listening and responding to cognitive, linguistic, and affective levels of communication.

2. Verbal Monitoring and Reflecting-Imitated (VMR-I) and Verbal Monitoring and Reflecting-Restated (VMR-R) are also INREAL strategies. During VMR-I, the supervisor listens to the communication partner and repeats, nonpunitively, what the partner has said, using the same words. The technique may be used to validate, reinforce, or emphasize the partner or the message, or to check semantic truth value. Paralanguage plays a very important role in using INREAL strategies. If the strategies are not used in a meaningful and sincere way, supervisors can sound like they are mimicking or parroting their partners. Most supervisors need practice to avoid giving this impression. Examples of successful use of VMR-I follow.

a. Semantic example:

SUPERVISEE: Chang just won't do what I tell him to.

SUPERVISOR: Chang just won't do what *you tell him to.* (*Used to affirm, acknowledge, or clarify that supervisee is being instructive rather than communicative.*)

b. Cognitive example:

SUPERVISEE: I don't seem to be understanding the concept of cognitive matching.

SUPERVISOR: You *don't* seem to be understanding cognitive matching. (*affirming*)

c. Affective example:

SUPERVISEE: I don't feel very comfortable having to confront Ingrid about not wearing her hearing aid.

SUPERVISOR: I can tell you aren't feeling comfortable about confronting Ingrid.

The VMR-R strategy is similar but is used to correct semantic truth value, while at the same time validating the partner. With VMR-R the supervisor listens to the partner and, nonpunitively, repeats correctly what the partner has said in error, using as many as possible of the partner's own words.

d. Semantic example:

SUPERVISEE: Chang just won't do what I tell him to.

SUPERVISOR: Chang just *won't* do what you tell him to? (*indicating that the word* can't *might be more accurate*)

e. Cognitive example:

SUPERVISEE: O.K. You see, I have him identify the toy I name by picking it up when I say, "Where's the car?" or "Where's the ball?"

SUPERVISOR: You're working at the *recognition* level by having him pick up the toy when you name it. (*indicating a recognition rather than an identification task*)

f. Affective example:

SUPERVISEE: I felt bad that she missed therapy today.

SUPERVISOR: You also felt relieved that she didn't show because then you had more time to prepare for your evaluation tomorrow.

3. Expansion-Elaborated (E-E) and Expansion-Restated (E-R) are additional INREAL strategies that can be used to facilitate a supervisor's listening and responding. When using E-E, the supervisor listens to the partner and responds by elaborating on the partner's own words. This strategy is used to validate, reinforce, or emphasize the partner or message and to add new information.

a. Semantic example:

SUPERVISEE: I'm beginning to see the scope of what we need to do in therapy with Carla.

SUPERVISOR: You do have a good scope of the therapy needed; now you need the sequence of categories. Scope and sequence go together.

b. Cognitive example:

SUPERVISEE: Dr. Stewart is the only team member who got to see Erin's repaired cleft.

SUPERVISOR: Dr. Stewart was the only team member to see Erin's repaired cleft, and he did it by forcing open her mouth, which may have traumatized Erin even more than she was when you saw her.

c. Affective example:

SUPERVISEE: I'm glad we decided to enroll Eric in therapy for a semester.

SUPERVISOR: You're glad we decided to enroll Eric as a preventive measure, and you've resolved your anger at Eric's mother for contradicting your original "let's wait and see" attitude.

With E-R, the supervisor listens to the partner and responds with a corrected and expanded version of the partner's own words.

d. Semantic example:

SUPERVISEE: I gave his dad all the information about the Medic Alert bracelets.

SUPERVISOR: You did give him the booklet, and now that we have the order form, you can give him that, too, since they aren't included in the booklet.

e. Cognitive example:

SUPERVISEE: I just don't know where to go next to find any more information about Moebius syndrome.

SUPERVISOR: You don't know where to find more information because you're focusing only on the medical aspects of the syndrome.

f. Affective example:

SUPERVISEE: I feel like such a failure at my first speech-language evaluation.

SUPERVISOR: You feel like a failure because you're being too critical of yourself. You got some good information about a very difficult client.

4. Paraphrasing is a listening-responding strategy in which the supervisor listens to the partner and then restates, in different words, what was just said. This skill is a component of the *Modeling* strategy used in INREAL. Modeling is the naturally conversational interpersonal communication strategy with which the supervisor listens to the partner and responds without using the partner's own words. Modeling can be used to counter an argument, to change, expand, or maintain a topic, or to respond to a direct or indirect request on a semantic, cognitive, or affective level.

a. Semantic example:

SUPERVISEE: Susie did really well in therapy today.

SUPERVISOR: You're saying that Susie initiated conversation, maintained her attention for 20 minutes, and demonstrated that she can use a crayon and paper appropriately for her age level. In other words, she accomplished the objectives you set for her therapy session. (*This clarifies what "did well" means.*)

b. Cognitive example:

SUPERVISEE: I decided to use an experiential language-learning model with Jody rather than the classical learning theory model, so I won't need to borrow your information on microunits.

SUPERVISOR: O.K. It sounds like you're applying some information from the Language Disorders class about bottom up–top down information processing.

c. Affective example:

SUPERVISEE: I'm feeling the need for some positive feedback. This hasn't been a good week for me.

SUPERVISOR: Let's go over the Therapy Observation Form I completed when I observed you yesterday. Maybe seeing in black and white the high quality skills you were exhibiting will give your self-confidence a boost.

5. Parasupporting, like Expansion-Elaborated, carries the partner's message a step further. Unlike the Monitoring and Reflecting, and Expansion strategies of INREAL, the *para*-strategies do not use the exact words of the partner. Paraphrasing and Parasupporting can be used to validate, reinforce, or emphasize the partner or message, check semantic truth value, and model a new way of saying similar ideas. In other words, Paraphrasing validates the speaker as a communication partner and acknowledges the speaker's thoughts and feelings, whereas Parasupporting goes on to advocate those thoughts and feelings (Stewart & D'Angelo, 1975).

Silence

Silence is a paralinguistic phenomenon that can be a significant part of communication. Silence and talk time can be valuable data in assessing features of an interaction, but like other features they comprise only a part of the whole. Some of the interpersonal functions served by silence include (a) punctuating or accenting, drawing attention to certain words or ideas; (b) evaluating, showing judgment of another's behavior, including favor or disfavor, agreement or disagreement; (c) attack (e.g., not responding to a comment, greeting, or written correspondence); (d) revelation, making some things known or keeping them hidden; (e) expression of emotions, such as disgust, sadness, fear, anger, or love; and (f) mental activity, showing thoughtfulness and reflection or ignorance through silence (Knapp, 1978a). The concept of *wait time* (also termed *pause time* or *reaction time latency*) is important in a supervisor's repertoire of communication abilities. A supervisor's wait time—the silence that occurs between the supervisee's turn and the supervisor's response—can have profound effects on the supervisee. Studies by Rowe (1986) on wait time, applied to supervision through the companion concept of the INREAL strategy of *Reaction Time Latency* (RTL), show that when a supervisor waits approximately 3–5 seconds after a supervisee's communication act, the following can occur:

1. The length of the supervisee's responses increases.
2. The number of unsolicited but appropriate supervisee responses increases.
3. The supervisee less often fails to respond.
4. Supervisee confidence, as shown in fewer inflected responses, increases.
5. The supervisee more often thinks speculatively.
6. Evidence, followed by or preceded by supervisee inference statements, increases.
7. The number of supervisee questions increases.
8. Contributions by "quiet" supervisees increase.
9. Supervisee utterances become more varied in type.
10. Supervisees exhibit greater response flexibility.
11. The number and kind of supervisor questions change.
12. Supervisor expectations for certain supervisees change.

Silence, then, can be as important in the communication process as are the verbal dimensions of the messages.

The vehicles for sending verbal and nonverbal messages back and forth between communicators are referred to as channels.

Channels

The communication channels used in Communication Disorders supervision are watching/moving, listening/talking, and reading/writing. The watching/moving channels of communication are discussed in detail in chapter 6, "Observation Competence," and the reading/writing channels in chapter 9, "Clinical Literacy." Supervisors should be competent in and use all six channels.

Aside from its technical, structured aspects, communication must also be considered from a functional perspective.

Functions

Basic communication functions are manifested in all supervisor interactions. Functions can be classified in many different ways, but the following five examples will illustrate the concept:

1. The *controlling* function involves the supervisor's or communication partner's attempts to direct or affect the behavior of the other, as well as responses to such attempts. Requesting, suggesting, warning, acknowledging, repeating, refusing, and assenting are examples of this function.
2. *Sharing feelings* includes communication acts such as praising, commiserating, ridiculing, approving, apologizing, and rejecting. All are messages used by supervisors and partners to express feelings to each other.
3. The *informing* function occurs when a supervisor and partner provide ideas and information to each other (e.g., by naming and giving examples) or respond to the information given (e.g., by answering, questioning, or denying).
4. When messages help sustain a supervisor-supervisee relationship, the function is

ritualizing. This one includes acts like greeting, thanking, introducing, and teasing.
5. The *imagining* function involves dealing creatively with reality through language; examples are speculating, fantasizing, storytelling, and dramatizing.

Knowing the function is not enough to capture someone's communicative purposes. The intent, or force, of a communication act may also need to be examined.

Intent/Force

Language functions may be used for different purposes. For example, someone may repeat (a controlling function) with the intent (also referred to as *force*) either to clarify or to emphasize. Someone may ask a question (an informing function) with the intent either to clarify or to seek additional information.

All the elements of communication presented thus far combine to form a communication system.

Communication Systems

In the simplest terms, a communication system is two or more persons in the process of relating to one another (Watzlawick, Beavin, & Jackson, 1967). (See chapter 3 for additional discussion of systems theory.) Each system operates in an environment, which includes anything or anyone that influences or is influenced by the system. A classroom, a supervisor-supervisee dyad, a clinician-client dyad, and a family are all examples of systems. Systems may be open or closed. An open communication system has the following characteristics: (a) the system operates as a whole unit, not simply as a collection of individuals; the actions of each member affect the actions of the others, and a problem for one system member is a problem for the others; (b) decisions and discussions are the joint effort of the members of the system;

even if each member does not participate in every decision or discussion, system members are encouraged to take part in these activities; and (c) feedback in the open system is positive; system members exchange encouragement, praise, and confirmation (Hubbell, 1981). Positive messages are related to healthy changes in supervisees and supervisors. Communication disorders supervision STYLES III and IV (described in chapter 3 and appendix B) are examples of bilateral, open communication systems.

The characteristics of a closed communication system include the following: (a) The system members operate more as individuals, each one with a prescribed status and role. The supervisors are authorities and decision makers on most matters. Supervisees are expected to act according to certain rules. The actions of one member of the system are treated as though they are separate from all others' actions; (b) Decisions in the closed system are based on predetermined rules and guidelines set by the supervisors. Supervisees are often told the results of such decisions. Decisions about what to do, what plans to follow, or who should do something are made on the basis of status (who is in charge, who has seniority, who has the highest degree, etc.); (c) Feedback in the closed system is negative. Criticism, suggestions, and rejection are characteristic of messages from one to another, usually from supervisor to supervisee. These messages help keep the system together by reinforcing the status quo. Relationships grow and develop with difficulty when negative feedback is the predominant mode of response. Communication Disorders supervision STYLES I and II are examples of unilateral, closed communication systems.

Systems can be formal or informal, and these differences in communication patterns are known as registers or codes.

Registers/Codes

Communication registers, or codes, occur as people adapt to the social and communication demands of situations. Registers are differences observable within speakers, across situations. The different registers allow speakers to convey their social position relative to that of their listeners while simultaneously communicating a message. Joos (1976) describes five registers or codes:

1. *Frozen:* the most distant, noninteractive form of communication code; it represents ritualistic language exchanges that may vary in content but rarely in form. This code may be used by Communication Disorders supervisors when interacting with ancillary professionals where contact is infrequent.
2. *Formal:* communication that informs with no participation from the listener (e.g., introductions, giving orders). Supervisors may use this code in situations of multi- or interdisciplinary or generic supervision.
3. *Consultative:* a form used with strangers; the speaker supplies background information (e.g., responds to an information-seeking question). This code is used in the Professional, Administrator, and Clinician roles (e.g., during family interviews or conferences).
4. *Casual:* a form used with acquaintances and friends in conversation; minimal background information is needed in the context. This is a common code for supervisors to use with supervisees.
5. *Intimate:* a form that excludes public information; each intimate group invents its own code. Some close-knit clinical staffs may use this type of code.

Joos states that a speaker is free to shift from one code to another even within one utterance; however, only neighboring codes can be used sequentially. It is considered inappropriate to shift two or more steps within a single utterance. For example, a speaker shifting from formal to casual presentation shocks the listener by changing the emphasis from what is said to how it is said, clouding the intent of the message. "Mr. Smith, I need to discuss your job description and salary with you" (formal); "Get the picture, Joe?" (casual).

Bernstein's sociolinguistic theory (1970) discusses *restricted* and *elaborated* codes. Restricted codes are the context-dependent modes of communication used with close friends and co-workers when details are unnecessary. Precise, detailed, context-independent statements that anyone can understand are elaborated codes. Supervisors interacting with supervisees use a range of restricted codes; when interacting with others, they must expand into more elaborated codes.

Most supervisors play many roles in society even within the course of a single day, and within the constraints of each role they must communicate their intentions. A woman can be a mother and a daughter, a supervisor and a supervisee, a stranger to some and an intimate to others. Even if the content of her message is identical across these multiple roles, she will use different verbal and nonverbal codes in each situation. For example, she might request supervision paperwork in the following ways:

"Excuse me, sir, do you have any of the supervision forms, F200?"

"Hon, please bring me the supervision forms from my briefcase."

"I see supervision forms all over this room! Get them picked up and bring them to my office within the next 5 minutes!"

Registers and codes can indicate relative power, persuasiveness, gender differences, the distance or closeness of relationships, telephone behavior, bonding among groups and subgroups, manners, conventionality, and conflict. We acquire specific registers or codes by hearing them in context and by practicing them.

The functional use of language in context is called pragmatics.

Pragmatics

Although the intent to obtain supervision forms is identical in the above examples, the verbal and nonverbal structures differ radically. A view of language that accounts for these variants is called *pragmatics*. One pragmatic theory argues that every communication act has three aspects: (a) the *illocutionary* intent of the sender to accomplish some goal, such as to inform, request, persuade, or promise; (b) the actual form of the communication act, the *locutionary* dimension, which consists of the syntax, semantics, and phonology; (c) the *perlocutionary* effect that the act has on the receiver (e.g., did the receiver comply with the request, understand the information?). The three requests for supervision forms are all similar in their illocutionary intent (or force) but differ in their realized locutions. It is obvious that the first example is used with a male stranger, the second with an intimate, and the third with a subordinate. If these utterances occurred in other contexts, they would be not only inappropriate but probably unsuccessful in their perlocutionary effect. Thus, variations in communication may be considered the pragmatic adaptations of language to the different social and contextual demands of each situation (Gleason, 1985).

Associated with the use of language in context is the idea that communicators have personal communication styles that must be adapted to a variety of contexts.

Communication Style

Communication style is a type of language variation that distinguishes individual speakers. For example, some supervisors tend to use a flowery, expressive style; others prefer a formal, grammatically correct style (*acrolect*); some choose a conversational, everyday style (*mesolect*); some will represent themselves through vulgar speech (*basolect*) (Muma, 1978).

Norton (1983) developed the *Communicator Style Measure* (CSM), a self-report tool that assesses how an individual communicates. The *CSM* consists of 51 items that are rated on a 5-point scale. The 11 styles subconstructs are: Friendly, Impression Leaving, Relaxed, Contentious/Argumentative, Attentive, Precise, Animated/Expressive, Dramatic, Open, Dominant, and Communicator Image. Stevens and Miller (1986) used the *CSM* to describe communication differences between direct and indirect styles of Communication Disorders supervision. Three subconstructs served to distinguish the direct from the indirect style: degree of precision, amount of dominance, and degree of contentiousness. As was noted in chapter 2, supervisors can self-administer the *CSM,* identify a personal style, and then work toward developing aspects of other styles that will allow them to be more flexible communicators.

Knapp (1978b) describes interpersonal communication style using a matrix that registers responsiveness and assertiveness. He states that interpersonal communication styles depend on whether individuals emphasize responsiveness (amiable, or "pleaser"), assertiveness (driver, or "dominator"), neither (analytical, or "computer"), or both (expressive, or "leveler").

One communication style that has been shown to be effective both in developing a relationship and then in maintaining a high level of interpersonal interaction and learning is *pacing and leading* (or simply *pacing*). Pacing, which uses the techniques of nonverbal mirroring, verbal matching of primary representational system (PRS) predicates, and meta-analysis (see p. 118). is employed in Neurolinguistic Programming (NLP) (Bandler & Grinder, 1979). It is based on the idea that "shared knowledge of style in such things as posture, gesture, eye contact, and the amount and kind of talk one should do ... is necessary if two people are able to communicate effectively face to face" (Erickson & Shultz, 1982, p. 7). Pacing is similar to the INREAL strategies (S.O.U.L., mirroring, self talk, parallel talk, verbal monitoring and reflecting, expansion, modeling, and reaction time latency) employed by Farmer (1984a, 1984b, 1984d) in the Interpersonal Communication Pacing (ICP) model of supervision conference communication. Other communication experts, using different terminology, have written about the effectiveness of various forms of interactional mutuality: *congruence*, or the compatibility of intra- and interpersonal verbal and nonverbal dimensions of messages in cognitive and affective domains (Tepper & Haase, 1978); *interactional synchrony*, or shared rhythmicity in movement and paralinguistics (Condon & Ogston, 1967; Kendon, 1980; LaFrance & Mayo, 1978; Long, 1978); *mirroring*, in which one person reflects another's linguistic and nonlinguistic dimensions of communication (Long, 1978; Bandler & Grinder, 1979); and *confluence*, a combination of the theories of mutuality and convergence (Buchheimer, 1963).

Companion concepts to metacommunication and pacing, as applied to supervision, are rhetorical sensitivity and cognitive complexity.

Rhetorical Sensitivity and Cognitive Complexity

Rhetorical sensitivity is the ability of a supervisor to adapt messages in response to a listener and a situation; cognitive complexity is an elaborated language code that minimizes ambiguity and reflects the supervisor's ability to take the listener's perspective (Dowling, 1986). Both are measures used in describing interpersonal communication. Hart and Burks (1972) describe five characteristics of rhetorical sensitivity. As applied to supervisors, they include the ability to:

1. Alter roles in response to the behavior of others, recognizing the complexity of humans.
2. Avoid stylizing communication into rigid behavior so that adaptation is possible.
3. Withstand the pressure and ambiguity of constant adaptation and learn to deal with different audiences.
4. Monitor communication with others to make it purposive rather than expressive; communicate directly rather than use emotion to manage problems.
5. Alter behavior in a rational and orderly way.

Hart, Carlson, and Eadie (1980) and Ward (1981) have posited three basic types of communicators, who can be envisioned on a continuum. At one end of the continuum is the noble self (NS), one who feels that total frankness and personal consistency are necessary. At the opposite end is the rhetorical reflector (RR), one who presumes that the satisfaction of others' needs is the primary goal of communication. At midline is the rhetorically sensitive (RS) individual who, when communicating, tries to balance personal needs with the desires of others. Rhetorical sensitivity and cognitive complexity are important elements in the use of registers or codes.

Life Scripts

Life scripts are routines or procedures an individual or a system follows in daily living and working (the routines of getting ready for work, eating a meal, celebrating a holiday, and so forth). It is important for supervisors not to assume that supervisees have the same scripts for supervision that they do. The use of S.O.U.L. can help a supervisor determine a supervisee's scripts so as to communicate in a way that will facilitate interactional mutuality.

Interactional mutuality is established through conversation. It is important for a supervisor to exercise conversational competence.

Conversational Competence

Conversations require the integration of verbal skills with nonverbal information, as well as prior and present contextual information. Conversationalists enter into an elaborate, unwritten social routine that includes rules about how to take turns, when to change topics, how to provide necessary information, and how to repair communication breakdowns. Adult conversational frames include (a) beginning in particular ways; (b) carrying out certain prearranged rituals for exchanging information; (c) acknowledging comments made by conversational partners; and (d) signaling the end of a conversation appropriately (Schegloff & Sacks, 1973). Grice (1975) described conversational events as rule-governed and as manifesting four basic expectations: (a) the *quantity* of information provided must be adequate to meet the listener's needs, but not excessive; (b) the *quality* of truthfulness must be substantiated; (c) topics must be *relevant*; (d) messages must be *understandable*. The units for analyzing conversations are the *turn* (a complete verbal and/or nonverbal communication act of one partner) and the *exchange* (one complete turn of each partner).

To be a good conversational partner, a supervisor should know about variables that affect conversation. Two of these variables are the gender of the communicators and the use of various types of questions.

Genderlect

One of the primary divisions in society is that between men and women. In adulthood individuals tend to adopt gender-associated speech styles. Speakers may choose deliberately to take on speech characteristics of the other gender, and in certain situations they are expected to. Professional women, in general, learn in professional situations to lower their pitch somewhat and also to lessen the range of pitch variation in their speech, traits characteristic of men (Kramer, 1974).

In American English, strong stereotypes exist concerning the sex-role appropriateness of particular speech patterns. Kramer (1974) has termed these sex-role-related variants *genderlects*. Some authors, according to Lynch (1983), contend that English is a masculine language, as reflected by the generic use of *he* and *men* to refer to both men and women. Such a condition tends to exclude women and to express male dominance. Because supervisors are predominantly women, stereotypic communication patterns are relevant to their success in all five supervision roles. Researchers concerned with feminist issues have observed that the use of certain masculine forms of communication tends to perpetuate sex-role stereotypes (Belenky, Clinchy, Goldberger, & Tarule, 1986; Gilligan, 1982; Lakoff, 1973; Langellier & Natalle, 1987; Lynch, 1983). Genderlects have been documented in the areas of vocabulary, conversational style, polite forms, and verbosity.

American women appear to use more standard phonetic forms than men; women are more likely to pronounce the final *-ing* of a word such as *working*, whereas men tend to pronounce it as *-in*. But the differences in genderlects are most often exhibited in frequency of usage of lexical items rather than in syntax or phonetics. Women are more likely to use intensifiers such as *so*, *quite*, *vastly*, or *such* and adjectives such as *adorable*, *cute*, or *lovely*. Women use a greater variety of color terms (i.e., shocking pink, lemon yellow), whereas men describe their environments with a limited, basic set of color names.

Conversational topics involving the economy, business, or jobs are often associated with men. Although women tend to introduce more topics into a conversation, a majority of the subjects are not sustained long enough to be discussed. In contrast, a majority of the subjects introduced by men become successful topics of conversation. Women are more likely to be interrupted during a conversation, and conversationalists are more likely to disagree with female speakers than with male speakers (Lynch, 1983).

Lakoff (1973) observed that women more commonly use polite forms, such as tag questions or requests, whereas men use more commands. Women are more likely to use polite speech forms such as *thank you* and *goodbye* (Greif & Gleason, 1980). Women tend to use more euphemisms and polite expletives such as *Oh dear!* or *My goodness!* Men, on the other hand, more commonly use swear words (basolect). Responses made with a rising intonation are often perceived as indicating characteristics thought of as feminine, such as lack of confidence, low aggressiveness, or susceptibility to influence. Lakoff (1973) proposed that these speech traits are linked to a particular sex because they signal either powerlessness or strength and anger. It may be that the powerful have no need to please.

It is also commonly believed that women talk much more and are more verbally fluent than men. However, this has not been substantiated in research. In fact, most studies have shown that men dominate the frequency, duration, and fluency of talk time. In Western societies, the powerful tend to speak while those who lack power listen (Lynch, 1983).

Langellier and Natalle (1987) summarized

TABLE 5–1
Comparison of three dimensions of feminine and masculine communication patterns

Item	Feminine Pattern	Masculine Pattern
Conversation Patterns (Maltz & Borker, 1982)	1. Create and maintain relationships of closeness and equality.	1. Assert a position of dominance.
	2. Criticize others in acceptable ways.	2. Attract and maintain an audience.
	3. Interpret accurately the speech of others.	3. Assert oneself when other speakers have the floor.
	4. Ask questions.	4. Make declarations.
	5. Facilitate.	5 Control.
	6. Use positive minimal response.	6. Tend to ignore other speakers.
	7. Use silent protest after an interruption.	7. Tend to interrupt more.
	8. Use *you* and *we* more.	8. Tend to challenge and dispute.
	9. Interpret minimal responses (*yes* and *mm-hmmm*) as indications that the other person is listening.	9. Interpret minimal responses as agreement with what the speaker is saying.
	10. View questions as part of conversational maintenance.	10. View questions primarily as requests for information.
	11. Tend to make explicit acknowledgement of previous comments and attempt to link to them.	11. Tend to ignore previous comments.
	12. Interpret verbal aggressiveness as personally directed, negative, and disruptive.	12. Interpret verbal aggressiveness as one conventional organizing structure for conversational flow.

studies of gender-related conversational patterns (Maltz & Borker, 1982), ethical styles (Gilligan, 1982), and forms of knowing (Belenky et al., 1986; Perry, 1970). Table 5-1 compares these three aspects of gender-differentiated communication in American society.

It is particularly important to be aware that during supervision conferences, head nodding may carry different messages for the sexes. Women tend to use head nodding as a supportive, nurturing function (Langellier & Natalle, 1987). Men, on the other hand, tend to nod with the intent to agree or confirm. Therefore, if a male supervisee interprets the female supervisor's head nodding as agreement or confirmation of his message, he may be very surprised

TABLE 5-1 *continued*

Item	Feminine Pattern	Masculine Pattern
	13. Tend to develop topics progressively and shift topics gradually.	13. Tend to define and develop topics narrowly, adhere to them until finished, and shift topics abruptly.
	14. Tend to discuss problems with one another, sharing experiences and offering reassurances.	14. Tend to view the discussion of a problem as an explicit request for solution. Respond by giving advice, acting as experts, lecturing their listeners.
Ethics (Gilligan, 1982)	*Ethic of Care:* 1. Weigh responsibility to self and others. 2. Show concern for relationships and the connection between people. 3. Communicate to solve problems.	*Ethic of Justice:* 1. Develop hierarchy of values. 2. Make impersonal judgments based on objectivity and fairness. 3. Work to protect individual rights.
*Forms of Knowing** (Belenky et al., 1986; Perry, 1970)	1. *Silence:* Women experience themselves as mindless, voiceless, and subject to the whims of external authority. 2. *Received knowledge:* Women think of	1. *Basic duality:* Men see the world in polarities: good/bad, right/wrong. Think of themselves as passive receptacles, depending on authority for knowledge. 2. *Multiplicity:* Men believe that author-

TABLE 5-1
continued

Item	Feminine Pattern	Masculine Pattern
	themselves as capable of receiving and reproducing knowledge from all-knowing external authorities but not of creating knowledge on their own.	ities are not necessarily right and everyone is entitled to an opinion.
	3. *Subjective knowledge*: Women think of truth and knowledge as personal, private, and subjectively known or intuited.	3. *Relativism subordinate*: Men believe that opinions need to be substantiated by evidence; take an objective, evaluative approach to the construction of knowledge.
	4. *Procedural knowledge*: Women invest energy in learn- and applying objective procedures for obtaining and communicating knowledge.	4. *Relativism*: Men realize that truth is relative and meaning depends on context; knowledge is constructed rather than given.
	5. *Constructed knowledge*: Women view knowledge as contextual, experience themselves as creators of knowledge, and value both subjective and objective strategies of knowing.	

*The lists in this section are developmental progressions.

when the supervisor responds with a negative verbal message. Awareness of genderlect can avert some of the miscommunication that may occur in supervision. The assumption is that if supervisor-supervisee gender communication patterns are congruent (masculine:masculine or feminine:feminine), a lower risk for miscommunication exists. Conversely, if the supervisor-supervisee patterns are incongruent (masculine:feminine or feminine:masculine), a higher risk of miscommunication exists. This assumption is irrespective of the sex of the supervisor or the supervisee. The concept of gender communication congruency emphasizes the importance of STYLE switching (similar to code switching in bilingualism) for supervisors.

COMMUNICATION COMPETENCE

TABLE 5-2
The effects of status and gender communication patterns on the risk for miscommunication between supervisors and supervisees

STYLE		Effect of Dominance Factor (DF)	Gender Communication Supervisor	Supervisee	Effect of Gender Congruence Factor (GCF)	Miscommunication Risk (MR)
I and II (Supervisor dominant)	1.	−	Masculine	Masculine	+	Medium Risk
	2.	−	Masculine	Feminine	−	High Risk
	3.	−	Feminine	Masculine	−	High Risk
	4.	−	Feminine	Feminine	+	Medium Risk
III and IV (Supervisor-supervisee equality)	5.	+	Masculine	Masculine	+	Low Risk
	6.	+	Masculine	Feminine	−	Medium Risk
	7.	+	Feminine	Masculine	−	Medium Risk
	8.	+	Feminine	Feminine	+	Low Risk

Code: + = positive effect on supervisor-supervisee communication
− = negative effect on supervisor-supervisee communication
DF + GCF = MR

As more studies show a definite difference in the communication patterns of men and women, the question arises whether other factors create possibilities of miscommunication between supervisors and supervisees. In a supervisor-supervisee relationship, status (dominant-subordinant) is a communication issue. Communication Disorders supervision STYLES I and II emphasize the dominance of the supervisor. STYLES III and IV assume a balance of status. Table 5-2 shows the possibilities for miscommunication between supervisors and supervisees when the elements of gender communication and status are both considered. As is evident from the table, two conditions (2 and 3) show high risk for miscommunication, four conditions (1, 4, 6, and 7) show medium risk, and two conditions (5 and 8) show low risk. The table emphasizes the variability of supervision communication from yet another vantage point.

Gender and its relation to communication remains an issue with which a majority of members of a female-dominated profession must contend, especially when operating in the Professional, Research, Educational, and Administrative domains of Communication Disorders supervision.

Question Types

Questions are interrogative expressions used most often in supervision to test knowledge and elicit information. It has been well documented that supervisors ask a preponderance of the questions when talking with supervisees (Blumberg, 1974; Roberts & Smith, 1982). Therefore, a detailed discussion of questioning is important.

Cunningham (1971) developed a useful classification system of question types.

Narrow or Closed-Ended Questions. These are questions that require low-level thinking, short factual answers, or other predictable responses including *yes* or *no*. The answers to narrow questions are predictable because they are specific, allowing for only a very limited number of acceptable answers. Their purpose is to collect information, to verify ideas and understanding of material, to understand materials, or to review previously studied material; they are used to identify, group, and note relationships.

a. Cognitive-Memory (C-M) questions. This kind of question calls for answers that reproduce facts, definitions, or other remembered information. When people respond to C-M questions, they may recall facts, define terms, identify things they have observed, or give answers they have learned by rote.

Examples:

Professional: What does CUSPSPA stand for?
Research: What is an interaction analysis tool?
Educational: What are the five communication disorders supervisor roles?
Administrative: What is the PPE?
Clinical: What is a clinical skill?

b. Convergent questions. Convergent questions are also narrow because they usually have one best or right answer, but they are broader than C-M questions because they require the person answering the question to put facts together and construct an answer. To respond to a convergent question, one is expected to explain, state relationships, associate and relate, or compare and contrast. The cue words (*how* and *why*) suggest explaining and are used often in convergent questions.

Examples:

Professional: How are CUSPSPA and ASHA related?
Research: What are the similarities between the Underwood Analysis System and the Blumberg Analysis System?
Educational: How do the five Communication Disorders supervision roles overlap?
Administrative: How can the C-BAM and the PPE be used together?
Clinical: Why has the concept of clinical skill versus clinical disposition become important?

Broad or Open-Ended Questions. These questions permit a variety of acceptable responses. They are not predictable and are designed to be thought-provoking. They call on the person responding to hypothesize, predict, or infer, and sometimes to express opinion, judgment, or feeling. Broad questions are not intended to elicit the one best answer; they are used to motivate people to explore a subject more deeply or to experiment. They may prompt new insights, ideals, appreciations, or desirable attitudes. They may be used to stimulate and guide interest in a new learning experience or problem-managing situation.

a. Divergent questions. A divergent question asks the respondent to organize elements into new patterns that were not clearly recognized before. In responding to divergent questions a person may perform the operations of predicting, hypothesizing, or inferring. Divergent questions encourage creative and imaginative responses.

Examples:

Professional: What are the advantages for your staff of belonging to CUSPSPA?
Research: How would you use an interaction analysis tool for research?
Educational: What are some good ways to prepare a supervisor for the five roles of Communication Disorders supervision?
Administrative: How would you introduce a new program concept to your staff?
Clinical: Define clinical competence in relation to clinical skills and clinical dispositions.

b. Evaluative questions. An evaluative question requires the respondent to judge, value, justify a choice, or defend a position. It is the highest level of questioning and involves all three of the other levels. An evaluative question causes respondents to organize their knowledge, formulate opinions, and take self-selected positions. To make judgments, they must use evidence. People judge what is good or bad, right or wrong, by applying learned standards. Because they can be either broad or narrow, evaluative questions are sometimes difficult to classify.

Examples:

Professional: What is your opinion of CUSPSPA?

Research: Which interaction analysis tool do you think is most useful?

Educational: Should all Communication Disorders programs have a supervision preparation component?

Administrative: How do you feel about using the PPE to plan for a supervision training program?

Clinical: Do you feel that clinical dispositions can be trained?

Studies of supervisors' communication behavior (Roberts & Smith, 1982) have shown that supervisors tend to ask primarily narrow or closed questions, which tend to reduce the amount and quality of the partners' responses. Concerns here are (a) the frequency with which supervisors ask questions, (b) the purposes for asking questions, (c) the types of question forms that are used, (d) the precision with which questions are asked, and (e) the alternative strategies.

It is not effective to try only to reduce the frequency with which questions are asked unless supervisors have alternative communication strategies to use. One possibility is to substitute statements that carry the request in a different form. For example, rather than asking, "What happened in therapy today?" a supervisor could say instead, "Tell me about today's therapy session." Changing grammatical forms is one way to decrease the frequency of questions but still be able to request necessary information. When questions are used they should be of various types, and they should be syntactically precise. According to Cunningham (1971), the four major problems with question phrasing are

1. A preponderance of narrow *yes* or *no* questions. (*Example*: "Should all Communication Disorders supervisors go through preparation programs?")
2. Ambiguous questions. (*Example*: "What about preparation in the supervision process?")
3. Spoon-feeding questions. (*Example*: "What is the acronym for Program Planning Evaluation?")
4. Confusing questions. (*Example*: What causes, or where could it be caused, more or less the traditional idea of supervision?)

For effective questioning, use the following strategies:

1. Have a purpose for requesting information. The purpose can guide the way the request is formed. For example, if the purpose of a question is to acquire correct or accurate information, a C-M question is appropriate; if organization of data is the purpose, then convergent questions can work best; analysis of reasons behind an action, evaluation of the quality of a relationship or of a conclusion, or divergent thinking require the explanatory, synthesizing/summarizing, judgmental, open-ended question forms (Frankel, 1973).
2. Ask fewer questions, with more balance between broad and narrow questions, direct questions and statements ("Tell me about . . ."); use sufficient pause time.
3. Create a better balance in group participation by calling on both willing volunteers and nonvolunteers and by using questions that both permit and encourage several people to respond.
4. Improve responses by using verbal prompts or follow-up questions that cause the respondent to correct, clarify, or extend the original answer.

Humor

Humor is a language function that includes cognitive, linguistic, and social dimensions of communication. It has a number of uses in supervision, including establishing rapport and developing camaraderie or social bonds; creating a relaxed atmosphere and decreasing anxiety or overcoming a stiff, formal style; encouraging communication on sensitive matters; furnishing insight into conflict or helping to diffuse conflicts;

stimulating problem solving, productivity, ingenuity, and creativity; improving job satisfaction and preventing burnout; and serving diagnostically and therapeutically in clinical situations. Application of humor to supervision requires unique communication skills that supervisors can develop as part of their overall communication competence.

The foregoing sections have dealt with 19 concepts that are important for supervisors to know and apply to different kinds of communication situations. Communication situations are classified into nine categories: intrapersonal, interpersonal, small-group, organizational, professional communication, interviewing, conferences, nontraditional communication, and conflict.

COMMUNICATION CATEGORIES

Intrapersonal Communication

Much of communication literature assumes that intrapersonal communication provides the base for communication behavior in interpersonal and person-to-group situations. Yarbrough (1981) states that it is difficult to know others without knowing oneself and that the way to know oneself is by identifying and acknowledging internal selves, or subpersonalities, that form a holistic community of identities in communication with each other (the theory of psychosynthesis). These subpersonalities make up what are also referred to as personal constructs, attitudes, beliefs, values, and biases. Knowledge and skill in intrapersonal communication is a basic building block for supervisors. (See chapter 2 for discussion of personal belief systems.) Eventually that knowledge and skill is applied to communication partners.

Interpersonal Communication

Interpersonal events are affected by intrapersonal ones and vice versa. Interpersonal communication is how people relate to one another in dyadic communication situations and in small groups. Both the encoder and decoder participate actively in formulating, perceiving, and negotiating codes to ascertain not only essential meaning but how meaning can be effectively conveyed. These communication transactions can often be described using the communication model of conversation, based on the conversational postulates of Grice (1975).

The anatomy of a conversation includes the following parts. The conversational partners (a) listen and talk, taking turns; (b) introduce a topic to talk about; (c) comment on what the other person has said; (d) do not change the topic of conversation until the other person has finished or permission has been granted to change the topic; (e) say what is thought to be true; (f) do not say more than needs to be said to have the listener understand; (g) attempt to make meanings understood; (h) request clarification if the partner's information is not understood; (i) acknowledge, respond to, and use nonverbal as well as verbal messages; (j) always learn something that was not known before; and (k) develop a conversational synchrony by waiting for each other to respond (Farmer, 1985).

The outcomes of interpersonal communication are largely affective, related to how the supervisor and a partner (or partners) feel about themselves and each other as a result of the communication event. Attention is focused on how relationships are initiated, nurtured, and maintained.

John Searle (Searle et al., 1980) wrote about sincerity and meaning in successful communication, and those two elements form the basis other authors use to explore the verbal and nonverbal dimensions of interpersonal communication. Most of the research has investigated verbal communication; however, more researchers are beginning to consider the nonverbal aspects. Recently, promising research on the combination of verbal and nonverbal dimensions of communication has begun to appear in the literature (Farmer, 1984a).

Berger and Calabrese (1980) discussed the *en-*

try phase of communication interactions and described the interactants' primary concern as reducing uncertainty or increasing the predictability of their behavior. In the report, the authors surveyed research on initial interactions and found that

1. Uncertainty decreases the amount of both verbal and nonverbal communication, the development of intimacy, and the rate of reciprocity while increasing the amount of dislike.
2. Similarities between persons reduce uncertainty; reduced uncertainty increases verbal and nonverbal communication, the level of intimacy, the rate of reciprocity, and the amount of liking.

Klevans and Volz (1976) and Mercer and Schubert (1974) placed importance on clinicians' nonverbal behavior. Mercer and Schubert found that differentiation of trainees into high (good) and low (poor) groups was paralleled by differences in nonverbal behaviors. Clinicians who were rated high by supervisors were those who used significantly more nonverbal behaviors that served as social reinforcers and signals (e.g., smiles, gazes, and positive head nods). Low-rated trainees, however, were found to use more distracting and self-manipulating behaviors.

Research has taught us much about the efficacy of various interpersonal communication styles, and the styles that reflect an integrative approach (those that address the cognitive, linguistic, social, pragmatic, and conversational components of language) appear to be efficacious in establishing and maintaining relationships. One such integrative model is Weiss's INter-REActive Learning (INREAL) model (Farmer, 1984a; Weiss, 1983). INREAL explicates the psycholinguistic strategies of Reactive Language, which include Reaction Time Latency, S.O.U.L, Mirroring, Self Talk, Parallel Talk, Verbal Monitoring and Reflecting, Expansion, and Modeling, and the positive effects of their use in changing communication and learning behavior. Weiss contrasts Reactive Language with Instructive Language and says that, although teaching and learning can occur with either strategy, the intent of Reactive Language is to *converse* or *interact*, with an emphasis on the *people* who are interacting, while the intent of Instructive Language is to *teach* or *test*, with an emphasis on the *information* being exchanged between the interactants. Thus, Reactive Language is empathic, person-centered, naturally conversational, and based on pragmatic principles. The interactants form a cooperative partnership in which growth is facilitated because learning is co-occurring and not unidirectional. INREAL has been applied to Communication Disorders supervision by Farmer (1984a, 1984b, 1984d). The strategies of Reaction Time Latency, S.O.U.L., Monitoring and Reflecting, and Expansion and Modeling were discussed earlier in this chapter, in the section on listening (see pp. 98–101). The other Reactive Language strategies include the following:

1. *Mirroring.* The primary method of nonverbal mirroring is direct matching of proxemics, kinesics (see p. 97), facial expressions, and gaze. When supervisors mirror, they purposefully imitate the head orientation, head movement, gaze, facial expressions, body orientation, trunk/torso movement, arm/hand positions, arm/hand movements, leg/foot positions, and leg/foot movements of their supervisees. A supervisor can mirror these movements and positions as they occur; this is termed *immediate mirroring*. The supervisor can also use the same behaviors a bit later; this is *delayed mirroring*. Both strategies help encourage interactions, establish turn taking, and create joint reference. Nonverbal synchrony is a well-documented phenomenon of genuine conversation. However, learning to use the mirroring strategy both intentionally and naturally can be difficult.

    a. Semantic example:

    Supervisee indicates that the therapy session went "O.K." (using the emblem, thumb and index finger forming a circle).

    Supervisor reproduces the emblem gesture.

b. Cognitive example:

Supervisee draws in the air (an illustrator) how her client produced (in reverse fashion) the letter *B*.

Supervisor reproduces the illustrator gesture.

c. Affective example:

Clinician nervously manipulates the pencil in his hand while he discusses a topic of sensitive nature to him.

Supervisor mirrors the nervous pencil movements.

2. *Self Talk*. The supervisor describes his or her actions, involvement, thoughts, or feelings about some aspect of the conversational topic. This strategy is a way of demonstrating topic/comment relationships in context. The supervisor links the self talk to what prompted it by matching the partner's Primary Representational System lexicon (see p. 117).

a. Semantic example:

SUPERVISEE: I just don't *see* another way to approach Craig's behavior problem. It's *clear* to me that he's just a spoiled brat!

SUPERVISOR: You have *painted* a *vivid picture* of your dilemma. I can understand why you *see* Craig as a spoiled brat. Can you *visualize* a way to approach the problem through Craig's mom? (*supervisor matches the supervisee's visual representational system*)

or

SUPERVISOR: I *hear* you. You're coming through *loud* and clear. I understand how frustrated you must *feel* by not being able to *tune* in to Craig's behavior problem. I guess he's just *marching* to the *beat* of a different drummer. (*Supervisor mismatches the supervisee's visual representational system by using both auditory and haptic representational systems in response.*)

b. Cognitive example:

SUPERVISEE: I guess I don't understand what he means by a "phonological disorder."

SUPERVISOR: Hmmmm, me either.

c. Affective example:

SUPERVISEE: I was so *nervous* during my first evaluation that I was shaking.

SUPERVISOR: I remember that *feeling*, too... and that was many years ago. (*haptic PRS used to match supervisee's*)

3. *Parallel Talk*. This strategy is used when the supervisor describes the partner's actions in a past or present experience. This strategy can be used to comment on the partner's involvement or to identify, clarify, or reinforce some aspect of the experience.

a 1. Semantic example (past):

In a recent therapy session, the supervisee sat on the right side of a stroke patient who exhibited right hemianopsia.

SUPERVISOR: In last Tuesday's session with Mr. Misner, you were side by side at the table and you were sitting on his right side.

a 2. Semantic example (present):

The supervisee has just explained how she was recording data in her client's fluency therapy.

SUPERVISOR: That system reflects detailed organization on your part and should provide us with the kind of information you just indicated was necessary to help Joe change his communication patterns.

b 1. Cognitive example (past):

The supervisee has written a description of

her client's behavior when he fell off his chair during therapy.

SUPERVISOR: The concrete examples you wrote down about Jeremy's eye movements, breathing, color, and facial expressions suggest petit mal seizures.

b 2. Cognitive example (present):

SUPERVISEE: Pepito sits like a frog, you know what I mean . . . with both legs out to the sides of his body.

SUPERVISOR: You just described an immature neurologic sitting pattern.

c 1. Affective example (past):

The supervisee laughed, clapped her hands, and bounced up and down when her 3-year-old hearing-impaired client said his first word in imitation.

SUPERVISOR: I remember how happy you were last January when Juan-Diego used the correct sign and said "ball" after he got his aid.

c 2. Affective example (present):

Having just completed her first communication evaluation, the supervisee is having a post-evaluation conference with her supervisor. She exhibits behaviors such as nervous laughing, frequent or rapid position changes, excessive paper shuffling, perspiring palms, and hesitant/dysfluent speech.

SUPERVISOR: I see you're anxious about our conference, and I bet you have butterflies in your stomach.

The antithesis of Reactive Language is Instructive Language. The consensus of the experts who write about Instructive Language (some use different terminology) is that it is less effective in developing or changing behavior, maintaining the behavior changes over time, or transferring behavior changes from one context to another (Cazden, 1979; Faber & Mazlish, 1980; Gazda, 1973; Ginott, 1965; Gordon, 1970, 1974; Spradlin & Siegel, 1982). Cazden's (1965) account of *school lesson* utterances defines the structure of Instructive Language that is predominant in academic settings: The teacher initiates, the student responds, the teacher evaluates. Instructive Language is characterized by suggestive or directive statements or questions intended to test or teach rather than to communicate.

Reactive Language is part of the broader concept of *pacing and leading*.

Pacing and Leading. Pacing and leading are terms used by Bandler and Grinder (1979) in their theory of Neurolinguistic Programming (NLP) to explain how an interactant can establish rapport with a partner through verbal and nonverbal communication and then lead the partner into some type of behavior change based on an understanding of the partner's world. (The terms *matching* and *modeling* are sometimes used in the literature as synonyms for *pacing* and *leading*.) Bandler and Grinder have written extensively on the techniques of NLP, especially in the verbal dimensions.

From linguistic analyses, Bandler and Grinder concluded that people use *representational systems*, or internal maps, to organize their individual realities. The maps are sensory (auditory, visual, haptic) and are, according to the authors, reflected in natural language and reflexive eye movements. The theory states that everyone specializes in one sensory system (the *Primary Representational System*, or PRS). By listening to the predicates a partner uses to describe an experience, the interactant can determine the PRS and then, by speaking the partner's "language," establish rapport quickly. Representational words such as (visual) *see, look, appears, show, focus, perspective, picture,* (auditory) *hear, sound(s), loud, ring, chime(s), resonate, listen,* (haptic) *feel, sense, gut reaction, grasp, handle, smooth, slow, move, ache* are examples of predicates that indicate PRS organization.

In the nonverbal dimension, Bandler and

Grinder suggest that reflexive eye movements also signal PRS orientation. For a right-handed person, visual and auditory *constructed* (imagined) images plus kinesthetic feelings (also smell and taste) are usually accessed by eye movements to the right; visual and auditory *remembered* images, plus phonological sounds or words, to the left. Farmer (1984a, 1984b, 1984d) and Carreras (1986) have applied the NLP theory of pacing and leading through PRS matching to the Communication Disorders supervision process.

The second verbal strategy that Bandler and Grinder have studied is their *metamodel*, based on transformational grammar theory. Transformational grammar is an explicit and complete model representing the structure of human language, which is itself a representation of the world of experience. According to the authors, meta-analysis provides a method of identifying, studying, and correcting surface and deep structure linguistic forms such as *deletions* (omissions of specific information important to the semantic truth value of the message); *lack of referential index* (failure to establish clear referents to which subsequent linguistic items refer, causing weak narrative cohesion); overuse of *unspecified verbs* (generic predicate forms such as *screwed up* instead of predicates that specify and delineate); *nominalizations* (which deny another person's perceptions and therefore enforce a personal view of the world); and *universal quantifiers* (assignments of characteristics to "everyone" or "no one," "everything" or "nothing," rather than to a specific person or thing to which the characteristic aptly refers). By identifying these grammatical forms, a supervisor can understand and enter a supervisee's world to create behavior change more effectively and efficiently.

In addition to the importance of linguistics in the communication process of pacing and leading, the concept of *cohesion*, or *cohesive harmony* (Halliday & Hasan, 1976) is also germane. Cohesive analysis explains why a text or conversation is interpreted in a certain way, including why it is ambiguous whenever it is so. Cohesive analysis explains the nature of conversational inferences, the meanings that the hearer gets out of a statement without the speaker having apparently put them in: presuppositions from the culture, from the shared experience of the participants, and from the situation. Cohesion is the component of the semantic system that provides the linguistic means for the presuppositions.

The basic concept Halliday and Hasan employ in analyzing cohesions is the *tie*. A tie is complex because it includes not only the cohesive elements but also whatever they presuppose. A tie is best interpreted as a relation between these two components. Five types of cohesion are used in analyses: reference, substitution, ellipsis, conjunction, and lexical cohesion. Cohesion, like the metamodel, has its foundation in transformational grammar. It is a linguistic mode of pacing and leading that supervisors can use to analyze and then manipulate their own or others' behavior.

Other theories of linguistic pacing and leading have been developed. Blank, Rose, and Berlin (1978) stress the importance of matching perceptions in discourse and present a 4-point scale of discourse abstraction. They suggest strategies for making simpler or more complex responses in order to match another's world knowledge more accurately.

Pickering (1987) suggests that supervisors and supervisees use metaphor frequently during supervision conferences and that it is important for a supervisor to join the supervisee's world by matching the metaphorical images.

Nonverbal pacing and leading also exists. Kendon (1980) and his colleagues, in studying interactional synchrony, found that shared rhythmicity in movement was most conspicuous at the beginning and at the end of interactions. Kendon stated that when people leave an encounter with a feeling of discomfort, or a feeling that rapport was not established, it may be due to asynchronous interaction. A limited amount of research has been done on interactional synchrony since it was first described by

Condon and Ogston (1967). Kendon argued that to move physically with another is to show that one is with the other in attention and expectations. Coordination of movement in interactions may be a very important way for people to signal that they are open to one another.

Erickson and Shultz (1982) labeled asynchronous interaction as *interactional arhythmia:*

> We can call the disturbance of regular rhythm interaction *arhythmia*.... The identification of arhythmia as an interactional phenomenon suggests that what is disturbing ... may be not so much that communication signals stop and start intermittently, but that they do so in a temporally unpredictable way, making it difficult for others to coordinate joint action with the person .... (pp. 113–114)

From additional research, Erickson and Shultz (1982) found that the maintenance of a stable pattern of interactional rhythm in the verbal and nonverbal behavior of both speaker and listener seems to enable partners to predict strategically salient next moments of interaction; interactants do not seem to understand each other well when arhythmia occurs.

In addition to movement synchrony, LaFrance and Mayo (1978) investigated posture and vocal synchrony. Scheflen (1966) showed that people often imitate each other's postures and suggested that such imitation may indicate shared viewpoints.

LaFrance and Broadbent (1976) studied the amount of posture sharing between students and professors. The results supported Scheflen's (1966) ideas about shared viewpoints and also showed that posture-sharing preceded rapport establishment when examined over time.

LaFrance and Mayo (1978) concluded, in reviewing the concept of *vocal synchrony* or *vocal convergence*—synchrony in length of speech, frequency of interruptions, pause length, speech rate, and vocal loudness—that "you adapt to the other because you wish to communicate. You converge when you wish to be involved ... you not only react to but you respond with" (pp. 76–77).

Researchers also describe *congruence*, a correlate of pacing and leading. Long (1978) reported that if facial expressions conflict, or if facial expressions and verbal content are not congruent with each other, then communication is counterproductive—it is an obvious display of nonunderstanding—and interaction is stopped.

Tepper and Haase (1978) reported that a balance between verbal and nonverbal dimensions of communication is crucial for the impact of a message. They cited studies to demonstrate that high-quality verbal empathic messages and genuineness are undermined by incongruent and inconsistent nonverbal cues.

Buchheimer (1963) discussed *confluence*, a combination of the concepts of mutuality and convergence. Confluence, Buchheimer believes, is necessary for the development of empathy, an essential in establishing rapport. Farmer's study of confluence (1984a) explored nonparticipant observers' ratings of the effectiveness of four conditions of the same Communication Disorders supervision conference: (a) *verbal matching*, in which the supervisor used pacing and leading by matching the verbal dimensions of the supervisee's communication; (b) *nonverbal mirroring*, where the supervisor used pacing and leading to match the nonverbal dimensions of the supervisee's communication; (c) *confluence* (also referred to as *interpersonal communication pacing*, or ICP), defined as the supervisor's simultaneous use of verbal matching and nonverbal mirroring; and (d) *incongruity*, which meant no intentional pacing and leading of verbal or nonverbal elements of the supervisee's communication. Raters judged the use of confluence to be the most effective, followed by nonverbal mirroring, verbal matching, and incongruity. Farmer concluded that (a) both the verbal and nonverbal elements of communication must be studied in supervision, together as well as separately; (b) congruence between verbal and nonverbal elements increases the effectiveness of a supervisor's communication; (c) confluence, or matching in both verbal and nonverbal dimensions of communication, provides the most effective supervisor communication behavior.

Schmitt and Gibbs (1984) investigated efficacy data for interpersonal skills in Communication Disorders supervision. They surveyed more than 250 studies to identify those that defined and described specific interpersonal skills considered important in a helping relationship. They used three criteria to identify the skills as potentially justifiable for emphasis by supervisors (pp. 2–3):

1. Discussion of the skill in more than one reference in the literature.
2. Inclusion of the skill in more than one clinical competence analysis system in speech-language pathology.
3. Evidence of research documenting the efficacy of the skill, either in clinical skills improvement by supervisees, in client outcome, or both. Six of 31 skills met the criteria: empathizing, praising, giving directions, confronting, creating immediacy of relationship, and communicating respect.

Clearly, there is evidence to support the idea that interpersonal communication generally and pacing/leading specifically are effective strategies for establishing rapport, exchanging information, and learning. However, it has also been argued that we need more efficacy data from studies of interpersonal skills as applied to Communication Disorders supervision.

Like dyadic communication, small-group communication requires that supervisors know and use intra- and interpersonal skills.

Small-Group Communication

Groups are a significant component of the supervision process, both personally and professionally. In supervision, a group is defined as a collection of three or more supervisors and/or clinicians who join together to accomplish goals through communication. The complexity of communication increases exponentially as the number of group members increases. Whereas in a dyad only 2 kinds of interchanges are possible, a triad increases the possible source/receiver combinations to 9. One more person increases the figure to 28. If we double the group to only eight persons, the total possible communication interactions reach 1,056 (Whitman & Boase, 1983). Competence in small-group communication is imperative for supervisors.

All group interactions have three major ingredients: content, group members, and the process of interaction. *Content* is the subject matter of the group's communication—what the group is talking about. The *process* is what happens among the group members while the group is working. Some variables of the process are morale, feelings, tone, atmosphere, influence, participation, roles, styles of leadership, leadership struggles, conflict, competition, cooperation, and so forth. In most interactions, little attention is paid to process. Since interactions among group members are critical in group supervision, awareness of them can help supervisors (a) to become more effective leaders and participants themselves, and (b) to help other group members become better group leaders and participants.

Process analysis is the procedure for studying content and process. Looking at both the work and personal dimensions, we can say that groups develop through three phases. During Phase I, the work issues center on goals and priorities and the personal issues pertain to level of personal involvement and how much to involve others. During this phase, leaders use communication strategies to "break the ice" and get active participation by organizing and clarifying. During Phase II, control, power, and responsibility emerge as issues. Work concerns center on group member roles and responsibilities; personal concerns hinge on controlling and being controlled by others. Communication strategies such as active listening and negotiating are used to settle differences among group members; tact and diplomacy are important when managing emotions. In Phase III the group is most cohesive. Work issues involve follow-through, or getting things done, and follow-up, making sure they are done right. Personal issues have to do with supporting and being supported by others. Communication strategies in this phase include rewarding the work of group members and building team spirit. Throughout the life of a group, the interaction pattern will shift from phase to phase as part of the group growth pattern. Eventually a group will develop a personality, or *syntality,* that synthesizes the personalities of group members into an integrated pattern of performance.

In some settings members who have a long history of working together become more efficient in decision making but less critical, losing their dynamic syntality and developing what Janis (1972) has termed *groupthink.* When a group is suffering from groupthink, they are no longer thinking as individuals but as one agreeable unit. Such singleminded cohesiveness can generate poor solutions. Therefore, it may be important to rotate group membership so that "new blood" can stimulate the group's critical thinking.

Organizational Communication

Supervisors always work in organizational systems; thus, organizational communication is an important part of Communication Disorders supervision. According to Goldhaber (1983), communication in an organization is a process through which the members of the organization exchange messages in a dynamic, continuous manner. To study message exchanges, researchers consider language modality, intended receiver, method of diffusion, and purpose of flow. They focus on role relationships, direction of message flow, and serial nature of message flow. Both formal and informal messages travel downward, upward, or horizontally through the network.

Downward communication consists of oral and written messages that flow from upper level personnel (e.g., administrators) to lower level personnel (e.g., staff or students). Downward communication has five purposes: (a) to provide job or task descriptions; (b) to provide job rationale; (c) to specify procedures and practices; (d) to give feedback; (e) to communicate goals.

Upward communication includes oral and written messages that flow from lower level personnel to upper level personnel. Upward communication has four purposes: (a) to describe what personnel are doing in specific tasks; (b) to describe unsolved work problems; (c) to suggest improvements; (d) to communicate how personnel think and feel about jobs, associates, and the organization.

The exchange of oral and written messages among people at the same organizational level of authority (e.g., among administrators, among staff, or among students) is called *horizontal* communication and has four purposes: (a) to coordinate tasks; (b) to employ problem management strategies; (c) to share information; (d) to manage conflicts within the organization.

Goldhaber (1983) stated that *informal* messages are not rationally specified, but develop through accidents of spatial arrangement, personality, and ability. The term *grapevine* refers to the informal message network. Research on the grapevine has shown that it is fast and accurate, that it carries much information, and that it passes the information by cluster. However, a negative aspect of the grapevine is *rumor,* information communicated without secure standards of evidence. Supervisors, especially in the Professional and Administrator roles, must be competent in organizational communication, formal and informal.

Supervisors are often called upon to speak in public when fulfilling the Professional, Researcher, Educator, and Administrator roles. Public speaking requires professional communication competence.

Professional Communication

Professional communication, more commonly known as public speaking, is fundamentally a utilitarian art. Supervisors need to be trained speakers who can publicly explain clearly and with confidence an intricate process, offer a realistic solution for an immediate problem, increase understanding and knowledge about an idea or concept, rekindle faith, or strengthen courage in times of stress. Professional communication includes the skills of *planning* a topic for a specific audience, *developing* it (gathering information and organizing the content), and *presenting* the speech in formal or informal style, to inform, to persuade, or to entertain. Supervisors can develop professional communication skills through college or university classes, community public speaking clubs, or private consulting organizations that provide training workshops. Although professional communication is more structured and formal than the intimate forms of communication, the same needs for competent communication exist on a large public scale as exist for organizations, small groups, or dyads.

Interviewing

Interviewing is a form of planned dyadic communication designed to accomplish specific goals, and supervisors may participate as either interviewers or interviewees. Interviews have three advantages over written communication: they allow for (a) immediate, efficient feedback; (b) adequate topic development; and (c) impromptu topics. Interviews have many different purposes (e.g., news gathering, counseling, employment, and conferences); this section will focus on the employment interview.

The employment interview itself involves just the listening/talking and watching/moving channels of communication. However, the complete process of interviewing includes the reading/writing channels in the form of job applications, resumes, and correspondence and thus requires communication competence in several different areas.

The supervisor as interviewer must consider the following aspects of the interview process. Interviews are generally done face to face, or sometimes over the telephone. Telephone interviews may be less expensive to conduct, but they require different communication skills on the part of the interviewer and the interviewee. Because there is no visual feedback from nonverbal dimensions of communication (e.g., facial expressions, dress, mannerisms, kinesics, proxemics), the oral communication must be more precise to convey the information necessary to make judgments about employment. Telephone interviews for employment are generally considered, by both interviewers and interviewees, more difficult to execute, less efficient, and less effective than the face-to-face interviews. Emerick and Haynes (1986) present a checklist of interviewing competencies that includes orienting the interviewee; using engendering communication, efficient questioning, informing, recording, and active listening strategies; monitoring nonverbal communication; and closing and analyzing the interview. Supervisors can use the checklist to develop interviewing competence or conduct employment interviews as part of their Administrative role.

Even with guidelines, interviewing problems still occur. The most common interviewing problems include the following:

1. Not providing or obtaining adequate information to make an informed decision.
2. Poor communication competence, including inability to handle emotional situations, memory failures, class or culture differences, to articulate thoughts and listen productively.

When a supervisor is on the other side of the table, i.e., the interviewee seeking a supervision position, different skills are necessary. According to interviewing expert R. A. Fear (1958), employers look for people who demonstrate three qualities: (a) mental abilities (intelligence, education, and mental aptitude); (b) motivation (enthusiasm and commitment to the job); and (c) maturity (the ability to manage different work and social situations in a careful, competent, productive manner). The interviewer will use the interview to evaluate these three *M*s. In addition, the interviewee must communicate a favorable impression that the interviewer will remember. The resume will document qualifications, but verbal and nonverbal performance during the interview will be the key factor in an interviewer's decision. In fact, some research has suggested that interviewers make decisions about employment within the first 5 minutes of an interview (Webster, 1964). A study done by Brandt (1979) identified five characteristics as contributing to an interviewer's impressions of an interviewee's competence and attractiveness:

1. *Unique impression.* The most important aspect of the interview is to present a unique personal impression early on.
2. *Openness.* The second goal is to share personal experiences and ideas voluntarily and sincerely.
3. *Attentiveness.* Active listening is as important for the interviewee as it is for the interviewer.
4. *Animation.* Enthusiasm manifested in hand gestures, facial expressions, proxemics, and mutual gaze makes a lasting impression on interviewers.
5. *Relaxedness.* A relaxed demeanor, shown in body position and paralinguistics, gives the impression of competence and confidence.

A key to being a good interviewee is self-control. Many applicants have good credentials, so the final decision about employment is often based on the communication competence of the interviewees.

The need for communication competence encompasses the written parts of the interviewing process, including resumes, pre- and postinterview correspondence, and job descriptions or contracts. A resume is a brief account of educational and professional experience. An effective resume is often the entree to personal interviews. Therefore a resume must be detailed enough to allow an employer to assess an applicant's qualifications. At the same time, it must be concise. To accomplish both objectives requires skillful writing.

Although resumes are usually written documents, the video resume is gaining in popularity. Video resumes have their own difficulties, however. Applicants, to present themselves in the best possible way, must be visually literate (see chapter 6). They must be familiar with marketing techniques, and they must understand the legal issues video resumes raise (e.g., Who owns them? Is it legal to require one? Can editing distort reality?). Video resumes should never replace written resumes, but can be used to supplement them. Video resumes can help employers screen potential applicants before inviting them for interviews and thus can be a cost and time efficient way of selecting the best person for the position.

Pre- and postinterview correspondence includes letters of inquiry, cover letters, and letters of thanks after the interview. Each letter has an appropriate format, style, and content. Competence in writing these letters can be advantageous to applicants.

Written communication also includes the job description and contract that the interviewee will have reviewed. If no job description exists, it should be negotiated and written by the employer and employee together. Job descriptions and contracts need to have precise language. All told, supervisors must be able to produce and interpret many different forms of writing in connection with the interview.

Supervision Conferences

The supervision conference is the main event of the supervision process; as a communication forum, it has received a great deal of research attention. Farmer (1987a) viewed conferences as hexagons composed of the dimensions *who, what, when, where, how,* and *why.* (See chapter 9 for a complete discussion of this model.)

From his work in supervisor training, Sperloff (1953) stressed that the primary tool of a supervisor is the communication skill used during conferences and that intended meanings will not get through unless there is a common referent for supervisor and supervisee. He also noted that verbal communication and overt actions (non-verbal communication) must be congruous and compatible. Sperloff trained supervisors in conference communication by means of role-playing, in which the supervisor assumed the role of the supervisee in order to understand the supervisee's reference state.

Although several writers in education have described models of supervision (Blumberg, 1974; Cogan, 1973; Goldhammer, 1969; Mosher & Purpel, 1972; Weller, 1971) and provided data to describe events that occur during supervision conferences in education (Blumberg, 1974; Michalak, 1969; Weller, 1971), comparable information in Communication Disorders is limited. Communication Disorders has drawn from the disciplines of education, medicine, communication studies, and psychology to conduct research on various methods of educating and training professionals to manage the needs of persons with communication disorders.

Research on Communication Disorders supervision conferences has yielded the following information. Four studies (Culatta & Seltzer, 1976, 1977; Irwin, 1975; Schubert & Nelson, 1976) used interaction analysis systems to describe conference behavior in speech-language pathology. All four studies examined supervisor and supervisee talk during Communication Disorders conferences and found that supervisors talked 6% to 30% more than did supervisees. Irwin (1975) and Culatta and Seltzer (1976, 1977) also examined changes in behavior over time. Irwin found no change in the percentages of talking time between the first and the second supervision session, and Culatta and Seltzer (1976, 1977) found no change in any of the supervision behaviors they studied over a 12-week period. In addition, Culatta and Seltzer (1976) and Irwin (1975) indicated that experienced supervisors, in contrast to inexperienced supervisors, used similar conference communication behavior with both experienced and inexperienced supervisees.

Dowling (1983) investigated whether academic and clinical preparation influenced the supervision conference communication of supervisors and supervisees. She found that, with training, the supervisors in her study modified their conference talk in response to the individual supervisees and the supervisees participated more actively in the conferences.

To improve research validity and reliability and to code behavior multidimensionally, Smith (1978) studied the content of supervision conferences using the Weller (1971) M.O.S.A.I.C.S. system. She found that Communication Disorders supervisors assumed a dominant role in the conferences through their initiating behaviors. Observer-judge perceptions of taped conferences indicated that when the supervisors' conference communication behavior was perceived as direct (authoritative), there were fewer total utterances, fewer utterances by supervisees, and less discussion in the affective domain. When the supervisors' conference communication behavior was perceived as indirect (non-authoritative), supervisors made more reflexive (reacting, responding) moves and there was more discussion in the affective domain.

Roberts (1979) performed a post hoc analysis of the Smith (1978) data and reported that supervisors set the content and interaction pattern for conferences and directed the dialogue. They focused on prescribing what supervisees should and should not do and on giving opinions and suggestions for future sessions; these patterns did not change over time. Roberts' study indicates that the verbal interactions of supervisors and supervisees, as a group, were not congruent with the clinical supervision model (Cogan, 1973) or with Communication Disorders supervision STYLE IV.

Pickering (1979) used a descriptive-qualitative approach and methodology to examine interpersonal communication in supervision conferences. She reported that supervisors frequently failed to attend to the students' feelings as expressed during conferences and that, in supervisors' journals, collaboration between supervisor and supervisee was often an issue.

Brasseur (1981) studied the direct and indirect

communication behaviors used by supervisors in conferences. Her subjects observed videotapes made from prepared scripts. Supervisor, graduate student, and undergraduate subjects perceived differences between direct and indirect supervision behaviors in the taped conferences. Sbaschnig, Sziraki, and Matecum (1986) found that observers preferred the indirect conferences over the direct.

Results from research by McCrea (1980) corroborated the finding of Pickering (1979) that supervisors showed underdeveloped interpersonal communication skills. McCrea also discovered that clients, not supervisees, were the main topic of supervision conferences and that the sessions usually did not include discussion of supervisee clinical behavior.

Casey (1980) and Underwood (1979) reported research that confirmed the 5-minute unit as being a representative sample of Communication Disorders supervision conferences. Casey also reported that the first 5 minutes adequately represented the communication patterns of the entire interaction. Therefore, the 5-minute *entry phase* of conferences appears to be a valid segment of conference time to use for analysis.

Farmer (1984a) also chose to study the entry phase, based in part on the work of Berger and Calabrese (1980), which showed that the first 5 minutes of an interaction are crucial for developing the dynamics of the rest of the encounter. Interpersonal Communication Pacing (ICP), described by Farmer, appears to be an effective strategy for reducing uncertainty and increasing predictability, the two variables Berger and Calabrese describe as the interactants' primary concerns in interpersonal encounters (see pp. 114–115).

Cumpata and Johnson (1983) examined student perceptions of group and individual Communication Disorders supervision conferences and found the following:

1. Supervisees across experience levels expressed more positive reactions to the group conference format than to the individual. However, subjects also tended to state a preference for the form they were involved with at the time. They believed the group conferences helped develop clinical and personal competence. Group conference participants believed that they had an opportunity to elicit others' opinions and suggestions and provide input themselves.
2. Less experienced supervisees wanted more guidance and direction than the more experienced supervisees did. More experienced supervisees responded negatively to the idea of having just one supervisor for all their clients in a particular setting.

To ensure successful conferences, supervisors need to plan *why* a conference is being held, *who* should attend, *what* will be discussed, *how* the conference will be conducted (i.e., in what supervision STYLE), *when* and *where* the conference will transpire. The *Advance Planner/Organizer* (Farmer, 1987a), is a helpful tool in planning conferences. The AP/O is used to organize conferences efficiently by grouping supervisees according to their readiness states, by the *kind* of conferences (planning, monitoring, managing, evaluating), the *purpose* (e.g., to establish goals and objectives, to plan an observation, to discuss clinician skills), the *form* (dyad or group), the *STYLE, duration, day, time,* or *place* of conferences. In addition, supervisors can implement the guidelines for conferences presented in Table 5–3.

Both supervisors and supervisees spend large amounts of time in conferences. Therefore, supervisors should conduct conferences effectively and efficiently using competent conference communication.

Nontraditional and conflict communication are areas of supervision that present special problems.

Nontraditional Communication

Three types of nontraditional communication deserve discussion as they relate to supervision:

TABLE 5-3
Guidelines for Communication Disorders supervision conferences

Before the conference
1. Identify the purposes for the conference (e.g., reporting, information sharing, problem management).
2. Announce the purpose and format of the conference in advance; inform group member(s) of what they should bring and be prepared to do.
3. Involve group member(s) in planning the conference (optional).
4. Set a time for the conference that is convenient for all.
5. Find a comfortable, relaxing, quiet place for the conference.
6. Invite all necessary people.
7. Send out notices of the meeting with return slips (optional).
8. Follow up on member(s) who do not return slips.
9. Prepare an agenda (optional).
10. Review records, data, notes.
11. Prepare specific materials (e.g., observation notes, clinical materials).

During the conference
12. Start the meeting on time.
13. Establish the ground rules early (regarding smoking, confidentiality, etc.).
14. Be friendly; establish a positive atmosphere.
15. Be flexible about following the agenda, if there is one.
16. Ask group member(s) about the specific client, program, problem, etc.
17. Make positive comments; talk about strengths as well as problems.
18. Be specific about the problems presented.
19. Vary conference activities (use videotape, discussion, role-playing, etc.)
20. Use language that group member(s) can understand.
21. Provide opportunities for group member(s) to speak as well as listen; be a good listener.
22. Work cooperatively with group member(s) on specific activities, tasks, ways of managing problems; clearly identify responsibilities.
23. Summarize the meeting; make sure supervisor and group member(s) are clear about the next steps.
24. Allow some time for informal interaction.

After the conference
25. Make a brief record of the content of the meeting.
26. Plan for follow-up.

(a) the communication patterns of different or varied linguistic systems (other than standard American English); (b) the communication patterns of minority language, multicultural populations; and (c) the communication patterns of lifelong (continuing education) learners.

Nonstandard American English. Nonstandard American English includes local and regional dialects not associated with any specific cultural or ethnic groups. These patterns are often referred to as *accents*. The southern drawl, the midwest twang, and the Boston /r/ are examples of dialectal patterns. Both speakers and listeners must make acoustic and phonologic adjustments if dialects interfere with communication.

Minority Language, Multicultural Communication. The American Speech-Language-Hearing Association has increased its efforts to address the issue of supervision in communication disorders in minority language users and multicultural contexts. Its Bilingual Language Learning System (BLLS) project produced the following statement (ASHA, 1982):

> Bilingual students need to be supervised by bilingual speech-language pathologists or audiologists in order to insure comprehensive assessments and to maximize the students' learning as future professionals. Bilingual supervisors are preferable to monolingual supervisors because they can more fully comprehend the assessment process and can provide insight and input into the total evaluation procedures. Feedback from the bilingual supervisors is critical, for once the students graduate, they frequently are the only bilingual-bicultural speech-language pathologists or audiologists within their work settings and communities. The bilingual students must demand from the bilingual-bicultural supervisors maximum supervision and academic guidance to insure breadth of knowledge and mastery of skill in effectively managing the minority-speaking speech-language and hearing disordered population. (p. 10)

With the dearth of bilingual-bicultural speech-language pathologists and audiologists in the profession, it is reasonable to assume that bilingual clinicians will rarely be supervised by a bilingual-bicultural supervisor, especially one who has been prepared in the supervision process. However, if supervision is provided by a monolingual English-speaking supervisor, will supervision management decisions be markedly different? If so, in what domains will they differ? To explore these questions, Farmer (1984c) conducted the only study to date in minority language supervision. Data analysis showed no statistically significant differences in how the bilingual and monolingual supervisors judged the clinicians' or the clients' behavior, or in the types of supervision process decisions they made. Individual supervisor judgments also showed no statistically significant differences. But the results should not be interpreted in a simplistic manner. All four supervisors were natives or longtime residents of multicultural Southwestern communities. They had prepared for supervision in a program that emphasizes critical observation of and competence in utilizing verbal and nonverbal communication (in English) during supervision. What may be more important than minority linguistic proficiency for supervisors in multicultural supervision is a sensitivity to the cognitive and social components of contextually based interactional communication. The study also strongly confirmed that conferences are a critical element in management decisions for Communication Disorders supervisors. In the conferences, supervisors, by communicating competently with minority language supervisees, can gain additional information that will help them plan and execute effective language intervention programs for minority language, multicultural clients who are communicatively handicapped. In short, when addressing the issue of minority language supervision in Communication Disorders, a monolingual English-speaking supervisor must have a minority language and multicultural sensitivity, as well as the ability to communicate with minority language, multicultural supervisees.

Lifelong Learners' Communication. With changing demographics in the United States, institutions of higher education and employment settings are adapting their educational and employment practices to meet the needs of older, nontraditional students. Some of these students have degrees and enter college for another; others are working toward their first degree. Some of these lifelong learners will enter the workforce as speech-language pathologists and audiologists. This fact is important to Communication Disorders supervisors because the communication and learning patterns of older nontraditional learners are different from those of younger college students and employees. Michalak and Yager (1979) define adult learning, or *andragogy* (Knowles, 1973) as "a learning process in which both the student and the teacher assume responsibility for what, when, how, and to whom information is taught" (p. 74). (Characteristics of andragogy were presented in chapter 2.)

Andragogy depends on supervisors using supervision STYLES III and IV, unlike *pedagogy*, which aligns with STYLES I and II. Much of the classroom and conference communication behavior in Communication Disorders training programs and subsequent worksites takes the form of pedagogy, which may not meet the needs of lifelong learners.

Conflict often occurs in interpersonal interactions, and its analysis combines all the previous communication concepts and categories. As a way of applying theoretical information, the next section will discuss conflict communication.

Conflict Communication

Wilmot and Wilmot (1978) define conflict as an "expressed struggle between at least two interdependent parties, who perceive incompatible goals, scarce rewards, and interference from the other party in achieving their goals" (p. 9). Conflict is viewed not as inherently evil but as an occurrence that must be managed carefully, creatively, and constructively. It is through *conflict communication* that conflicts are recognized, expressed, experienced, and managed. The supervisor, with a substantial background in communication theory, a repertoire of verbal and nonverbal communication strategies, and the skills to employ those strategies, can learn to "do" conflict in a manner that is productive, rather than destructive, for all parties.

Conflicts are inevitable and significant dimensions of human relationships. Everyone experiences conflicts, and every encounter brings the potential for conflict (Stewart, 1982). Ironically, it is a basic societal assumption that conflicts are abnormal, unnatural, wrong, or bad. As a result, many individuals fear conflicts and believe that they should be prevented. This belief prevails primarily because many conflicts result in damage either to relationships or to the work in hand, or both. Conflict is not inherently detrimental and may be productive. Thus, since conflict cannot be prevented, people need to learn to *manage* conflicts in productive rather than destructive ways. Productive conflict management, as defined by Katz and Lawyer (1983), is "a process of diagnosing a conflict situation and engaging the appropriate problem-solving approach to generate a solution that satisfies the interests of all parties involved" (p. 32).

By its nature, conflict is an active process; therefore, we describe interactants' behavior from the perspective of their "doing conflict." Conflicts can involve supervisors in all five roles and with all types of interactants, including clients/patients, students, colleagues, parents, families, significant others, primary caregivers, and administrators.

Although both supervisor and supervisee must be skilled in conflict management for productive conflicts to emerge, generally the supervisors must develop and then help the supervisees develop the required attitudes and skills.

The study of conflicts has shown that they need not be destructive; other basic principles of conflict management include the following:

1. Conflicts and disagreements are not the same.
2. Harmony and conflict are both normal conditions of being; conflict is not pathological nor the result of "personality problems."
3. Conflicts do not need to be "resolved"; they should be "managed" in a constructive manner.
4. Conflicts are ongoing rather than episodic.
5. Conflicts are not nebulous, ambiguous phenomena; they have definite structures, goals, systems, strategies, tactics, styles, and power types.
6. Conflicts have both a content and a relational level. Many conflicts are identified as goal-centered when in fact they are relationship-centered.
7. Individuals have a predominant *conflict style* that they use when engaged in conflict.
8. In general, children and adults are not taught alternative strategies to manage conflict productively (e.g., to maintain, reduce, or esca-

late it) but instead are encouraged to resolve or avoid conflict.
9. If information about conflict is presented in a work system, the information is usually addressed only to managers or supervisors, not the low power people.
10. In general, males are expected to "do conflict" differently from females; certain conflict management strategies are acceptable for males but not for females and vice versa.
11. Same-sex interactants generally use different conflict tactics from opposite-sex interactants.
12. Same-age interactants generally use different conflict tactics from different-age interactants.
13. Same-status interactants generally use different conflict tactics from different-status interactants.
14. Conflict is done differently intra- and interculturally.
15. Humans are naturally biased; that is, they have preferences based on neurologic perceptions and contextual experiences.
16. Because of the complexity of communication in general, and within conflict specifically, communication variables other than amount of talk play major roles in conflict management. It is imperative, then, that supervisors become skilled communicators.

Supervisors can learn productive conflict management by studying and analyzing various aspects of conflict such as intra- and interpersonal, verbal and nonverbal dimensions of communication; conflict styles; power; structure; goals; strategies and tactics; intervention; and education or training.

Intrapersonal conflicts, a supervisor's unclearly defined personal constructs, attitudes, beliefs, values, and biases, have a direct impact on interpersonal communication. As Yarbrough (1981) pointed out, the basic requirement for quality interpersonal communication is a substantial repertoire of communication strategy choices or responses. Increased choice assumes internal awareness; repressed or ignored intrapersonal conflicts decrease the supervisor's awareness of self and partners. Mismanaged intrapersonal conflict not only decreases the chances for quality interpersonal communication between the supervisor and partner, it increases the chances for less productive interpersonal conflicts. Often this results in less satisfactory service to clients or patients. When supervisors do productive conflict, their communication behavior will fit Yarbough's (1981) description:

> The partners engage in supportive feedback, describing rather than evaluating behavior of the other, owning feelings and responses rather than blaming the other, being empathetic with the other's position; are aware of relational and content issues; and have a repertoire of styles with which to respond to the conflict. (p. 648)

Styles. Kilmann and Thomas (1975) described five characteristic approaches (conflict styles) used in interpersonal confrontations. The five styles relate to the interpersonal styles discussed by Knapp (1978b). The styles are based on a four-cell matrix of high and low assertiveness (concern for self) and cooperativeness (concern for other); the fifth style (compromise) holds a neutral, median position on the matrix (see Figure 5-1). The four cells of the Interpersonal Styles and Conflict Styles matrix correspond directly with the four cells of the Communication Disorders supervision STYLES matrix (see Figure 3-5, p. 63).

A supervisor who demonstrates the *competition/driver* attitude believes that someone must win and someone must lose in a conflict. Using this style, a supervisor exhibits strong concern for self (high assertiveness) and weak concern for the supervisee (low cooperation), as evident in verbal and nonverbal behaviors such as gesture and vocal emphasis, abrupt greetings and departures, domineering statements, impatience, high energy, frequent interruptions, blaming, asserting, confronting, and ordering. Supervisees tend to respond to the competition style with submission, nervousness, or rebellion.

FIGURE 5-1
Conflict styles and interpersonal styles matrix.

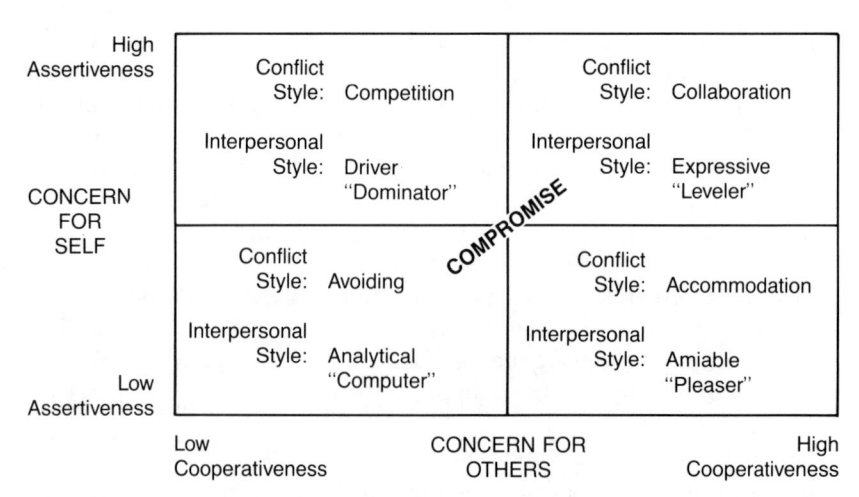

	Low Cooperativeness	High Cooperativeness
High Assertiveness (Concern for Self)	Conflict Style: Competition / Interpersonal Style: Driver "Dominator"	Conflict Style: Collaboration / Interpersonal Style: Expressive "Leveler"
Low Assertiveness	Conflict Style: Avoiding / Interpersonal Style: Analytical "Computer"	Conflict Style: Accommodation / Interpersonal Style: Amiable "Pleaser"

COMPROMISE lies at the center. Horizontal axis: CONCERN FOR OTHERS.

Adapted from "Interpersonal Conflict: Handling Behavior as Reflections of Jungian Personality Dimensions" by R. Kilman and K. Thomas, 1975, *Psychological Reports, 37,* pp. 971–980, and from *Social Intercourse: From Greeting to Goodbye,* by M. Knapp, 1978, Boston: Allyn & Bacon.

A supervisor who uses an *avoiding/analytical* style does not openly pursue personal concerns or those of the partner. The supervisor exhibits weak concern for self and weak concern for the supervisee, as evident in verbal and nonverbal behaviors such as brief greetings and departures, minimal use of voice, reserved responses, patience, low energy, silence, deliberation, requests for facts and details, technical orientation, equivocation, and indecision. Supervisees, when doing conflict with a supervisor who is employing this style, tend to respond with frustration and frequent attempts to elicit responses from the supervisor.

The *accommodation/amiable* style requires a supervisor to neglect or give up personal concern(s) in order to satisfy the concern(s) of the supervisee. When the accommodation style is used, a supervisor exhibits weak concern for self and strong concern for the supervisee, as evident in verbal and nonverbal behaviors such as animated, expansive greetings and protracted departures, frequent eye contact, sitting close, leaning forward, touching, infrequent interruptions, letting the supervisee talk, questioning, smiling, indecision, and concern about what the supervisee thinks of the supervisor. Supervisees tend to respond to the accommodation style with friendliness, talk, and dominance.

With a *compromise* style, both the supervisor and the supervisee neglect or give up their concern(s) and use statements such as "Not everyone can get his or her own way; you have to be satisfied with part of the pie."

When a supervisor uses the *collaboration/expressive* style, supervisor and supervisee together develop new solutions creatively through transactive communication in order to maximize goals for both. The supervisor who uses a collaboration style exhibits strong concern for self as well as strong concern for the supervisee, using verbal and nonverbal behavior such as gesture and vocal emphasis, responsive listening, balanced talking and listening, friendliness, asserting and questioning, direct body orientation, and frequent eye contact. Supervisees, when doing conflict with a supervisor who is employing the collaboration style, tend to respond with friendly sharing of ideas. Although this style affords maximum opportunities for productively managing conflicts, it is the most complex and difficult style to develop and use. Yarbrough

(1981) listed five steps to acquiring a successful collaboration style: awareness, acceptance, coordination, integration, and synthesis.

The rules of conflict management governing four of the styles (competition/driver, avoiding/analytical, accommodation/amiable, and compromise) are grounded in a win/lose structure. In intrapersonal conflict, the supervisor's subpersonalities are viewed as opposites; one subpersonality's gains are perceived as another's losses, and because of lack of trust among the subpersonalities, various means of control (e.g., suppression of subpersonalities) need to be devised. In interpersonal conflict, the supervisor and the supervisee are seen as opposites; one individual's gains are perceived as the other's losses, and again lack of trust leads to the use of control methods.

With the collaboration style, however, conflict changes from a win/lose to a win/win perspective. Intrapersonally, the goal of conflict changes from one subpersonality winning at the expense of other subpersonalities to integration and synthesis of the subpersonalities. At the interpersonal level, the goal of conflict is not the supervisor winning at the expense of the supervisee, but integration of the goals of both interactants into a constructive relationship that can produce positive interactions.

Although the collaboration conflict style has the greatest potential for productive conflict management, this is not to say that the other four styles should never be used. For example, the avoiding style may be appropriate when excessive change in the life of the supervisor or the supervisee makes it impossible to deal with every conflict. Supervisors should develop the flexibility to use and respond to different conflict styles and to employ the one(s) that will lead to productive management of any given confrontation.

Power. Duke (1976) believes that power is the core of conflict theory. Power is influence, and it is used in conflict to move interactions along to some kind of management. As Wilmot and Wilmot (1978) point out, power is not a thing that people have, but a product of the social relationship. Deutsch (1973) describes power in this way: "Power is a relational concept; it does not reside in the individual but rather in the relationship of the person to his environment. Thus the power of an agent in a given situation is determined by the characteristics of the situation" (p. 15). In order for supervisors to transact productive rather than destructive conflicts, they need to know about power and its bases. French and Raven (1960) discuss five types of power.

1. *Reward* power occurs when a supervisor is in a position to control the rewards a supervisee will attain; the supervisor has something of value that the supervisee wants. For example, the supervisor could have reward power over the supervisee because the supervisor could promote the supervisee or provide a merit pay raise.
2. *Coercive* power is the reverse of reward power. The supervisor has some form of punishment that can be leveled against the supervisee if the supervisee does not do what the supervisor wants. For example, the supervisor could have the coercive power of negative evaluation or grading if the supervisee does not follow the supervisor's instructions.
3. *Legitimate* power stems from the supervisor's position in a social system that the supervisee accepts. For example, a supervisee accepts a person as a Communication Disorders supervisor. The supervisor then has a legitimate power base.
4. *Referent* power arises when a supervisee identifies strongly with a supervisor. If a supervisor is highly admired by a supervisee because of superb supervision competence, then the supervisor has referent power.
5. *Expert* power occurs because an individual has some special knowledge or expertise that is useful to others. For example, if only one member of a supervision staff has education

and training in the supervision process, that person has an expert power base in clinical supervision staff meetings.

As conflict is defined by Wilmot and Wilmot (1978), the interdependency of the interactants presupposes that each has some base(s) of influence in the relationship. To manage conflict productively a supervisor needs to analyze the power of both parties. A basic tenet of productive conflict management is that conflict partners have a better chance of developing a constructive relationship if the power is distributed equitably. One-sided power relationships tend to lead to destructive conflict. It is a difficult task to equalize the power in a supervision relationship in order to have a more productive interaction. In some instances supervisors must relinquish some power base(s); in other cases they may need to point out sources of power that supervisees have available but are not using to advantage.

Power is at the heart of conflict, and it influences the choices that supervisors and supervisees make during conflict. Power is relational; it arises because supervisors and partners are interdependent and can mediate the goal attainments of each other. When supervisors become aware of power relations, they can balance the power bases in interactions and create new options for managing conflicts.

Structure. When a supervisor and a supervisee are involved in a communication transaction, the verbal and nonverbal actions of one influence the choices (responses) of the other. The choices of each party within a conflict, coupled with the rewards that follow those choices, are termed the *structure* of the conflict. Conflict structure is most often studied using two types of theories: game theories (Berne, 1964; Kadushin, 1968; Rapoport, 1970; Sleight, 1984) and Transactional Analysis (Harris, 1967).

One type of game theory is concerned with games of strategy where the best course of action depends on what one participant expects the other to do. In all types of strategic games, the rewards for playing depend on how well one player outwits the opponent; each strategy is a conditional choice, conditional on the choices made by the opponent (Rapoport, 1970). In a destructive supervision conflict, the supervisor intends to maximize his or her gains and minimize the losses, which results in a win/lose situation. Verbal and nonverbal communication moves or strategies can be plotted or calculated until the supervisor wins the conflict. Although strategic game theory has been used for conflict analysis, its most serious limitation for this purpose is that it often underrates or misrepresents communication as a transactive phenomenon. A truly communicative interaction cannot be predicted; it must grow from the uniqueness of each interactional context.

Berne (1964) discussed real-life games that people play and defined games as "on-going series of complementary ulterior transactions progressing toward a well-defined, predictable outcome" (p. 48). Kadushin (1968) discussed game-playing in supervision, and Sleight (1984) described game-playing specifically in Communication Disorders supervision. Again, truly communicative supervision interactions cannot be considered games.

A second way of looking at the structure of conflicts is the Transactional Analysis (TA) model (Harris, 1967). Transactional Analysis (I'm OK—You're OK) combines intra- and interpersonal communication theory. Behavior and attitudes in dyads, according to TA, are influenced by three personality ego states: the *Parent* ego (critical, prejudicial, advisory, nurturing); the *Child* ego (inadequate and powerless in a world of competent people); and the *Adult* ego (examining all the evidence of a given problem and utilizing the best powers of reasoning). All three ego states are operational in supervisors and supervisees and are identifiable in their verbal and nonverbal communication. Harris also outlines four possible *life positions:* I'm Not OK—You're OK, I'm Not OK—You're Not OK,

I'm OK—You're Not OK, and I'm OK—You're OK.

When supervisors and supervisees engage in conflict, the nonconstructive behavior of the Child is often apparent in one participant or the other or both, accompanied by an overt display of emotion. The supervisor may also display the Parent who knows what is right and wrong, thereby closing off viable alternatives. The Adult ego state, the one that reflects OK feelings about self and others, will consider the issues inherent in the conflict, attempt to reduce the negative feelings, and reflect on the past behavior that was instrumental in initiating the conflict. After examining all of the alternatives at both the content and the relationship levels, the Adult will then select and incorporate these new ways of thinking, feeling, and acting into his or her behavior. The new ideas, feelings, and behavior must then be tested in the conflict context to determine their efficacy in constructing a productive relationship.

When analyzing the TA structure in conflicts, supervisors can examine their own and the supervisee's operating ego states and life positions. To manage conflict productively within the supervision process, supervisors must be aware of the ego states and life positions that are operating and act accordingly.

The topic of goals often emerges as researchers analyze style, power, and structure in conflicts.

Goals and Issues. Realistic, well-negotiated goals allow for productive conflict management. Hawes and Smith (1973) discuss three types of goals: *prospective* goals, statements made prior to the conflict and generally predictive in nature; *transactive* goals, those that develop or change as a result of the communication transaction and may be predictive or explanatory in nature; and *retrospective* goals, statements that make sense after the conflict takes place and serve an explanatory function.

When examining issues and goals it is important to explore the level(s) on which the conflict is operating. Most, if not all, conflicts have two levels: *content,* the subject matter or surface structure of the conflict, and *relational,* the affective deep structure of the conflict participants' feelings toward themselves and each other. It is important for both supervisors and supervisees to identify the conflict level accurately, because that knowledge will aid in determining how the conflict can be managed most productively.

For example, the supervisor and supervisee may need to decide whether the conflict is about using the supervisor's therapy strategy rather than the supervisee's (content level) or whether the issue is that the supervisor does not respect the supervisee as the competent colleague she is (relational level). Once the focus is decided, goals for managing the conflict can be established. If each partner is focused on a different level, mutual goals for productive management cannot be obtained.

Intervention. Conflict intervention, the process of entering into and negotiating a conflict, involves a number of procedures, beginning with *confrontation.* A supervisor may initiate a conflict with a supervisee in one of the following ways: direct challenge, pointing out the supervisee's behavior, changing his or her own behavior, self-disclosure, metacommunicating, or withdrawal of reinforcement (Egan, 1973). Any of the methods can be carried out in a positive or a negative way, but positive confrontation generally leads to more productive conflict management.

Another type of confrontation that is important, both to the analysis of conflict and to the development of productive conflict management skills, is *self-confrontation.* Self-confrontation is generally done through videotape analysis. Farmer (1982, 1987c) discussed the importance of training in self-confrontation for supervisors and supervisees. (See chapter 6, "Observation Competence," for videotape analysis techniques.)

One central requirement for accurate analysis of communication interactions is *critical obser-*

vation skill. Farmer (1982, 1987c) discussed the importance of training in critical observation. Supervisors and supervisees must be able to identify verbal and nonverbal communication behaviors, communication systems (open or closed), and communication flow (downward, upward, both [vertical], or horizontal/lateral). In addition, they must differentiate accurately among observed behaviors, interpretations, judgments, and opinions.

Once supervisors are competent in confronting both self and others, and competent in the communication strategies that can lead to productive conflict management, they can implement those strategies in specific intervention tactics and techniques.

Tactics are planned methods of conducting conflict interactions (Wilmot & Wilmot, 1978). The purpose of using tactics is to keep a conflict moving by changing its direction so that it does not deadlock. Four categories of tactics exist, each of which includes specific techniques: *avoidance, escalation, maintenance,* and *reduction*. It is important to recognize that the most beneficial way to work with a conflict situation may not be to avoid or reduce it (which is the tendency for most untrained conflict participants) but to maintain it for more thorough management or escalate it for clearer understanding of the issues, levels, and goals.

Tactics of conflict management can be used either by those actively involved in the conflict or by an outside party. Two types of third party interventionists exist: the *mediator,* who has no power to make decisions but must have the necessary communication skills to guide the conflict to productive management, and the *arbitrator,* who not only guides discussion through skilled communication but also is empowered to make decisions for conflict interactants.

Techniques of intervention are more specific and can be used by supervisors within the general tactic areas. Wilmot and Wilmot (1978) discuss the following techniques which are reflected in the Interpersonal Communication Pacing (ICP) model (Farmer, 1984a, 1985). The principles apply to participants, mediators, and arbitrators.

1. Direct the feedback process (Filley, 1975).
    a. Be descriptive rather than judgmental; focus feedback on observed behavior rather than on individuals or on inferences.
    b. Encourage specificity.
    c. Address things that can be changed.
    d. Encourage feedback when it is requested.
    e. Give feedback as close as possible to the behavior being discussed.
    f. Encourage feedback whose accuracy can be checked by others.
    g. Speak only for yourself.
    h. In giving feedback, describe behavior in terms of *more* or *less* rather than in terms of *either-or*.
    i. Focus feedback on sharing ideas and information and on exploring alternatives, rather than on giving advice, answers, and solutions.
    j. Focus feedback on the value it may have to the recipient, not on the release that it provides to the person giving the feedback.
    k. Give the amount of information the recipient can use, rather than the amount that could be given.
2. Engage quiet individuals in a nonthreatening way.
3. Limit the agenda and keep the interactants to it.
4. Set and enforce time limits.
5. Compare positions.
6. Restate positions.
7. Reverse roles when appropriate.
8. Recognize the limitations of the mediator and arbitrator roles.
9. Encourage the interactants to have a range of positions.
10. Summarize and get commitment.
11. Establish superordinate goals.
12. Equalize power.

13. Produce graduated tension reduction.
14. Use the institutions or individuals who specialize in conflict management.
15. React constructively to criticism.
    a. Be honest; everyone has faults.
    b. Mentally assume the critic's position.
    c. If the criticism is unfounded, say so; don't harbor resentment.
    d. Don't apologize unnecessarily.
    e. Don't whine during or after criticism.
    f. Talking should stop when stress levels rise.
    g. Disarm the critic by asking how something could be done better or differently.
    h. Focus efforts on improvement.

If conflict in supervision is to be viewed as an inevitable, ongoing, normal, growth-producing aspect of human communication, then it must no longer be regarded as a pathological phenomenon grounded in gender, age, status, and cultural differences that foster fear and avoidance. Supervisors can adjust their attitudes by learning more about the nature of conflict as its complexity unfolds through scholarly research.

For the kind of learning that leads to productive change of a conflict system's rule structure ("second-order" change, as defined by Watzlawick, Weakland, & Fisch, 1974), supervisors must engage in serious self-study and personal development. As more and more individuals in a supervision system learn about basic communication and conflict management, the quality of interactions will improve. Conflicts that have been managed in adversarial terms can become collaborative, and participants can attempt to negotiate disputes to produce win/win outcomes. Training in communication and conflict management can lead to personal and systemic change.

This chapter has introduced many communication concepts that supervisors must understand and use. Therefore, supervisor training programs should include such concepts so that speech-language pathologists and audiologists can learn about and practice the many aspects of communication. The next section discusses assessment and preparation in four areas: personal, interactional, organizational, and interview.

COMMUNICATION ANALYSIS

Personal Analysis

Personal analysis was described in chapter 2. The Personal Communication Disorders Supervision Characteristic Profile (Table 2–6, p. 43) can be used to summarize personal analysis results. However, before supervisor trainees can select specific tools for personal assessment, they need to have a global picture of communication as it operates in the teaching-learning process.

Johari Window. The Johari Window offers a useful way of understanding how known and unknown information about supervisor trainees and their instructors fits into supervision preparation and implementation. The Johari Window was developed by Joseph Luft and Harry Ingham and gets its name from the first names of its authors (Luft, 1961; Sergiovanni & Starratt, 1979). Kennedy, McCready, and Shapiro (1987) applied the concept of the Johari Window to the dynamics of change in supervisors, supervisees, and clients.

Figure 5–2 shows the teaching-learning relationship between the supervisor trainee and the instructor in a supervisor preparation program.

In the first cell, the *Open Self,* the supervisor trainee's knowledge of personal communication behavior and other aspects of professional practices corresponds with the instructor's knowledge. This is the area in which communication occurs most effectively and in which the need for the trainee to be defensive is minimal. The instructor works with the trainee to broaden or enlarge this cell.

In the second cell, the *Hidden Self,* the trainee knows about aspects of personal communication

	What the supervisor trainee knows about self	What the supervisor trainee does not know about self
What the instructor knows about the supervisor trainee	OPEN SELF (Information known to self and others)	BLIND SELF (Information known only to others)
What the instructor does not know about the supervisor trainee	HIDDEN SELF (Information known only to self)	XXXXXX XXXXXX UNDISCOVERED SELF XXXXXX XXXXXX (Information known neither to self nor to others)

XXXXXX
XXXXXX
XXXXXX = Area of mutual insight
XXXXXX

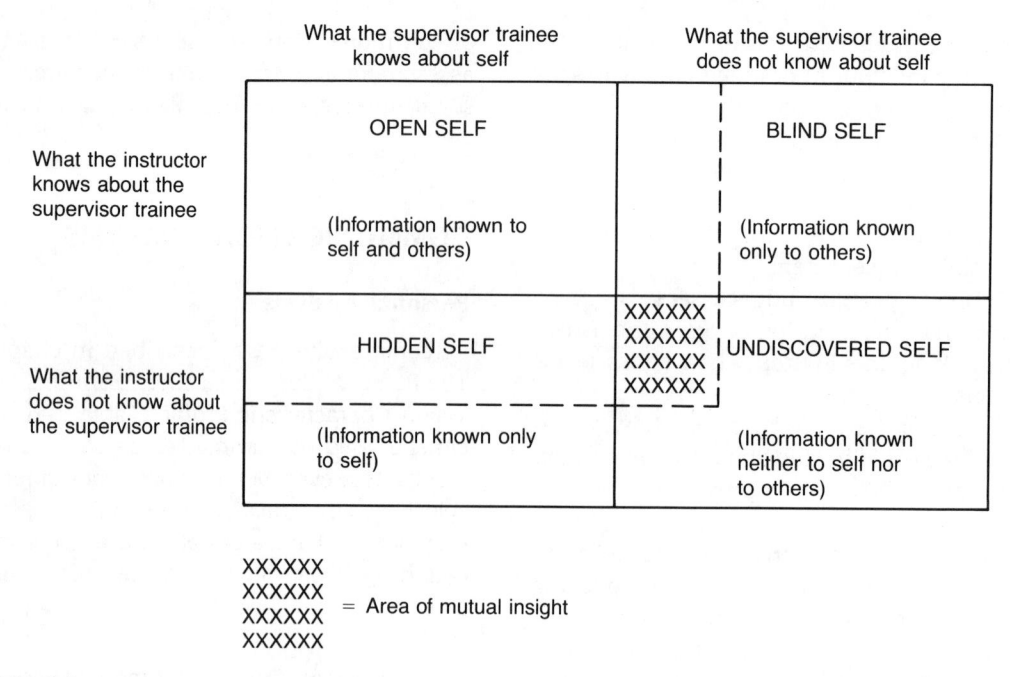

FIGURE 5-2
Johari Window. Adapted from *Of Human Interaction* by J. Luft, 1969, New York: National Press Books.

behavior and professional practice that the instructor does not know. Often the trainee conceals this knowledge from the instructor for fear that the instructor might use it to punish, hurt, or exploit the trainee. The second cell suggests how important a climate of trust and credibility is to the success of supervision training and implementation. In situations represented by this cell, the trainee is encouraged to reduce the size of the cell.

In the third cell, the *Blind Self,* the instructor knows about aspects of the trainee's communication behavior and professional practice of which the trainee is unaware. This cell, though large initially, is reduced considerably as learning develops and matures. This is the cell most often neglected by traditional evaluation-of-learning methods.

In the fourth cell, the *Undiscovered Self,* are aspects of the trainee's communication behavior and professional practice not known to either the instructor or the trainee.

As shown in Figure 5-2, an area of mutual insight develops as a result of increasing the Open Self and decreasing the Hidden Self, the Blind Self, and the Undiscovered Self. Mutual insight grows for both the supervisor trainee and the instructor as they both learn more about the trainee through the process of personal assessment discussed in chapter 2.

The Johari Window can be applied to the supervision process as well as to the supervisor training process. On the matrix, the supervisee replaces the supervisor trainee; the supervisor replaces the instructor. Through competent communication, the supervisor can help the supervisee enlarge the *Open Self* quadrant by reducing the other three. Such development results in supervisor-supervisee mutual insight, the cornerstone of quality supervision.

Interaction Analysis (IA)

Instruments used to record and analyze supervisor and supervisee communication behavior during conferences are termed *interaction analysis instruments*. Although hundreds of IA tools exist, six are used most often to analyze the communication behavior of Communication Disorders supervisors in dyadic interaction with supervisees: the *Content and Sequence Analysis System* (Culatta & Seltzer, 1977); the *System for Analyzing Supervisor-Teacher Interaction* (Blumberg, 1974); the *Underwood Category System for Analyzing Supervisor-Clinician Behavior* (Underwood, 1979); *McCrea's Adapted Scales* (McCrea, 1980); the *Oratio Transactional System* (Oratio, 1977); and the *Multidimensional Observation System for the Analysis of Interactions in Clinical Supervision (M.O.S.A.I.C.S.)* (Weller, 1971). Note that analyzing a supervisor's communication alone is not productive. One must examine it in tandem with the supervisee's to make accurate judgments about the appropriateness of the transaction. Interaction Analysis in supervision has four uses: (a) self-analysis for the supervisor, the supervisor trainee, or the supervisee; (b) peer analysis for the same three; (c) joint analysis for supervisor and supervisee, supervisor and supervisor trainee, or supervisor trainee and supervisee; and (d) research in supervision conference communication.

Interaction analysis systems are classified in several ways. In a *frequency*-based system, every behavior is recorded into a category. In a *time*-based system, behaviors are recorded and categorized at specified intervals. Some systems look at *content*, whereas others document *process*; some are *unidimensional*, whereas others are *multidimensional*, looking at several dimensions of the same behavior. Different IA systems look at *affective, linguistic,* or *cognitive* domains. Most instruments have been developed for dyadic analysis, although a few accommodate group interaction. Most are hand-analyzed, but the option of computer analysis is slowly emerging. Of the six instruments mentioned above, none addresses nonverbal communication, and as a result interpersonal communication confluence (verbal plus nonverbal) is not addressed.

According to Anderson (1980), some advantages of IA systems are that they

1. provide a shorthand for gathering selective data about a process without having to record every event.
2. encourage objectivity by limiting observations to specific behaviors, inhibiting instant, subjective evaluation, and documenting series or patterns of behavior from which to draw inferences later.
3. document specific behavior over time.
4. provide a means for self-analysis and measurement of change.
5. provide data for research.

Disadvantages of the IA instruments are that they

1. generally lack good reliability and validity standards.
2. produce quantities of data that often become unmanageable and are used unproductively.
3. may be overused and/or misused.
4. generally address a limited range of communication behaviors, providing a simplistic picture of the very complex process of communication.
5. reflect the biases of the developer.

Herbert and Attridge (1975) state that the methodological problems in using IA systems are extensive and results must always be viewed critically. Some of the problems include sampling, use of context and inference by observers, observer selection and training, and the critical questions of validity and reliability. Anderson (1980) and her colleagues analyzed each of the six tools using the Herbert and Attridge criteria and briefly described them, giving their advantages and disadvantages.

Smith and Mawdsley (1987) offered examples of nonstandardized methods for analyzing group management rotation rates, response rates, talk time, and question types in clinical and supervisory interaction. Other discrete language analysis systems, computerized and noncomputerized, are discussed in chapters 10 and 11.

It is also important to be able to analyze interaction within Communication Disorders supervision groups. One type of group analysis is a communication network that tracks who talks to whom. Another approach documents the different kinds of contributions each member makes, as does the M.O.S.A.I.C.S. Two interaction analysis instruments designed specifically for examining groups are discussed next.

Proana 5 (Lashbrook & Lashbrook, 1972) is a tool for network analysis, recording who talks to whom and how often. (Proana 5 was originally developed as a computer program to analyze small-group interaction; the name is an abbreviation for "process analysis of a 5-person group.") On a network chart such as the one in Figure 5-3, the frequency with which each line is used shows how often each group member talked and to whom he or she directed communication.

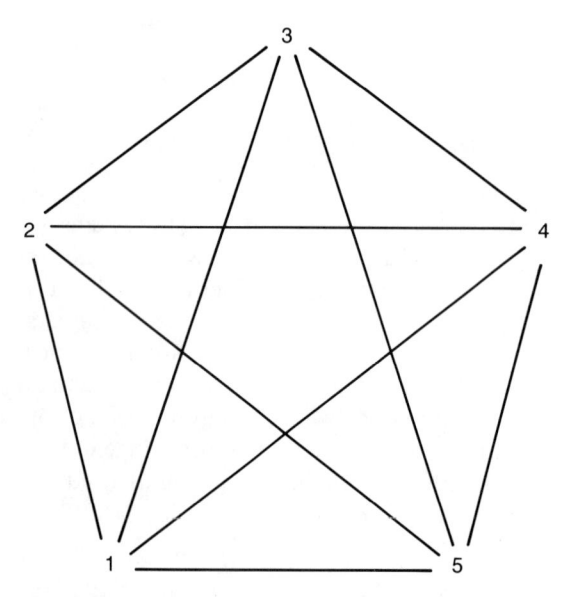

FIGURE 5-3
Interaction network

For a five-member group, 10 lines of communication are possible (1-2, 1-3, 1-4, 1-5, 2-3, 2-4, 2-5, 3-4, 3-5, 4-5). Arrows at the midpoint of each communication line indicate the direction of flow (i.e., who initiated the interaction). Record communication line usage by making a mark on the appropriate line(s) each time a member talks. In productive groups, all lines will be used, but not necessarily equally. The tallies at the end of the group interaction will show a variety of patterns. Two people speaking only to each other constitute a clique or coalition; an individual with no marks is an isolate, someone excluded from the flow of communication by choice (withdrawal) or by other members of the group. Likewise, dominance can be detected if one person talks more than any two others combined. Proana 5 may be useful in recording communication during group supervision. However, in group interactions it is sometimes difficult to identify to whom the speaker is directing comments.

Although Proana 5 is useful for measuring the frequency of talk in a group, it does not account for the content, or what was said. IPA (Interaction Process Analysis), developed by Bales (1950), provides a mechanism for documenting what kinds of comments individuals make. Figure 5-4 shows a matrix for Bales's IPA categories.

The IPA is based on the idea that members contribute to the group process in accord with the task and also with personal needs. Some remarks are made to facilitate the task, others for socioemotional purposes.

According to a profile of typical group discussions (Goss, 1983), members of most groups tend to give suggestions, opinions, and orientation more frequently than they ask for them (56% as compared to 10% of the contributions). In addition, most groups spend more time talking about task (66%) than about relationships (34%). Like the Proana 5, IPA can be used to identify leaders, isolates, and dominant members. Used together, the Proana 5 and Bales's IPA analysis systems can provide a complex diagram of group discussion. To date no research has been published that analyzes Communication Disorders group supervision using either of these two systems.

Supervision systems are parts of larger organizational systems. Researchers can study communication flow in supervision systems in terms of how these systems fit into the larger organization.

Organizational Communication Audit

One way to examine the communication system within an organization is to conduct a *communication audit* that tracks the flow of information from its source through the system. Two instruments for recording this flow are the *Episodic Communication Channels in Organization (ECCO)* and the *Organization Communication Development (OCD)* analysis instruments.

ECCO analysis was developed by Keith Davis in 1952 as an instrument to analyze and map communication networks and to measure rates of flow, distortion of messages, and redundancy. *ECCO* is a convenient, fast, reliable field instrument. It records concrete messages rather than perceptions or attitudes. Its major disadvantage is that it sometimes takes several weeks for a message to be totally diffused within an organization, and this lag time may affect respondents' recall of the facts (Goldhaber, 1983).

The *OCD* procedure was developed by Osmo Wiio and Martii Helsila of Finland (Goldhaber, 1983). The questionnaire calls for responses on a 5-point scale, providing data for statistical analysis in the areas of mode of message transmission (oral or written), type of communication (formal or informal), and direction of communication (upward, downward, or horizontal). The questionnaire also asks two open-ended questions:

1. What is especially bad about the communication in this organization?
2. What is especially good about the communication in this organization?

The communication audit can benefit the Communication Disorders supervisor, particularly in the Administrator role. Farmer (1987b), using modified versions of the *ECCO* and *OCD* instruments, audited a Communication Disorders training program. Results suggested that, overall, the program's communication system was ineffective. Specific results from 16 items were used in setting goals and objectives to improve communication and strengthen the academic and clinical programs for undergraduates, graduates, and faculty members.

Interview Analysis

The *Interview Analysis System (IAS)* (Farmer, 1980), a modification of the *Conover Analysis System* (Conover, 1974) has been used successfully in training verbal interviewing skills. The *IAS* uses only the most basic categories to yield maximum information about kinds of significant verbal interaction between interviewer and interviewee. Its brief, easily learned coding system is a useful tool to facilitate the interviewing ability of Communication Disorders supervisors or supervisor trainees.

The Molyneaux/Lane Interview Analysis (Molyneaux & Lane, 1982) is designed to help investigate the nature of interactions in an interview. It can be used to analyze individual interviews, pinpoint personal proficiencies and areas of weakness, document interviewee and/or interviewer change, or facilitate research. With practice, professionals can use the three-digit coding system comfortably either with a verbatim typescript of the interview or while listening to the tape itself. For computer research, an additional coding system identifies feelings expressed in interviews. Categorizing, coding, and analysis with this tool may be too difficult and time-consuming for frequent use. However, some such means of documenting interviewers' verbal behavior for analysis and comparison over time can help supervisors develop their interviewing ability.

AREAS	COMMUNICATION FUNCTIONS	INTERACTION PATTERNS*									
		1-G	1-2	1-3	1-4	1-5	2-G	2-1	2-3	2-4	2-5
(A) Social-Emotional area: positive reactions	1. Shows solidarity, raises others' status, gives help, rewards										
	2. Shows tension release, jokes, laughs, shows satisfaction										
	3. Agrees, shows passive acceptance, understands, concurs, complies										
(B) Task area: attempted answers	4. Gives suggestion, direction, implying autonomy for other										
	5. Gives opinion, evaluation, analysis; expresses feeling, wish										
	6. Gives information, orientation, repeats, clarifies, confirms										
(C) Task area: questions	7. Asks for information, orientation, repetition, confirmation										
	8. Asks for opinion, evaluation, analysis, expression of feeling										
	9. Asks for suggestion, direction, possible ways of action										
(D) Social-Emotional area: negative reactions	10. Disagrees, shows passive rejection, shows formality, withholds help										
	11. Shows tension, asks for help, withdraws out of field										
	12. Shows antagonism, deflates others' status, defends or asserts self										
	TOTALS										

Interaction Pattern Analysis:

Part I

(Check appropriate problems)
- 6:7 = Problems of Communication
- 5:8 = Problems of Evaluation
- 4:9 = Problems of Control
- 3:10 = Problems of Decision
- 2:11 = Problems of Tension Reduction
- 1:12 = Problems of Reintegration

FIGURE 5-4
Group interaction process analysis

INTERACTION PATTERNS*

3-G	3-1	3-2	3-4	3-5	4-G	4-1	4-2	4-3	4-5	5-G	5-1	5-2	5-3	5-4	TOTALS

Part II
(percentages) %

A (1 + 2 + 3) = Positive Reactions _____
B (4 + 5 + 6) = Attempted Answers _____
C (7 + 8 + 9) = Questions _____
D (10 + 11 + 12) = Negative Reactions _____

*Interaction Patterns: 1–G = Group member 1 initiates or responds to interaction with group (G); 1–2 = Group member 1 initiates or responds to interaction with group member 2, etc.

Adapted from *Interaction Process Analysis* by R. Bales, 1950, Chicago: University of Chicago Press.

COMMUNICATION COMPETENCE AND INCOMPETENCE

All of the concepts and types of communication discussed so far can be synthesized into a final concept: *communication competence.* Communication competence means both having and using the knowledge of who can say, write, or sign what, in what way, where and when, by what means, and to whom. Competent communication must be functional; functional communication must work for those who are exchanging information. Communication is functional if a speaker displays (a) fluency, coherence, and effectiveness of control, (b) a low degree of egocentricity, and (c) communication flexibility in many different contexts and roles. Researchers have pinpointed specific communication characteristics that violate these three basic criteria and thus result in incompetent communication (Simon, 1979).

In Communication Disorders supervision, incompetent communication occurs when

1. the supervisor does not take the supervisee's perspective into consideration when giving information or instructions (incongruence). For example, when the age, gender, and background of the supervisee are not considered, the complexity of the message (its structure and vocabulary) is not keyed to the supervisee's ability to comprehend and respond; the supervisor does not give the proper amount of information to convey communication intent.
2. messages are not clearly organized into main points and subordinate information.
3. messages are not well planned or structured. Experiences and events are not related sequentially, but uttered in freely associated thoughts that sound incoherent. Fluency of expression is marred by verbal mazes (false starts) while the supervisor is deciding where to begin or how to structure the content, or searching for the right word (arhythmia).
4. the flow of meaning is interrupted. Cluttered words or slurred speech can lead the supervisee to make inaccurate assumptions about the supervisor's intent. The supervisee may also have difficulty interpreting indirect or "tactful" statements (i.e., polite, rather than direct linguistic forms). The problem with these indirect statements, such as sarcasms, is that the surface meaning is often different from the intended meaning, and the supervisee may not perceive the disjunction.
5. the language system does not adapt flexibly to varying communication needs. In such cases social aspects of language may be adequate but the cognitive and affective components are inadequate. The supervisor is unaware of the limitations of the restricted code being used (e.g., when using acronyms or professional jargon with a beginning supervisee who doesn't know what they mean).
6. deficiencies in oral language often affect written and read communication.

With these kinds of communication incompetence in mind, supervisors can implement the following plan to increase communication competence in supervisory systems.

DEVELOPMENT OF COMMUNICATION COMPETENCE

Developing competence in communication may not be easy for many supervisors and supervisor trainees. Some research indicates that supervisors' communication behavior changes minimally over time (Culatta & Seltzer, 1976, 1977; Roberts & Smith, 1982). To maximize successful attempts at this developmental journey, a number of steps must be taken.

Step 1. Supervisors need to begin by developing comprehensive personal profiles using the assessment procedures discussed earlier. From such a profile, goals and objectives can be written to facilitate change.

Step 2. The second step is to set goals and objectives. Goals are long-term and must include skills *and* dispositions. For each goal, include the following elements:

1. Time (when goal will be attained)
2. Direction (what is to be done; an outcome)
3. Measureability (criteria for judging change)

Objectives are the steps that lead to goals; they, too, must include both skills and dispositions and contain the same three elements.

Without well-developed goals and objectives it is difficult to establish a long-range, realistic, and meaningful program for change. Examples of Communication Disorders supervision role-related goals and objectives are shown in Table 5-4.

Step 3. Acquiring communication competence involves second-order change. Individuals must need and be prepared to change, and they must have a supportive system within which to practice newly learned behaviors, or second-order change will not take place. (See chapter 3 for a discussion of change.)

Step 4. In the final step, supervisors use available programs to facilitate change in communication patterns, or develop new ones. The *Verbal and Nonverbal Interpersonal Communication Pacing Facilitation Program* (Farmer, 1984d) is a systematic method of developing pacing and leading skills for professional use. Role-playing and role reversal in psychologically comfortable contexts are effective ways to practice new communication behaviors. Other academic and continuing education programs in communication skills development abound, in the form of seminars, workshops, or college and university courses.

TABLE 5-4
Sample goals and objectives for five Communication Disorders supervision roles

Role	Goal	Objective
Professional	By the end of the year 19_____, to improve my public speaking ability while presiding at the (state) supervision meetings; improvement will be judged by increased scores on the _____ rating form to be completed by a colleague. The proficiency will be utilized in all subsequent public speaking situations.	On January _____, June _____, and December _____, 19_____, a colleague will evaluate my public speaking ability at the (state) supervision meetings using the _____ rating form. Each rating will be higher than the baseline rating of _____.
Researcher	By the end of the year 19_____, to have submitted for publication two articles pertaining to Communication Disorders supervision. This schedule will be continued for the next 5 years.	By March_____, and July_____, 19_____, two articles will have been submitted to *The Clinical Supervisor* and the *Journal of Communication Disorders*.

TABLE 5-4 *continued*

Role	Goal	Objective
Educator	To improve my conference communication with Level I supervisees by the end of spring term 19_____. Bi-term monitoring using the *Underwood Category System for Analyzing Supervisor-Clinician Behavior* will be done for the next 3 years, by which time all of the areas of my personal profile will have been addressed.	By April_____, 19_____, I will have had a minimum of five improved conferences in the area of supervisor's questions. I will ask fewer questions and, specifically, fewer narrow questions.
Administrator	To increase my communication with supervision personnel during weekly staff meetings by the end of (month) as measured on a communication network using Proana 5.	After each staff meeting during the month of _____, I will analyze my group interaction using the Proana 5. Using data from the first meeting as baseline, I will then have more frequent communication with more staff members during each subsequent meeting. The level of communication interaction attained by the end of the month will be maintained for the remainder of the year.
Clinician	To improve my Reaction Time Latency during therapy sessions with language-impaired preschoolers. Judgements will be made by INREAL specialist colleagues during the next evaluation term.	By _____ I will have received positive feedback from INREAL specialist colleagues that my Reaction Time Latency with four language-impaired preschoolers was appropriate for each child and the context. This proficiency will be maintained for the duration of therapy with each child.

SUMMARY

Supervisors need to be competent communicators because the foundation of Communication Disorders supervision is communication. All other aspects of supervision (e.g., leadership, power, authority, models, or theories) are based on various combinations of the dimensions of communication discussed in this chapter. Ultimately the success of the supervision system depends on the communication competence of the supervision staff. Therefore, institutional preparation programs and continuing education offerings need to be of a quality that will facilitate the development of communication competence in Communication Disorders supervisors, present and future.

APPLICATIONS

Discussion Topics

1. Discuss whether it is important to have a supervisor with native-speaker proficiency in the relevant foreign language supervise the therapy of minority language clients.
2. Discuss the importance of the supervisor-supervisee conference in changing the supervisee's clinical behavior.
3. Discuss the components of a communication audit. How could it be done with a staff of supervisors? Why might it be done?
4. Discuss the variables that can affect conferences, including who is involved, communication style of the supervisor, preparation of the supervisee, reason for the conference, environment, time of day, level of the clinician, gender of the participants, and ranks of the participants.
5. Discuss video resumes: their advantages, their disadvantages, and what preparation is necessary for a supervisor to produce or to review one.

Laboratory Experiences

1. Identify five good ways for a supervisor to encourage a quiet member of the supervision group to participate; five good ways to keep an unusually vocal supervisee from dominating the group.
2. Identify your predominant subpersonalities and list how they might affect your supervision.
3. Do an interaction analysis of a supervision conference in which you were the supervisor. Use the IA tool of your choice.
4. Role-play a supervision conflict and apply the information about productive conflict management as you participate. Play the roles of both the supervisor and the supervisee.
5. Develop your Personal Communication Disorders Supervision Profile (see Table 2-6, p. 43).

Research Projects

1. Research the In Absentia model of group supervision using Bales's IPA analysis system.

2. Research the patterns of conflict communication within a specific Communication Disorders supervision setting.
3. Conduct a study of the nonverbal qualifiers (intonation, pitch, quality) associated with the sincerity feature of genuine communication.
4. Conduct a survey of beginning supervisees' life scripts that influence the Communication Disorders supervision process.
5. Design a replication study of Farmer's (1984c) research on bilingual supervision.

REFERENCES

American Speech-Language-Hearing Association. (1982). *Bilingual Language Learning System (BLLS)*. Rockville, MD: Author.

Anderson, J. (Ed.). (1980). *Proceedings of the Conference on Training in the Supervisory Process in Speech-Language Pathology and Audiology*. Bloomington: Indiana University.

Bales, R. (1950). *Interaction process analysis*. Chicago: University of Chicago Press.

Bandler, R., & Grinder, J. (1979). *Frogs into princes*. Moab, UT: Real People Press.

Belenky, M., Clinchy, B., Goldberger, N., & Tarule, J. (1986). *Women's ways of knowing: The development of self, voice, and mind*. New York: Basic Books.

Berger, C., & Calabrese, R. (1980). Some explorations in initial interaction and beyond: Toward a developmental theory of interpersonal communication. In B. Morse & L. Phelps (Eds.), *Interpersonal communication: A relational perspective* (pp. 50–62). Minneapolis, MN: Burgess.

Berne, E. (1964). *Games people play*. New York: Grove Press.

Bernstein, B. (1970). A socio-linguistic approach to socialization: With some reference to educability. In F. Williams (Ed.), *Language and poverty* (pp. 25–61). Chicago: Markham.

Blank, M., Rose, S., & Berlin, L. (1978). *The language of learning: The preschool years*. New York: Grune & Stratton.

Blumberg, A. (1974). *Supervisors and teachers: A private cold war*. Berkeley, CA: McCutchan.

Brandt, D. (1979). On linking social performance with social competence: Some relations between communication style and attributions of interpersonal attractiveness and effectiveness. *Human Communication Research, 5*, 223–237.

Brasseur, J. (1980). The observed differences between direct, indirect, and direct/indirect videotaped supervisory conferences by speech-language pathology supervisors, graduate students, and undergraduate students. *Dissertation Abstracts International, 41*, 2131B. (University Microfilms No. 80-29, 212)

Buchheimer, A. (1963). The development of ideas about empathy. *Journal of Counseling Psychology, 10*(1), 61–70.

Carreras, N. (1986). *A pilot study to determine the effect of eye-movement mirroring and/or predicate matching on variables of rapport*. Unpublished master's thesis, New Mexico State University, Las Cruces.

Casey, P. (1980). The validity of using small segments for analyzing supervisory conferences with McCrea's Adapted System. *Dissertation Abstracts International, 41,* 1729B. (University Microfilms No. 80-24, 566)

Cazden, C. (1965). *Environmental assistance to the child's acquisition of syntax.* Unpublished doctoral dissertation, Harvard University.

Cazden, C. (1979). Peekaboo as an instructional model: Discourse development at home and at school. *Papers and Reports on Child Language Development, 17,* 1-29.

Cogan, M. (1973). *Clinical supervision.* Boston: Houghton Mifflin.

Condon, W., & Ogston, W. (1967). A segmentation of behavior. *Journal of Psychiatric Research, 5,* 221-235.

Conover, H. (1974). *Conover Analysis System.* Unpublished manuscript, Ohio University, Athens.

Culatta, R., & Seltzer, H. (1976). Content and sequence analysis of the supervisory session. *Asha, 18,* 8-12.

Culatta, R., & Seltzer, H. (1977). Content and sequence analysis of the supervisory session: A report of clinical use. *Asha, 19,* 523-526.

Cumpata, J., & Johnson, K. (1983, November). *Student perceptions of group and individual clinical-supervisor conferences.* Poster session presented at the annual convention of the American Speech-Language-Hearing Association, Cincinnati, OH.

Cunningham, R. (1971). Developing question-asking skills. In J. Weigand (Ed.), *Developing teacher competencies* (pp. 81-130). Englewood Cliffs, NJ: Prentice-Hall.

Deutsch, M. (1973). Conflicts: Productive and destructive. In F. Jandt (Ed.), *Conflict resolution through communication* (pp. 155-197). New York: Harper & Row.

Dowling, S. (1983). Teaching clinic conference participant interactions. *Journal of Communication Disorders, 16,* 385-397.

Dowling, S. (1986, November). *Supervisory training: Impact on cognitive complexity and rhetorical sensitivity.* Paper presented at the annual convention of the American Speech-Language-Hearing Association, Detroit.

Duke, J. (1976). *Conflict and power in social life.* Provo, UT: Brigham Young University Press.

Egan, G. (1973). Confrontation. In *Face to face* (pp. 106-134). Monterey, CA: Brooks/Cole.

Emerick, L., & Haynes, W. (1986). *Diagnosis and evaluation in speech pathology* (3rd ed.). Englewood Cliffs, NJ: Prentice-Hall.

Erickson, F., & Shultz, J. (1982). *The counselor as gatekeeper.* New York: Academic Press.

Faber, A., & Mazlish, E. (1980). *How to talk so kids will listen & listen so kids will talk.* New York: Avon.

Farmer, S. (1980). Interview Analysis System. *SUPERvision, 4*(4), 8.

Farmer, S. (1982, March). *Visual literacy: Information and training program for communicative disorders specialists.* Paper presented at the American Speech-Language-Hearing Association South Central Regional Conference, Colorado Springs, CO.

Farmer, S. (1984a). Supervisory conferences in communicative disorders: Verbal and nonverbal interpersonal communication pacing. *Dissertation Abstracts International, 44,* 2715B. (University Microfilms No. 84-00, 891)

Farmer, S. (1984b, November). *Facilitating interpersonal communication competence in supervisory conflict systems.* Miniseminar presented at the annual convention of the American Speech-Language-Hearing Association, San Francisco.

Farmer, S. (1984c). *Bilingual supervision: Does it make a difference?* [Machine readable data file No. ED 239-805]. Las Cruces, NM: ERIC/CRESS (Producer). Arlington, VA: U.S. Department of Education, Educational Resources Information Center (ERIC) (Distributor).

Farmer, S. (1984d, November). *Verbal and nonverbal interpersonal communication pacing (ICP): A facilitation program.* Videotape program presented at the annual convention of the American Speech-Language-Hearing Association, San Francisco.

Farmer, S. (1985). Relationship development in supervisory conferences: A tripartite view of the process. *The Clinical Supervisor, 3*(4), 5-22.

Farmer, S. (1987a). The art and science of conferences: Tessellations. In S. Farmer (Ed.), Clinical supervision: A coming of age. Proceedings of a national conference on supervision (pp. 176-190). Las Cruces: New Mexico State University.

Farmer, S. (1987b). An organizational communication audit of a communication disorders training program. *SUPERvision, 10*(4), 28-30.

Farmer, S. (1987c). Visual literacy and the clinical supervisor. *The Clinical Supervisor, 5*(1), 45-71.

Fear, R. (1958). *The evaluation interview.* New York: McGraw-Hill.

Filley, A. (1975). *Interpersonal conflict resolution.* Glenview, IL: Scott, Foresman.

Frankel, J. (1973). *Helping students think and value: Strategies for teaching the social studies.* Englewood Cliffs, NJ: Prentice-Hall.

French, J., & Raven, B. (1960). The bases of social power. In D. Cartwright & A. Zander (Eds.), *Group dynamics: Research and theory* (2nd ed.) (pp. 601-623). New York: Harper & Row.

Gazda, G. (1973). *Human relations development.* Boston: Allyn & Bacon.

Gilligan, C. (1982). *In a different voice: Psychological theory and women's development.* Cambridge, MA: Harvard University Press.

Ginott, H. (1965). *Between parent and child.* New York: Macmillan.

Gleason, J. (Ed.). (1985). *The development of language.* Columbus, OH: Charles E. Merrill.

Goldhaber, G. (1983). *Organizational communication* (3rd ed.). Dubuque, IA: Wm. C. Brown.

Goldhammer, R. (1969). *Clinical supervision.* New York: Holt, Rinehart & Winston.

Gordon, T. (1970). *P.E.T.—Parent Effectiveness Training.* New York: New American Library.

Gordon, T. (1974). *T.E.T.—Teacher Effectiveness Training.* New York: Peter H. Wyden.

Goss, B. (1983). *Communication in everyday life.* Belmont, CA: Wadsworth.

Greif, E., & Gleason, J. (1980). Hi, thanks, and goodbye: More routine information. *Language in Society, 9,* 159-166.

Grice, H. (1975). Logic and conversation. In P. Cole & J. L. Morgan (Eds.), *Syntax and semantics: Vol. 3. Speech acts* (pp. 41-58). New York: Academic Press.

Halliday, M. (1973). *Explorations in the functions of language.* London: Edward Arnold.

Halliday, M., & Hasan, R. (1976). *Cohesion in English.* London: Longman.

Harris, T. (1967). *I'm OK—You're OK.* New York: Harper.

Hart, R., & Burks, D. (1972). Rhetorical sensitivity and social interaction. *Speech Monographs, 39,* 75-91.

Hart, R., Carlson, R., & Eadie, W. (1980). Attitudes toward communication and the assessment of rhetorical sensitivity. *Communication Monographs, 47,* 1-22.

Hawes, L., & Smith, D. (1973). A critique of assumptions underlying the study of communication in conflict. *Quarterly Journal of Speech, 59,* 423-433.

Herbert, J., & Attridge, C. (1975). A guide for developers and users of observation systems and manuals. *American Educational Research Journal, 12,* 1-20.

Hubbell, R. (1981). *Children's language disorders: An integrated approach.* Englewood Cliffs, NJ: Prentice-Hall.

Irwin, R. (1975). Microcounseling interviewing skills of supervisors of speech clinicians. *Human Communication, 4* (Spring), 5-9.

Janis, I. (1972). *Victims of groupthink.* Boston: Houghton Mifflin.

Joos, M. (1976). The style of the five clocks. In N. Johnson (Ed.), *Current topics in language: Introductory readings* (pp. 152-56). Cambridge, MA: Winthrop.

Kadushin, A. (1968). Games people play in supervision. *Social Work, 13,* 23-32.

Katz, N., & Lawyer, J. (1983). Communication and conflict-management skills strategies for individual and systems change. *Phi Kappa Phi Journal, 63,* 31-33.

Kendon, A. (1980). Movement coordination in social interaction: Some examples described. In W. von Roffler-Engel (Ed.), *Aspects of nonverbal communication.* Bath, England: Pitman Press, Swets & Zeitlinger B.V.-Lise.

Kendon, A., & Ferber, A. (1973). A description of some human meetings. In R. P. Michael & J. H. Crook (Eds.), *Comparative ecology and behavior of primates* (pp. 591-668). London: Academic Press.

Kennedy, K., McCready, V., & Shapiro, D. (1987). Dynamics of change in supervisors, supervisees, and clients. *SUPERvision, 11*(2), 26-32.

Kilmann, R., & Thomas, K. (1975). Interpersonal conflict: Handling behavior as reflections of Jungian personality dimensions. *Psychological Reports, 37,* 971-980.

Klevans, D., & Volz, H. (1976, November). *The nonverbal behavior systems: A procedure for evaluating clinical interaction.* Poster session presented at the annual convention of the American Speech and Hearing Association, Houston.

Knapp, M. (1978a). *Nonverbal communication in human interaction* (2nd ed.). New York: Holt, Rinehart & Winston.

Knapp, M. (1978b). *Social intercourse: From greeting to goodbye.* Boston: Allyn & Bacon.

Knowles, M. (1973). *The adult learner: A neglected species.* Houston: Gulf.

Kramer, C. (1974). Woman's speech: Separate but unequal? *Quarterly Journal of Speech, 60,* 14–24.

LaFrance, M., & Broadbent, M. (1976). Group rapport: Posture sharing as a nonverbal indicator. *Group and Organizational Studies, 1,* 328–333.

LaFrance, M., & Mayo, C. (1978). *Moving bodies: Nonverbal communication in social relationships.* Monterey, CA: Brooks/Cole.

Lakoff, R. (1973). Language and woman's place. *Language and Society, 2,* 45–80.

Langellier, K., & Natalle, E. (1987). Communication, gender perspectives, and the clinical supervisor. In S. Farmer (Ed.), *Clinical supervision: A coming of age. Proceedings of a national conference on supervision* (pp. 14–37). Las Cruces: New Mexico State University.

Lashbrook, W., & Lashbrook, V. (1972). *Proana 5: A computer analysis of small group discussion.* Minneapolis, MN: Burgess.

Long, L. (1978). *Listening/responding: Human relations training for teachers.* Monterey, CA: Brooks/Cole.

Luft, J. (1961). The Johari Window. *Human Relations Training News, 5,* 6–7.

Lynch, J. (1983). Gender differences in language. *Asha, 4,* 37–42.

Maltz, D., & Borker, R. (1982). A cultural approach to male/female miscommunication. In J. J. Gomperz (Ed.), *Language and social identity: Studies in international sociolinguistics* (pp. 196–216). Cambridge, MA: Harvard University Press.

McCrea, E. (1980). Supervisee ability to self-explore and four facilitative dimensions of supervisor behavior in individual conferences in speech-language pathology. *Dissertation Abstracts International, 41,* 2134B. (University Microfilms No. 80-29, 239)

Mercer, A., & Schubert, G. (1974, November). *Nonverbal behaviors of speech pathologists in the therapy setting.* Paper presented at the International Communications Convention, New Orleans.

Michalak, D. (1969). Supervisory conferences improve teaching. *Florida Educational Research and Development Council Research Bulletin, 5.*

Michalak, D., & Yager, E. (1979). *Making the training process work.* New York: Harper & Row.

Molyneaux, D., & Lane, V. (1982). *Effective interviewing: Techniques and analysis.* Boston: Allyn & Bacon.

Mosher, R., & Purpel, D. (1972). *Supervision: The reluctant profession.* Boston: Houghton Mifflin.

Muma, J. (1978). *Language handbook: Concepts, assessment, intervention.* Englewood Cliffs, NJ: Prentice-Hall.

Myers, G., & Myers, M. (1973). *The dynamics of human communication: A laboratory approach.* New York: McGraw-Hill.

Norton, R. (1983). *Communicator style: Theory, applications, and measures.* Beverly Hills, CA: Sage.

Oratio, A. (1977). *Supervision in speech pathology: A handbook for supervisors and clinicians.* Baltimore, MD: University Park Press.

Parks, M. (1980). Relational communication: Theory and research. In B. Morse & L. Phelps (Eds.), *Interpersonal communication: A relational perspective* (pp. 287–296). Minneapolis, MN: Burgess.

Perry, W. (1970). *Forms of intellectual and ethical development in the college years.* New York: Holt, Rinehart & Winston.

Pickering, M. (1979). Interpersonal communication in speech-language pathology clinical practicum: A descriptive humanistic perspective. *Dissertation Abstracts International, 40,* 2140B. (University Microfilms No. 79-23,892)

Pickering, M. (1987). Metaphoric expression in supervisory conferences. In S. Farmer (Ed.), *Clinical supervision: A coming of age. Proceedings of a national conference on supervision* (pp. 125–131). Las Cruces: New Mexico State University.

Rapoport, A. (1970). Conflict resolution in the light of game theory and beyond. In P. Swingle (Ed.), *The structure of conflict* (pp. 1–43). New York: Academic Press.

Roberts, J. (1979). *The supervisory conference in speech-language pathology.* Unpublished manuscript, Indiana University, Bloomington.

Roberts, J., & Smith, K. (1982). Supervisor-supervisee role differences and consistency of behavior in supervisory conferences. *Journal of Speech and Hearing Research, 25,* 428–434.

Rowe, M. (1986). Wait time: Slowing down may be a way of speeding up. *Journal of Teacher Education, 1,* 43–50.

Sbaschnig, K., Sziraki, D., & Matecum, S. (1986). *An analysis of preference in supervisory styles.* Unpublished manuscript, Wayne State University, Detroit.

Scheflen, A. (1966). Natural history method in psychotherapy: Communication research. In L.A. Gottschalk & A. H. Auerback (Eds.), *Methods of research in psychotherapy* (pp. 206–222). New York: Appleton-Century-Crofts.

Schegloff, E., & Sacks, H. (1973). Opening up closings. *Semiotica, 8,* 289–327.

Scherer, K. (1980). The functions of nonverbal signs in conversation. In R. St. Clair & H. Giles (Eds.), *The social and psychological contexts of language* (pp. 225–244). Hillsdale, NJ: Lawrence Erlbaum.

Schmitt, J., & Gibbs, D. (1984, November). *Interpersonal skills in clinical supervision: An investigation of efficacy data.* Paper presented at the annual convention of the American Speech-Language-Hearing Association, San Francisco.

Schubert, G., & Nelson, J. (1976, November). *Verbal behaviors occurring in speech pathology supervisory conferences.* Paper presented at the annual convention of the American Speech-Language-Hearing Association, Houston.

Searle, J., Kiefer, F., & Bierwisch, M. (Eds.). (1980). *Speech act theory and pragmatics.* Boston: Kluwer.

Sergiovanni, T., & Starratt, R. (1979). *Supervision: Human perspectives* (2nd ed.). New York: McGraw-Hill.

Simon, C. (1979). *Communicative competence: A functional pragmatic approach to language therapy.* Tucson, AZ: Communication Skill Builders.

Sleight, C. (1984). Games people play in clinical supervision. *Asha, 26,* 1, 27–29.

Smith, K. (1978). Identification of perceived effectiveness components in the individual supervisory conference in speech pathology and an evaluation of the relationship between ratings and content in the conferences. *Dissertation Abstracts International, 39,* 680B. (University Microfilms No. 78–13, 175)

Smith, K., & Mawdsley, B. (1987). Analysis in the supervisory process. In S. Farmer (Ed.), *Clinical supervision: A coming of age. Proceedings of a national conference on supervision* (pp. 164–176). Las Cruces: New Mexico State University.

Sperloff, B. (1953). Empathy and role-reversal as factors in industrial harmony. *Journal of Social Psychology, 37,* 117–120.

Spradlin, J., & Siegel, G. (1982). Language training in natural and clinical environments. *Journal of Speech and Hearing Disorders, 47*(2), 2–6.

Stevens, L., & Miller, L. (1986, November). *Communication and linguistic differences between directive and non-directive supervisory styles.* Paper presented at the annual convention of the American Speech-Language-Hearing Association, Detroit.

Stewart, J. (Ed.). (1982). *Bridges not walls* (3rd ed.). Reading, MA: Addison-Wesley.

Stewart, J., & D'Angelo, G. (1975). *Together: Communicating interpersonally.* Reading, MA: Addison-Wesley.

Tepper, D., & Haase, R. (1978). Verbal and nonverbal communication of facilitative conditions. *Journal of Counseling Psychology, 25*(1), 35–44.

Underwood, J. (1979). *Underwood category system for analyzing supervisor-clinician behavior.* Unpublished manuscript, University of Northern Colorado, Greeley.

Ward, S. (1981, November). *Rhetorically sensitive supervisory communication: A situational analysis.* Paper presented at the annual convention of the Speech Communication Association, Anaheim, CA.

Watzlawick, P., Beavin, J., & Jackson, D. (1967). *Pragmatics of human communication.* New York: Norton.

Watzlawick, P., Weakland, J., & Fisch, R. (1974). *CHANGE: Principles of problem formation and problem resolution.* New York: Norton.

Webster, E. (1964). *Decision making in the employment interview.* Montreal, Canada: McGill University Industrial Relations Center.

Weiss, R. (1983). *INREAL Training Evaluation Model (ITEM)* (revised). Unpublished interaction analysis system used in INREAL training. University of Colorado–Boulder.

Weller, R. (1971). *Verbal communication in instructional supervision.* New York: Teachers College Press, Columbia University.

Whitman, R., & Boase, P. (1983). *Speech communication: Principles and contexts.* New York: Macmillan.

Wilmot, J., & Wilmot, W. (1978). *Interpersonal conflict.* Dubuque, IA: Wm. C. Brown.

Wood, B. (1981). *Children and communication: Verbal and nonverbal language development* (2nd ed.). Englewood Cliffs, NJ: Prentice-Hall.

Yarbrough, E. (1981). Intrapersonal conflict management. In A. Goldman (Ed.), *Psychology of public communication* (pp. 628–650). Huntington, NY: Robert E. Krieger.

6
Observation Competence

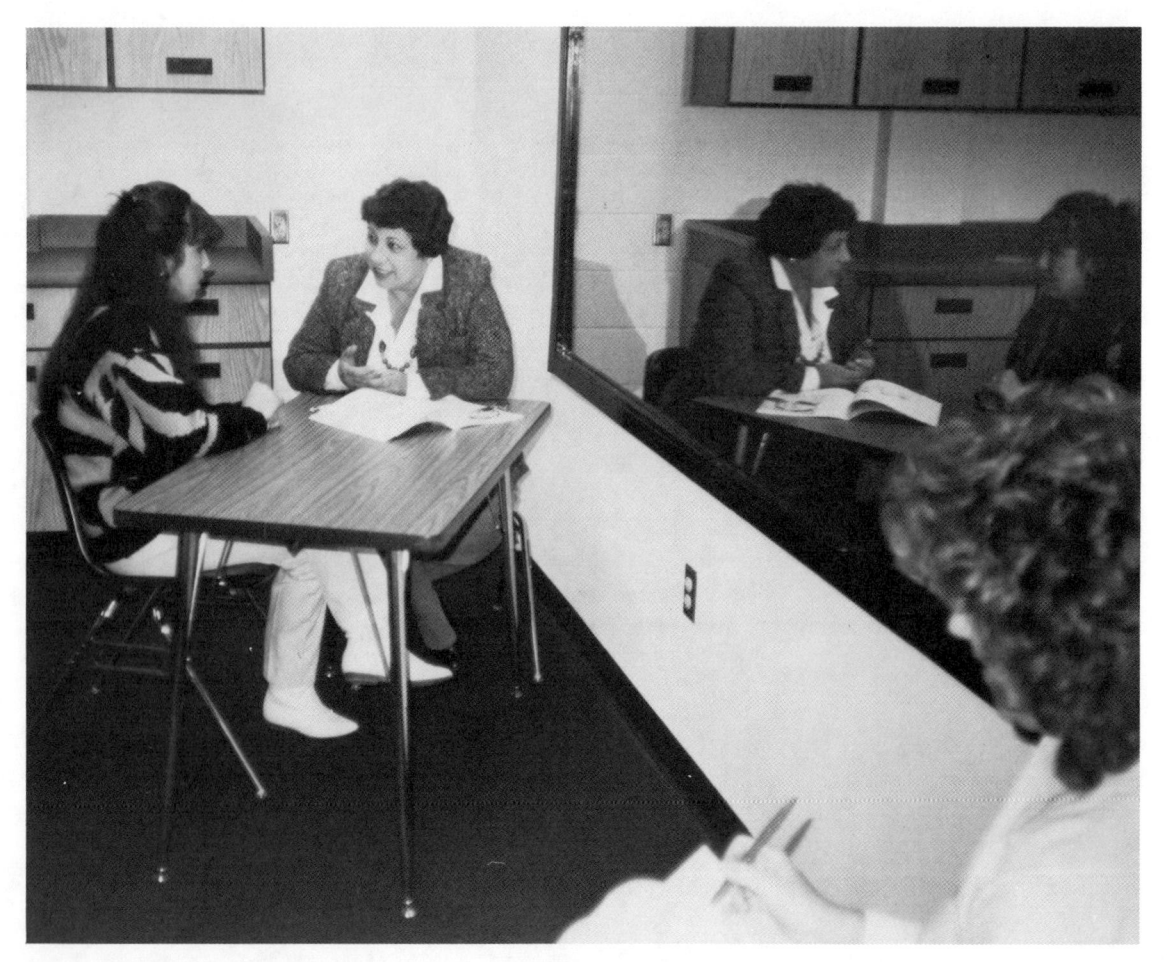

CRITICAL CONCEPTS

- Being competent in observation is important for Communication Disorders supervisors.
- Supervisors can become competent observers by learning to apply observational knowledge and skills to all dimensions of behavior in all supervision roles.
- Visual literacy is a component of observation that requires specific training, including knowledge, skill development, and practice.
- Supervisors may use various forms or modes of observation, patterns or systems of observing, and recording methods depending on the purpose for observing.

OUTLINE

INTRODUCTION
VISUAL LITERACY
    Elements of a Visual Literacy Training Program
OBSERVING NONVERBAL BEHAVIOR
OBSERVING VERBAL BEHAVIOR
MODES
    Live Observation
    Closed Circuit Television
    Telecommunication
    Audiotape Recording
    Videotape Recording
    Interactive Video Discs
    Written Plans
SYSTEMATIC OBSERVATION
    Frequency
    Duration
    Prearranged versus Spontaneous
    Focused
    Guided versus Solo
OBSERVATION RECORDING SYSTEMS
    Ratings
    Narrative Data
    Checklists
    Timing
    Tallying
SUMMARY
APPLICATIONS

INTRODUCTION

Observation competence, the ability to apply observational knowledge and skills across the dimensions of behavior, is essential for the Communication Disorders supervisor to perform the roles of supervision effectively. Becoming competent in observation is an ongoing process of synthesizing *knowledge* of observation, developing *skills* through clinical application and supervision experience, and formulating *dispositions* from continued information, academic training, and opportunities to practice and self-evaluate. This chapter presents ideas and concepts about observation in supervision and highlights skills necessary for the development of observation competence. The chapter has emerged from two assumptions: (a) observation is a science, with systematic methods for gathering, recording, analyzing, and reporting data; and (b) observa-

---

This chapter was contributed by Judith L. Farmer, New Mexico State University.

tion competence is a synthesis of learned behaviors and therefore can be taught.

The importance of observation competence has been repeatedly emphasized in many professions. Diagnosis and treatment in medicine, social work, and clinical psychology are particularly dependent on the observational skills of the clinician. Training programs in observation have long existed in law and law enforcement professions. Educators are increasingly stressing the observation skills needed for effective teaching, training teachers to observe their students' styles of learning and to create learning environments and instructional objectives based on those observations.

Long recognized as important in developing clinical skills, observation for the Communication Disorders student has been considered a prerequisite for participation in clinical practicum and an essential tool for diagnostic and therapeutic functions (Kunze, 1967). ASHA's training program requirement that students complete 25 clock hours of supervised clinical observation before beginning active participation in clinical practicum mandates the period of directed observation (ASHA, 1984). Observation competence is necessary in all aspects of the Communication Disorders profession: evaluation, therapeutic management, administration, research, professional development, education, and clinical supervision.

Although the importance of observation is well established, the development of observation skills has received minimal attention in the past. Too often it has been assumed that with clinical experience, feedback, and self-evaluation, observers will "naturally" progress toward observation competence. Studies of the process of observation, however, have drawn attention to the need for specific training in observation. Methods of teaching observation skills to classroom teachers have been detailed by Rowen (1973), Cartwright and Cartwright (1974), Stubbs and Delamont (1976), Stallings (1977), and Boehm and Weinberg (1977). Jaggar and Smith-Burke (1985) offer guidelines for observing language performance within the classroom. In Communication Disorders, preservice courses in training observation skills have been included in university training programs, and varied pedagogical and clinical application formats have been proposed (Golper, McMahon, & Gordon, 1976; Gonzales, 1985; Guinty & Scudder, 1980; Klevans, Volz, & Friedman, 1981; Kunze, 1967). Harris (1979) found a self-teaching, programmed approach, using videotapes and a manual, to be an efficient method for training preclinical students to identify the goals and associated procedures of therapy sessions. Dowling (1981) introduced the emphasis on using specific procedures to examine observational data. Grijalva (1982) studied the observation skills of preclinical Communication Disorders students and concluded that (a) before clinical practice, students need to be trained to observe specific behaviors exhibited in therapy sessions, and (b) an observation training program using videotaped therapy sections is an effective way to train the observation skills of preclinical students. Dowling (1984) reported the observation skills of graduate student clinicians who were evaluating their therapy to be as precise as those of their clinical supervisors; she suggested that clinical training programs may wish to direct their observation competency goals toward those clinicians who have not reached minimal competency levels rather than provide identical training for all clinicians. Gonzales (1985) studied the need to train observation skills in undergraduate beginning clinicians and tested a model training program; she concluded that beginning clinicians need observation training and that her model program taught improved observation skills that were retained over time.

Supervisors need observational knowledge and skills beyond those of an observant clinician. The quality of supervisory feedback for clinicians depends on supervisors' critical observation abilities. Supervisors are expected to use observation in meeting the ASHA minimum requirement of direct supervision of at least 25% of therapy sessions and at least 50% of diagnostic sessions (ASHA, 1984). The sixth task of supervision identified by the ASHA Committee on Supervision, assisting the supervisee in observing and analyzing assessment and treatment sessions, requires the following competencies: selection and use of data collection procedures; data recording, analysis, and interpretation; and revision of plans based on data obtained (ASHA, 1985) (see appendix A). Rassi (1985) gave supervisors the opportunity to discuss aspects of clinical instruction and observation. She summarized supervisors' comments about observation in regard to methodologies, documentation, feedback, modes, data recording, student stress, ASHA requirements, and off-campus sites. Supervisors' responses in each of these areas emphasized the importance of competent observation in the supervision process.

Observation skills training is a basic dimension in programs that offer preparation for supervision. Anderson (1981) noted the need for supervisors in clinical education to become competent in observing the behaviors of clients, supervisees, and themselves and urged researchers to study the components of the supervision process. Harvey (1980) developed a program for training graduate student clinical supervisor trainees to observe and studied its effectiveness; her results indicated the importance and feasibility of having an observation skill development module in Communication Disorders supervision graduate training programs. More recently, researchers in supervision have provided input that is useful for planning training components. Runyan and Seal (1985) emphasized the importance of training supervisors' observation skills in their comparative study of supervisors observing a videotaped therapy session. Smith and Mawdsley (1987) drew attention to the observation/analysis/interpretation process of supervision by summarizing data collection approaches and presenting specific observation recording tools to be used in developing self-assessment skills in supervisees. Lougeay-Mottinger, Harris, and Stillman (1987) presented data to support the use of a videotape coding system to analyze students' and supervisors' clinical behavior. In their study of supervisors' written narrative comments on student clinical performance, Peaper and Mercaitis (1987) noted that written comments were more evaluative than feedback given during supervisory conferences. They stressed the importance of using various types of feedback after a clinical observation. Emphasizing the importance of training observation skills in supervisors, Anderson (1988) provided detailed observation information on strategies, methods of data collection, and analysis systems.

In each of the five supervisory roles of Professional, Researcher, Educator, Administrator, and Clinician, observation competence is a primary requirement. The Professional draws on observation skills in leadership, organizational record keeping, and public relations; a trained observer will be more sensitive to the dynamics of group interaction and will have alternative methods to present for maintaining and analyzing logs, data, or records. The Researcher, given the current emphasis on contextually-based, naturalistic modes for studying communication, finds critical observation skills increasingly important; a trained, competent observer will obtain reliable and valid information and will have the interpretation bases for data analysis. The Educator relies on visual feedback from students in the classroom, uses observation competencies in all direct supervision of clients and supervisees, and is coming to depend increasingly on varied modes for direct clinical supervision, videotapes for classroom instruction and in-service presentation, and more time efficient observation recording systems. The Administrator uses observation competencies when interviewing prospective employees, evaluating staff members, conducting meetings, or publicizing programs and services. The Clinician employs observation competencies in all clinical

FIGURE 6-1
Components of observation competence

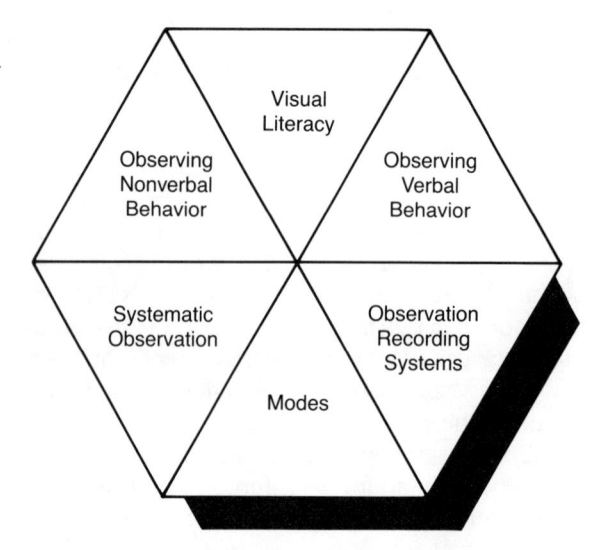

contacts and services, demonstrates observational reliability as an expert witness in the courtroom, and uses observation skills to interact with colleagues and other professionals. Thus, observation competence is a goal for all supervisors.

Competence in observation includes the following components: visual literacy, observing nonverbal behavior, observing verbal behavior, modes of observation, systematic observation, and observation recording systems (see Figure 6-1). A discussion of the components begins with visual literacy.

VISUAL LITERACY

Visual literacy is the knowledge, skills, and dispositions involved in recording, interpreting, integrating, utilizing, and reporting visual experiences. Supervisors should be familiar with visual literacy tools and should know how to apply the grammar and syntax of visual language, read and write visuals, and translate back and forth between visual and verbal language.

The concept of visual literacy in supervision has been introduced and detailed by Farmer (1987). Using television, and particularly videotape, Farmer (1981) devised and implemented a training program for visual literacy awareness for Communication Disorders specialists. He reported the importance of becoming visually literate, the necessity for training in order to become visually literate, and the elements of a viable training program. Communication Disorders supervisors use visual literacy in all supervisory roles and therefore need specific training in visual literacy.

Elements of a Visual Literacy Training Program

A visual literacy training program should cover the concept of visual literacy; the role of television in learning; the uses of television in supervision; the processes of videotape recording and videotape analysis; observer biases; the choice of visual focus for observation; the limits of assumptions and inferences based on visual information; and how to record, interpret, and report visual experiences.

The Concept. The concept of visual literacy is the starting point for a visual literacy training program. Visual literacy is acquired through awareness, practice, and experience. It includes becoming aware of visuals, learning to respond to visual images, interpreting and remembering visual images, using visual language to describe what one sees, documenting visual occurrences, and developing the ability to describe an incident or person so that someone else will visualize it in essentially the same way.

Learning from Television. Understanding the role of television in learning is part of visual literacy. People are accustomed to using television for learning as well as for entertainment. For many, television has replaced other visual media such as newspapers, books, and magazines as the primary source of information and entertainment. Sales of videocassette units for home use have exceeded all marketing expectations, as have rentals of videotapes. Commercial videotapes provide instruction in every dimension of life. Many students have been raised in an environment where learning from television is a daily habit and easily respond to learning technical information via videotape. Some individuals, however, are so accustomed to having a television as auditory and visual background that they may have difficulty using television actively or interactively. *TV watchers* tend to view television as a passive activity, a relaxing form of entertainment; *TV learners* respond to television by gaining information, talking about what they are viewing, and connecting material presented on television with that in printed visuals, their experiences, and their actions. TV watchers can become TV learners by being guided in watching (when, for example, parents watch children's programs alongside their children, talking about, copying, or acting out what they are seeing, or when supervisors guide supervisees through videotaped observations). Supervisors need to know how to use television for learning and how to teach supervisees to learn from television.

Television and Supervision. Whether in the form of live closed circuit television, regular network programming, or videotape, television has many uses in Communication Disorders supervision. These include classroom instruction (presenting commercially prepared or instructor-prepared information about various disorders, conditions, syndromes, diagnostic tests, intervention techniques, and educational and employment opportunities), research, inservice and professional presentations, and community/parent/family instruction. Academic and clinical settings equipped with closed circuit television systems allow for live video monitoring of clinical practicum and therapeutic services as well as for transmission of live and recorded sessions to classrooms and conference rooms. Instructional teleconferences on national and state levels widen resource bases for supervisors. Network programs that feature stories or information about communication, disorders, or handicapped individuals may supplement regular class assignments. Videotape equipment provides relatively low-cost opportunities for supervisees or supervisors to tape a session and observe and evaluate it immediately afterward or later, permitting active learning and allowing for self-confrontation, self-analysis, interaction analysis, and contextual analysis.

Videotape Recording and Analysis. Videotape recording in supervision has unlimited possibilities, and it has in many clinical settings replaced the traditional audiotape recording. Videotapes in classroom settings have largely replaced the traditional 16 mm educational films, which have been well established as a useful part of training in observation (Irwin & Nickels, 1970). Tables 6-1 and 6-2 detail the advantages and disadvantages of clinical use of videotape recording.

Since for many people videotaping is not initially comfortable, special procedures may be required in the clinical setting. In supervision, videotaping can lead to both positive and negative experiences with self-confrontation.

Self-confrontation, the process of being one's own critical audience, is not easy for supervisor, supervisee, or client. Learning to self-evaluate requires skills as well as experiences. If unprepared to view themselves and if without specific constructive purpose, observers may find critical

TABLE 6-1
Advantages of clinical videotape recording

1. Videotaping heightens sensitivity to kinesic behavior. Time and motion studies have been shown to increase observers' awareness of movement.
2. Videotaping is used therapeutically.
   a. Physical and psychological characteristics of the current environment are important determinants of behavior and need to be analyzed; this can be done with videotaping.
   b. Perceptions, including interpersonal perceptions, are generally accurate if partial representations of the environment. Therefore, the environment needs to be an integral part of the behavioral analysis.
   c. Behavior can often be modified by increasing the range of information about the environment to which the individual can respond.
   d. Younger children are often excited and pleased about seeing themselves; videotape recording may be more successful with young children than with older clients.
   e. Videotaped vicarious desensitization can lower anxiety in both group and individual settings.
   f. Videotaping can help participants understand interactions, which in turn promotes a more egalitarian relationship.
   g. Videotaping provides immediate playback.
   h. Videotaping, which includes sound and visual images, can make complex interactions more concrete. Abstractions can be better understood and can also be retained longer.
   i. Videotaping allows participants to take some responsibility for themselves because they can see themselves from the outside.
   j. Videotaping allows supervisors to select short, edited segments, which are most effective for confrontation analysis.
   k. Videotaping can provide additional reinforcement for selected behaviors.
3. Videotaping allows for splitting audio and visual channels. It is frequently important to look at verbal and nonverbal behaviors separately.
4. Libraries of videotapes are being developed. Videotape libraries are important teaching resources.
5. Exercises for developing verbal and nonverbal communication skills can be evaluated through videotaping.
6. Comparative analyses may be done through videotaping.
7. Learner participation and interest can be increased through videotaping.
8. Videotape replay is an inexpensive self-instruction tool.
9. Videotape materials can be updated and kept current inexpensively.
10. Audiences are enlarged. Videotape recording expands dissemination for topics of general interest that are originally presented in smaller meetings.
11. Videotape facilitates identification of *multiple messages*—incongruence of verbal and nonverbal messages.
12. Videotaping allows for *focused feedback*, which requires a performer to be actively involved, leading to higher gains in self-awareness.
13. Stopping the videotape at intervals to permit discussion or participation can enhance the learning process.
14. Various viewer participation techniques can enhance learning. Responding aloud or silently to questions on the tape, mentally reviewing the material while the tape is running, and writing responses are effective learning strategies.
15. Review of taped performances over succeeding days enhances the learning process.
16. Videotapes provide enhanced observational opportunities.
17. Videotapes can easily integrate many teaching techniques, such as verbal explanations, diagrams, and clinical examples.
18. Performers can review the tapes as often as they wish and at their own convenience.
19. Performers can view videotapes at their own speed, allowing for self-paced instruction.
20. Videotapes prepared in a training institution can be shared in other parts of the country, making the expertise of teaching staff available to a wider audience.

Source. "Visual Literacy and the Clinical Supervisor" by S.S. Farmer, 1987, *The Clinical Supervisor,* 5(1), pp. 53–55.

TABLE 6-2
Disadvantages of clinical videotape recording

1. Anxiety and self-consciousness may arise from videotaping.
   a. Anxiety is reported to be highest in persons who are inexperienced, lack information, or need to master a new role.
   b. Older children, adolescents, and physically impaired individuals may be concerned about the way they look to others; they may use denial to cope with self-perceptions. The supervisor must exercise caution when using videotaping with these groups.
   c. Adults tend to perceive self-observation as a social situation calling for self-criticism. Their discussions are more abstract, cognitive, and self-conscious. They may struggle to control "giveaways" of underlying self-images.
   d. Humans' fear of the machine can reduce the encounter to a series of calculated manipulations. Poor-quality productions can result from lack of training or fear of using the equipment.
   e. In most instances, adequate preparation and goal setting for people involved will reduce the anxiety and self-consciousness to a level that does not interfere with learning. However, "adequate" is different for each person, so a sensitivity to each person's needs is a necessity for instructors.
2. Legal issues arise from videotaping. Photographic/electronic recording of the behavior of clients, clinicians, and others creates the possibility that these recordings could be played back in settings outside the control of the subjects. Conceivably such playback could be against the interests of those who were filmed and those who did the filming. Thus, it could be considered an invasion of privacy and legal action could ensue. Or the potential threat of privacy invasion could contribute to one's anxiety about being taped.
3. Distortions can arise from videotaping.
   a. Technical misuse of video equipment can distort a person, an interaction, or a context so that the message is difficult to interpret or is deceptive. Learning how to operate the equipment correctly will allow filming of situations in the most accurate way possible.
   b. Highlight segments may be missed because of technical mismaneuvers. Many programs are amateurish because of a poor sense of the visual.
4. The Hawthorne effect (or *novelty effect*) may have some bearing on the results of videotaping. Initially, the novelty of using new equipment or trying a new procedure can create changes in behavior or conditions that do not last when the novelty wears off.
5. Rapid changes in technology may make video systems a continuing problem.
6. Some people believe that videotape instruction reduces direct personal contact.
7. There may be a lack of opportunity for immediate feedback.
8. Production costs of videotape recording may be high.
9. Video script writing, as well as video transcription, is difficult and time-consuming.
10. Videotape recording equipment is not easy to use and often it requires extensive preparation on the part of instructors and trainees.
11. It does not necessarily save class or individual time. In role-playing with discussion, for example, replay can easily consume two to three times the number of hours required for role-playing without videotape.
12. Since videotape recording often involves both the instructor and trainees on a personal and highly emotional level, it may be difficult to use objectively.

Source. "Visual Literacy and the Clinical Supervisor" by S.S. Farmer, 1987, *The Clinical Supervisor,* 5(1), pp. 55–57.

self-observation unproductive at best or ego-damaging at worst. But when the observer is prepared with information and tools to evaluate various aspects of a taped session and is familiar with the basics of visual literacy, self-confrontation can be a powerful learning medium.

The supervisor needs to be prepared to deal with the observer's anxiety, both in tape preparation and in post-taping analysis. Although some people respond naturally to recording sessions and comfortably to critical self-observation, many express apprehension and concern and are therefore unable to perform at their best or typical levels. A supervisor experienced in videotape use and self-confrontation can help someone who is apprehensive about being videotaped by using desensitization exercises (e.g., practice recording sessions, role-playing, rehearsal) and playback activities (e.g., playback done by the individual alone or with a supportive peer, playback within a supportive group, discussion in dyads).

Once the observer is comfortable with being videotaped and with the concept of self-confrontation, specific analytical approaches can be introduced. Depending on the purpose for videotaping, the supervisor and supervisee may select various aspects of the session to examine critically (e.g., nonverbal behaviors, verbal behaviors, the client, the clinician, how materials are being used, how tests are being administered). They may select self-analysis (critical examination of one's own behavior or performance), interaction analysis (study of the interaction between two individuals, the messages being conveyed between them, the communication exchanges), contextual analysis (focus on the simultaneous and sequential relationships of behaviors within the social and environmental setting), or transactional analysis (contextual analysis that also looks at the choices people make about their communication behavior in light of the responses of others). A suggested sequence of training is summarized in Table 6–3.

Equipment Use. Learning to use the tools of visual literacy is important to the user as well as to the maintenance of the equipment. Proficiency in the use of videotape recording systems (camera, lighting, microphones, monitors, tapes, playback systems) is critical. Also important is the ability to manage the equipment using basic filming techniques (focusing, framing the subjects, knowing when to zoom in or out, panning the area, highlighting certain aspects such as facial expressions) and taping in a variety of settings (in a studio, in clinic/school/hospital/office, on site, in the home). Familiarity with various brands of equipment will facilitate the supervisor's using or selecting new equipment. Technical proficiency is only half of competent equipment use; attitudes toward the medium and its use affect communication with others involved and will strongly influence the outcome. If a supervisor believes that videotape recording is a constructive training tool, the participants can use this aspect of visual literacy as a powerful instrument for learning.

Biases. Visual literacy training programs should teach about biases, personal preferences of

---

TABLE 6–3
Suggested sequence of training for self-confrontation

1. Trainee observes videotape alone.
2. Performer trainees and instructor (or experienced confederate) observe together; an occasional positive comment about what is being viewed is appropriate.
3. Instructor (or confederate) models specific, productive comments about the *instructor's* verbal and nonverbal behavior.
4. Trainees use productive communication strategies to comment positively about their *own* verbal and nonverbal behavior.
5. Instructor (or confederate) models specific, productive strategies for commenting about aspects of the *instructor's* verbal and nonverbal behavior that require modifying.
6. Trainees use productive strategies to comment about aspects of their *own* verbal and nonverbal behavior that require modifying.
7. Trainees employ observation/communication skills within a group setting.

Source. "Visual Literacy and the Clinical Supervisor" by S.S. Farmer, 1987, *The Clinical Supervisor,* 5(1), pp. 57–63.

which one may or may not be aware. Observers can begin to manage their biases by knowing that biases are present in all individuals, that they affect human behavior and particularly observation, that it is important for observers to recognize their own biases, and that biases affect decision making.

Supervisors should first identify their own biases (e.g., by listing three to five things that they like to do in therapy, the positive biases, and the same number of things they do not like to do in therapy, the negative biases). Next, supervisors should have opportunities to experience the natural tendency to watch for or concentrate on aspects of a situation that are positive biases and to ignore those that are negative biases. Note that the positive biases take one's attention away from the negative biases. Following this recognition exercise, supervisors would do well to try to identify all biases (observing various clients, ages, disorders, and sites; discussing preferences with peers; making a list of positive and negative biases) and to determine their own approaches to the management of biases. Supervisors may find it beneficial to set specific observational goals and objectives that take positive and negative biases into account, perhaps trying to counteract negative biases by concentrating on aspects not usually noted first.

Awareness of attributional biases is particularly important in supervision. Causal attributions, or beliefs about causes of performance, are significant from the viewpoint of the supervisor, who may be relating to a session as an observer and comparing data with the supervisee who is relating to the session as the actor/participant. Roberts and McCready (1987), in a study of differences in causal attributions made by supervisees taking actor and observer roles in hypothetical therapy sessions, reported that attributions differed for actors and observers in good and poor therapy sessions. Actor-observer biases may be brought to the supervisee's attention through role-playing activities, videotape analyses, and group discussions.

Recognizing and accepting biases, knowing that they will affect observations, judgments, and decisions, and managing them appropriately will significantly improve the quality of observation (Farmer, 1982).

Focus. All observations should be guided by a purpose. The purpose of an observation will suggest the direction for focus, the act of concentrating on or tuning in to particular aspects of the visual field. Unless awareness and use of focus are included in observation training, supervisors may unsystematically focus on the particulars suggested by their biases.

The view when observing is often physically restricted by the mode of observation, such as through a small observation window, the camera of a closed circuit television system, or the seating location selected by the observer. This restriction may be unintentional, if a supervisor did not consider focus in planning for the observation, or intentional, when planning has determined that a particular focus will yield the desired information. Depending on the purpose for the observation, the supervisor may decide to focus just on the supervisee, only on nonverbal behavior, on several of the techniques being used, on the client's responses to the test being administered, on the parents' responses to the supervisee's suggestions, and so forth. More typically, however, the supervisor will spend designated times during the session focusing on different aspects and will follow a pattern of converging on specifics and diverging to a broader picture.

Like the lens of a camera, which zooms in and out to focus on certain aspects of the total picture, the supervisor uses different degrees of visual concentration. A wide view of the observation is a *macrofocus,* visually absorbing the total picture; when the view narrows, becoming more defined, the observer zooms in to a *microfocus* (Farmer, 1982). Each kind of view provides different information and is a valuable part of the total observation. A macrofocus yields low agreement between observers, a high degree of inference, more opportunities and information

TABLE 6-4
Comparison of macrofocus and microfocus methods of observation

Variable	Macrofocus	Microfocus
Agreement between observers	lower	higher
Degree of inference	higher	lower
Ability to generalize	easier	more difficult
Subjectivity	higher	lower
Portion of the therapeutic process viewed	more	less

for generalizations, a higher degree of subjectivity, and a more complete picture of the total therapeutic process. Conversely, a microfocus produces higher agreement between observers, a low degree of inference, less information from which to generalize, a lower degree of subjectivity, and a less complete picture of the total therapeutic process. Table 6-4 compares macrofocus and microfocus across five variables.

Supervisors use both macrofocus and microfocus during an observation, since each brings in different information, to gain a complete picture. Experienced supervisors will develop a focusing pattern in which they systematically macrofocus and microfocus during an observation; the pattern will vary according to the specific purpose of the observation. Activities to help supervisors learn the skill of focusing include guided observation (in which the instructor designates the appropriate focus orally or in writing during the observation); group discussions of focus; practice in focused record keeping (e.g., tallying the number of times the supervisee said "Okay?"); and writing narrative descriptions of observed events.

Assumptions. Assumptions are discussed in a visual literacy training program to help the supervisor learn about both the benefits and the hazards of taking something for granted without sufficient supportive evidence. Whereas observations can be documented by what the observer has seen, assumptions cannot. To assume that a supervisee has administered a diagnostic evaluation tool according to standardized procedures simply because that individual has completed a course in diagnostic evaluation is to risk not knowing for sure whether the supervisee is applying what was learned. To observe the supervisee administer the test is to document those skills through observation. Trainees can become aware of the tendency to make assumptions through visual literacy activities such as (a) watching selected videotaped portions of a therapy session, writing hypothetical assumptions about the entire session, and discussing what is being observed and what is being assumed; (b) debating within dyads the assumptions they might make in response to pictures of interactions; or (c) critiquing peers' narratives of therapeutic scenarios, noting assumptions versus observations.

Inferences. Inferences, or conclusions drawn from facts seen, should also be considered in visual literacy training. Observations can be documented by what was seen; inferences result from seeing only a part of the picture and making conclusions based on just that portion. To infer following a 5-minute observation period that a young client who is uncontrollably charging around the therapy room is always uncooperative, or that the supervisee is unable to manage the child, may result in inappropriate supervisor response (particularly if the client is momentarily reacting to sensitivities to the sugar just consumed in a candy bar and the supervisee is charting the child's reactions, as requested by the child's pediatrician). Activities to train supervisors in awareness and management of inferences might include (a) practice in contrasting observed information with inferred information about pictures (*inference:* "The boy's mother is angry today"; *statement:* "The woman is pointing at the boy who is climbing on the drinking fountain"); (b) identification of prepared statements (*inference or descriptive statement?* "The supervisee did not get enough sleep the night before the meeting"; "The supervisee's head drooped and her eyes closed on three occasions during the meeting"); or (c) role-playing of intervention activities during which the supervisor stops the action periodically to discuss inferences.

Additional Visual Literacy Skills. The final element of a visual literacy training program is the recording, interpreting, and reporting of visual information. Being able to read, write, and interpret visuals requires (a) comprehension and use of descriptive vocabulary (seeing the same picture the writer saw; creating an accurate picture for readers through words); (b) interpretation of visual symbols (understanding the meanings of pictures, images, or spatial relationships and explaining them to others); (c) use of visually-oriented vocabulary ("You saw the value of that activity"; "He has visions of controlling his parents"); (d) understanding of directionality (identifying laterality in mirror images, such as in indirect laryngoscopy or in reverse images on videotapes); and (e) skills of visual memory (immediate and long-term recall of visual information). Activities aimed at strengthening each of these areas, if included in a visual literacy training program, will encourage supervisors to apply visual literacy skills in supervision.

Thus, visual literacy, a major component in observation competence, results from having knowledge about visuals, gaining the skills through training to observe and document visuals, and developing the dispositions of a visually competent observer. Communication Disorders supervisors rely on visual literacy in all roles and need a basis in visual literacy to develop competence in observing nonverbal and verbal behavior.

OBSERVING NONVERBAL BEHAVIOR

Though generally recognized as functionally interrelated and interdependent, nonverbal and verbal communication behaviors may be separated for the purpose of training observation skills. First, nonverbal behavior, a term "commonly used to describe all human communication events which transcend spoken or written words" (Knapp, 1978, p. 38) will be discussed in relation to the supervisor's own performance across the roles of supervision.

Easily taken for granted and often more difficult to observe and record systematically than verbal or linguistic behavior, nonverbal communication may be conveying as much as 80% of the meaning of a message (Thompson, 1973). Nonverbal behaviors may be regarded as positive or negative, obvious or obscure, accurate or inaccurate, essential or confusing. They may be interpreted in many different ways and therefore may significantly affect the outcome of intervention (Goldberg, 1976; Klevans & Volz, 1976). Supervisors monitor their own nonverbal communication while observing the nonverbal behavior of supervisees. Research suggests that supervisees who are rated high use more nonverbal behaviors than supervisees who are rated low and that advanced supervisees use more positive nonverbal communication than do beginning supervisees (Schubert, 1978). Competence in using and observing nonverbal behavior should be emphasized in supervisor training and reviewed at the professional, in-service level.

Supervisory preparation programs should lead students to (a) become aware of nonverbal behavior, (b) gain academic information about nonverbal communication, (c) practice observing nonverbal behaviors in their own environment, (d) practice observing in the clinical environment, (e) practice observing as supervisor trainees, and (f) use observation of nonverbal behavior to effect clinical change as supervisors. The wide range of information available on specific aspects of nonverbal communication should be applied to the client and family, supervisee, and supervisor within each relevant setting or environment.

Awareness and academic study of nonverbal communication include the traditionally studied specific areas of nonverbal behavior: paralinguistics, kinesics, tactile perception, proxemics, chronemics, color, olfactory sense, gustatory sense, objects and artifacts, atmosphere or ambience, silence, organismics, and situation or environment (see chapter 5 for further discussion of nonverbal communication). The following brief notations describe each of these areas in which the supervisor needs to develop observation competence:

- *Paralinguistics:* symbols communicated in variations of vocal quality; auditory nonverbal signals. Includes prosodic features or vocal effects of variations of pitch, loudness, duration, quality, and timing; noticeable changes in intonation, such as teasing, whining, sarcasm; sounds of yawning, crying, laughing.
- *Kinesics:* use of movements to convey messages. Includes body movements and postures, gestures, and facial expressions and eye movements.
  Body movements and postures: positioning of body parts in action and at rest; position shifts; speed and rhythm of movements; movements toward or away from someone or something; body responses that show likes, dislikes, approval, disapproval; posture in general, when sitting, when walking; movements in response to another person.
  Gestures: expressive movements of head or limbs, such as yes/no head shakes or hand clapping, nervous mannerisms such as leg kicking or finger tapping. May support or contradict speaker's verbal message; may encourage or discourage, confuse or clarify, help or hinder.
  Facial expressions and eye movements: posturing of the face to convey a message. Includes smiles, frowns, raised eyebrows, grimaces, winces, lip quivering; relaxed or tense, animated or stoic, concentrating or daydreaming expressions; a receptive, nonjudgmental facial expression maintained during counseling; eye gaze, directed or undirected, mutual, avoiding, or searching; widening or narrowing of pupils.
- *Tactile communication:* communication through touch; developmentally the most primary sense. Touch can be used as a modality inroad in therapy; as a relaxing, calming stimulus; for support, as in a pat on the back; to convey warmth, anxiety, protection, friendliness, or fear; to show desire to touch and be touched, or not to touch or be touched. Includes touching oneself and touching others.
- *Proxemics:* the manipulation of space to send messages between individuals. Includes size and arrangement of setting or room; size and shape of furniture; proximity of individuals (intimate, social, or public distances); combination of seating arrangements; respect for personal space; crowded versus open spacing.
- *Chronemics:* time as a conveyer of messages. Includes time orientation, understanding, and organization; use of and reaction to time pressures; our innate and learned awareness of time; wearing or not wearing a watch; arriving, starting, and ending late or on time.
- *Color:* the use of color in the setting (walls, floor, furniture), in clothing, or in other materials to convey messages.
- *Olfactory sense:* smells used to transfer messages. Includes aromas or odors within the environment, of foods, of seasons; olfactory memory; personal aromas such as body smells, perfumes and deodorants, odors from certain diseases. Smell is used as a sen-

sory inroad in intervention approaches; the accuracy of the sense decreases with aging.
- *Gustatory sense:* signals sent via taste. Includes increased or decreased nutritional intake; gustatory memory; pleasant and unpleasant interpretations. Accuracy of the sense decreases with aging.
- *Objects and artifacts:* message carriers such as clothing, jewelry, eyeglasses and hearing aids, personal possessions, items a client brings to therapy, or professional markers such as name plates or uniforms. May function as supports or distractions.
- *Atmosphere or ambience:* overall communication in a setting; combines the perceived attitudes of the occupants with proxemics, colors, sounds or silence, olfactory messages, and object messages.
- *Silence:* use of oral quiet and body inactivity to transmit messages. May be for listening, waiting, observing, gaining attention, thinking; may express anger, frustration, signal inability to talk or respond; may be used as a counseling response; may convey boredom, discomfort, hostility, reverence, agreement, grief; may be appropriate or inappropriate.
- *Organismics:* the effects of relatively unalterable physical attributes on communication. Includes physical characteristics such as height, weight, eye and skin color, body dimensions, gender, race, age; physically apparent disabilities such as various syndrome characteristics, neurological and orthopedic handicaps, or physical deformities.
- *Situation or environment:* the effects the immediate setting has on communication. Individuals behave differently in different settings; the perceived expectations in a particular setting (home, school, or work) produce characteristic communication patterns.

In all aspects of nonverbal behavior, cultural, gender, and regional differences and patterns abound. Supervisors need to become familiar with the patterns in a particular setting before initiating intervention that interprets or manipulates nonverbal communication. A nonverbal message may be unintentional or unconscious or may be carefully orchestrated. The supervisee may be sending too many or too few nonverbal messages or may be using nonverbal communication that is inappropriate for the context. Agreement between verbal and nonverbal messages is important; the nonverbal message may be more reliable when the two are in conflict. Whereas verbal communication is the primary mode for conveying information, nonverbal communication is the primary mode for the affective component of the meaning. Nonverbal communication provides clues to help the listener interpret the verbal message.

Depending on the purpose for observation, the supervisor may select particular elements of nonverbal behavior to observe. The resulting information, when synthesized with observations of verbal behavior, provides the supervisor with a total picture from which to give supervisees specific feedback.

OBSERVING VERBAL BEHAVIOR

As important as observing nonverbal behavior is learning skills to observe *verbal behavior*. Verbal behavior, the transfer of messages via spoken or written words, is recognized as functionally interrelated and interdependent with nonverbal communication but may be isolated for the purpose of training observation skills.

Observation of verbal behavior receives continual emphasis in clinical training programs, particularly for purposes of identifying or treating specific communication disorders (e.g., "Does the client's speech sound like he has a hearing loss?" "Describe the child's pattern of articulation errors." "Is the client's language age-appropriate in phonology and syntax?"). In supervision training, verbal behavior is observed not only in clients, but also in supervisees (their competence in verbal language, particularly for communication as professionals) and in supervisors themselves (their verbal competence in performing the roles of supervision). (See chapter 5 for a detailed discussion of verbal behavior.) Supervisors should observe the following aspects of verbal behavior in themselves, supervisees, and clients and across the roles of supervision:

- *Quantity of verbal behavior:* the amount of talking within a given time or session. Includes the amount of each person's talk time in relation to that of the others; the amount of listening time in relation to talking time; verbal dominance or equality; use of repetition or reiteration; appropriate or inappropriate length of utterances; consistent or inconsistent quantity.
- *Rate of verbal behavior:* the speed of delivery of verbal language. May be appropriate or inappropriate for the individuals or situation; rapid, slow, varied, or consistent; may enhance or interfere with meaning.
- *Verbal behavior skills:* include articulation, voice, and fluency; morphology, semantics, pragmatics, and syntax; presence or absence of communication disorder. May be appropriate or inappropriate for individuals and situation.
- *Clarity of verbal behavior:* includes clear or vague connotations and denotations; simple or complex forms of the message; complete or incomplete messages.
- *Accuracy of verbal behavior:* includes reporting facts as given rather than altered; distinguishing observations from inferences and assumptions; reporting events in correct order or sequence.
- *Positive/negative attitudes conveyed:* includes positive versus negative forms of statements (*negative:* "Don't sit on the table"; *positive:* "Sit on the chair"); expressed interest or disinterest, support or lack of support; sympathy, empathy, ridicule, acceptance, nonacceptance, judgment, criticism, help, candor.
- *Use of titles or names:* how individuals address each other. Includes markers of respect, formality/informality, culture, age, profession, role or relationship (e.g., "teacher," "father"); may show influences of setting (e.g., school, hospital, handicamp).

As with nonverbal behavior, observers consider cultural, gender, and regional differences and patterns when observing verbal behavior. Verbal language observed may be recorded via audiotape or videotape, and the resulting transcriptions may be analyzed through various handwritten or computer systems. Interaction analyses, in which exchanges between two or more people are identified and systematically studied, produce the most usable information when they include both nonverbal and verbal behaviors (Schubert, 1978). Thus, supervisors combine nonverbal and verbal behavioral information to develop a whole picture on which to base supervision strategies.

MODES

Modes of observation include live observation, closed circuit television, telecommunication systems, audiotape and videotape recording, and written plans for programming. Supervisors use various modes, selecting each according to the purpose of the observation and including all over a period of time to obtain a complete picture of the supervisee and the intervention program.

Live Observation

Live observation, observing the occurrence on site at the time it happens, may be done inside the room or through an observation window. When observing in the room, the supervisor elects to be a participant or nonparticipant, depending on the purpose of the observation. As a participant, the supervisor becomes a part of the therapy interaction and can thus influence directly or even control the situation; the participant can model responses, demonstrate techniques, or support the supervisee. During certain audiological assessments, the supervisor may need to be situated physically close to the supervisee to provide immediate intervention (Rassi, 1987). As a nonparticipant, the supervisor sits apart from the therapy situation, trying not to distract the client, and is not included in the interaction; this approach gives the supervisor a better opportunity to record information and prepare written feedback, although the supervisee and client may perceive themselves as being under close scrutiny ("Be careful, the boss is watching"). Because both participant and nonparticipant approaches are intrusive, supervisees and clients alike may behave atypically, demonstrating clinical reactivity. This factor of clients and supervisees responding to the presence of the supervisor is significant in the evaluation of observation data (Anderson, 1988). Observing within the room, however, whether as participant or nonparticipant, gives the supervisor specific information that would not be obtained from outside the room. Thus, live observation within the room is an important supervision tool for gaining a total picture of the supervisee's therapeutic program.

Live observation through an observation window (one-way mirror) provides a broad view of the physical area, does not disturb the session, allows the supervisor to focus on specifics without having to rely on the positioning of a camera lens, permits detachment from the ongoing situation, makes written recording easier, and lets the supervisor comment on the session to other supervisees or the client's family who may also be observing. In addition, the supervisor may give oral feedback while audiotape recording the session from the observation room, thus providing the supervisee with feedback recorded simultaneously with the session. If participants prefer immediate feedback, the supervisor may use an FM transmitter to communicate with the supervisee, who wears a compatible receiver. Hagler and Holdgrafer (1987) used this approach to demonstrate the effectiveness of immediate feedback for supervisees; they advocated using immediate as well as delayed feedback to help supervisees change behavior. Poor equipment quality or maintenance may limit the supervisor's observation. Although an observation window provides reliable visual information, auditory input is only as good as the sound system, and supervisors may need to supplement their data with live in-the-room observation.

Closed Circuit Television

Closed circuit television (CCTV) is an increasingly popular mode of observation. A well-designed CCTV system can be a nonintrusive vehicle for live observation and for automatic or unattended videorecording. The supervisor may receive the live session on a monitor located in an office, in a room where the client's family is simultaneously conferencing, or in the classroom where a large group of students can observe. CCTV can be used to observe more than one function at a time; the supervisor can switch channels back and forth between a case history interview and the simultaneous examination of the client, watch the audiology student's testing procedures and the client's responses on a split screen, or observe several different therapy sessions scheduled at the same time. Unless the system provides a means of direct communication between the supervisee and supervisor, such as a telephone, intercom, "bug-in-the-ear," or FM system, the supervisor cannot provide on-site suggestions or demonstrate techniques and must rely on some form of delayed feedback. Many supervisees prefer the CCTV mode to having the supervisor interrupt the session by coming into the therapy room. The attitudes of supervisors toward the CCTV system (is it "a 'Big Brother' surveillance" or "an effective, efficient, and helpful mode of observing"?) are the most significant variables in its acceptance by clients and supervisees. The supervisor should monitor the supervisees' explanations of the purposes of the system to clients and their families and should ensure that appropriate permission-to-videotape forms have been signed by client and/or family and supervisee. For automatic or unattended videorecording, some CCTV systems can be programmed to record during certain times in specific locations, providing the supervisee and supervisor with systematically obtained observation records. The advantages of CCTV systems are many; the most frequently expressed disadvantages include restriction of focus (the camera lens generally provides a macrofocus, single-position view unless a focusing remote control is used by the clinician or supervisor), limitation of space that can be used within the room (the clinician may need to confine the client to a particular area in order to stay on camera), and dependence on electronic equipment that may fail periodically.

Telecommunication

Telecommunication is the newest mode in clinical supervision, although long-distance, two-way auditory and visual communication has long been used in Communication Disorders to deliver academic information and clinical services (Vaughn, Kramer, Lightfoot, Faucett, & Tidwell, 1982). Telecommunication for observation is necessary given the growing needs of Clinical Fellowship Year supervision, corporate and private practice supervisors who must travel long distances to supervise employees, regional satellite centers that provide services under the direction of a centrally located administrator, and geographically widespread off-campus practicum students. Training in the use of telecommunication devices is now mandatory in preservice programs. The supervisor and supervisee may maintain contact and exchange information through direct telephone conversations, computer interactions via modem, satellite television transmissions, or a combination of these modes. A supervision conference on the telephone is enhanced when the supervisee visually transmits the audiogram, the page of data, the lesson plan, or a videotaped segment of the client to the supervisor during the conversation. A supervisee in a rural area may depend on satellite to transmit a speech sample and view of an oral mechanism to the supervisor, who responds in consultation or makes a copy to relay to a cleft palate team for additional review. Training in the use of telecommunication for supervision includes use and maintenance of the equipment as well as observation competence.

Audiotape Recording

Audiotape recording (ATR) continues to be a convenient, inexpensive, widely and frequently used mode of observation recording for supervisee and supervisor, particularly in evaluation (e.g., speech and language sampling), therapy (sampling, analysis, maintaining data for pre- and postprogram comparison), and record keeping. In training programs, an audiotape submitted with written lesson plans for intervention sessions provides an additional basis for supervisory feedback. The supervisor learns to sample sessions on audiotape and receives valuable supplementary information from listening to parts of sessions. Some supervisors choose to respond orally, directly on the submitted audiotape, giving the supervisee another type of input. Audiotape recording allows supervisors to listen to sessions at convenient times and to replay them over and over (particularly useful when recording data). Audiotape helps listeners focus on verbal behavior, eliminating most nonverbal data. Tapes are conveniently small and lightweight.

Disadvantages supervisors report in audiotape use include difficulty in reconstructing the context unless the supervisee has used glossing (telling about the environment or events as they are happening, clarifying oral language that might be unclear without nonverbal behaviors accompanying it); restriction to only the auditory channel for analysis; and limitations of tape and recorder quality. Commercial audiotapes continue to be helpful, particularly in teaching beginning Communication Disorders students to recognize particular disorders. For geographically isolated supervisees who wish to send supervisors a taped sample of a communication disorder or a particular session for consultation or feedback, audiotapes are easy to record, convenient to mail, and economical.

Videotape Recording

With the growing presence of videocassette recorders in professional, business, and home settings, the relatively low cost of cameras, playback systems, and tapes, and the ease of management of VHS equipment, videotape recording (VTR) has become the most desired mode of recording communication behavior. The standard 1/2-inch VHS system, which at present is more easily available and more frequently used than the Beta, 3/4-inch, and camcorder systems, can meet the needs of supervisors and has unlimited potential in supervision.

For record keeping, supervisors may wish to videotape conferences with supervisees for later analysis (self-confrontation, verbal or nonverbal behavior analysis, interaction analysis) or record maintenance (particularly for supervisees who are having difficulties in clinical practicum or for those whose records need to show that they have been given specific information). A videofile of clients sampling various disorders, ages, and sites is a valuable resource for clinical education and administration and may be used in supervisory staff meetings, in-service programs, and classrooms. Also useful for supervisees in university settings are videotapes contributed by alumni detailing their employment sites, professional endeavors, and research projects; requests for such videotapes from alumni employed in a variety of settings often meet with enthusiastic response.

Supervisors may use videotape to maintain a record of their own professional accomplishments, whether to demonstrate that they have met specific goals or objectives or for an eventual video resume to supplement their written resume. As an administrator, the supervisor may screen candidates for a position by viewing videotapes they have prepared (see p. 123). The supervisor may even distribute a videotape of the facility, staff, and environs to publicize an available position or to locate only those candidates who would be seriously interested in a personal interview. Sending a similar videotape to a prospective employee before an interview will familiarize the candidate with the setting and staff and will enhance the quality of the interview.

Supervisors find numerous public relations uses for VTR, including publicity and support for programming, public education (dispersing information about communication disorders or using a videotaped tour of a setting to inform the public of available services), and fundraising. In addition, supervisors may find that a video record is a time efficient way to inventory the contents (equipment, materials, and furniture) of an office, department, clinic, or practice for insurance purposes.

Videotape recording is essential for establishing data bases in clinical supervision. Indispensible in analyzing supervisory conferences, videotape records allow researchers to observe nonverbal as well as verbal behavior and can provide frame-by-frame comparisons. VTR is an important self-analysis tool for supervisors, particularly for examining supervisee-supervisor interaction over time. Maintaining longitudinal records of clients (e.g., taping a 5-minute segment of a cerebral palsied child's communication every month over 5 years) will provide valuable material for future in-service programs or other clinical education activities. Supervisees will develop self-analysis skills and self-confidence by keeping videotape records of their clinical growth; when they begin clinical practicum they should record 15 to 20 minutes of their interaction with a client, then add to the tape at the end of each semester of their preparation program. In the Administrator role, supervisors may tape newly developed programs, different supervisee styles, or portions of staff meetings for a longitudinal record. In the Professional role, supervisors may want to maintain videotapes of their presentations at professional meetings over the years, charting their individual professional development, or may establish videotaped records of the history of an organization, including officers, financial status, and programs.

Supervisors depend on VTR for interactive teaching; video equipment can help train supervisees and supervisors in verbal and nonverbal communication at both the preservice and in-service levels. For clinical education at the preprofessional level, videotapes supplement instructor demonstrations and allow for group or individual self-paced learning. Possible topics include clinical observation, hearing assessment, hearing amplification selection and fitting, administration of speech and language assessment tools, phonetic transcription, therapy techniques, and management and clinical decision making. At the in-service level, commercial videotapes of information about new techniques, tests, and therapy kits, new surgical or medical treatments, or newly identified syndromes may be used for staff meetings or in-service programming or may circulate among the staff for individual viewing.

Interactive Video Discs

Video discs are in limited use in supervision, although video disc technology is beginning to emerge in the clinical process. Projects for using interactive video discs with lipreading learners, hearing-impaired children, and mentally handicapped children have been directed toward educational functions (Behrmann, 1984). Possible uses in observation include training supervisors in observation skills, recording and storing observed clinical information (e.g., samples of various disorders), and long-distance sharing of supervisory information. The present high cost of video disc equipment, especially in the production of discs, limits the usefulness of this mode, particularly when compared with the cost of VHS equipment and tapes.

Written Plans

Finally, supervisors can obtain information about a supervisee's competence in observation or a client's status through written plans: program plans, daily or weekly lesson plans with evaluative information, anecdotal notes from diagnostic sessions, progress notes, charts. Does the supervisee record observation information objectively? Has the supervisee recorded the visuals as clearly and succinctly as possible? Supervisees who tend to be stronger in using auditory information than in using visual information may need particular guidance in developing appropriate lesson plan formats. As recommended by Anderson (1988), joint supervisor-supervisee planning during a conference can provide the foundation for the observation and result in higher quality written plans.

The modes of observation presented here give supervisors several options for obtaining observation information. Each mode has advantages and disadvantages; each provides different types of information. Thus, the mode or modes appropriate for a particular observation depend on the kind of information the supervisor is seeking.

SYSTEMATIC OBSERVATION

In addition to selecting the appropriate modes for observation, Communication Disorders supervisors choose a systematic approach for observing events and behaviors to gain the most thorough, accurate, and representative information. Like the mode, the system or method of observation selected depends on the purpose of the observation. An observation plan includes time elements (frequency and duration of observation), whether the event is to be prearranged or spontaneous, the scope and pattern of focus, and whether the observation should be guided or solo. To learn to select the most appropriate system for observing a particular supervisee, event, or site, supervisors need specific training that will help them set the observation plan, lead them to practice various patterns of observing, and give them experience in critical observation.

Frequency

Frequency of observation, or how often the supervisor observes the supervisee, depends on the setting, the supervisee's clinical competence, the supervisor's assessment of the supervisee's training needs, and the purpose of the observation. A supervisor who is primarily functioning as an administrator may observe a certified audiologist or speech-language pathologist only once or twice a year, whereas in a clinical preparation program a supervisor will meet or exceed the ASHA minimal standard of observing 25% of clinical management activities. The purpose of the observation directly dictates the frequency. For example, to see whether a supervisee is maintaining a specific behavior over a 6-week period, the supervisor would want to observe every week. A training program supervisor concerned about a particular supervisee and the resulting quality of service might observe every session. An administrator who wished to observe before completing an annual employee performance evaluation might schedule an observation once a year.

Duration

Duration of observation, how long the supervisor observes during a particular session, also depends on setting, the supervisee's clinical competence, the perceived needs of the supervisee, and especially the purpose for observation. An on-site visit or a videotape viewing may last from a few minutes to the whole session. If the supervisor simply wishes to get a sense of what is going on during the session, then 3 to 5 minutes is sufficient (Schubert, 1978). If information is needed about a particular behavior, such as how often the supervisee uses verbal positive reinforcement, then the entire session may need to be observed. Any time during the session is appropriate for spot-checking except the first and last 5 minutes; however, if the supervisor wants information about the sessions' openings and closings, then those are the portions that should be observed. The longer the duration of the observation, the more data are obtained in a quantitative sense, but shorter observations are likely to yield data similar in quality, especially when the frequency is regular. As with frequency, requirements of the setting may dictate the duration of observation, particularly in clinical preparation programs where ASHA standards of direct supervision must be met.

Prearranged versus Spontaneous

Both prearranged and spontaneous observations are important in the supervisor's information gathering, because each type yields different information. If the supervisor arranges to observe a particular session or portion, the session may reflect what the supervisee thinks the supervisor wants to see (therapy done in a particular way, reinforcement reflecting the supervisor's philosophy, audiological tests sequenced in the order that the supervisor uses) when at other times the supervisee may be using another, perhaps even more effective, approach. Because the supervisee is prepared, however, the supervisor may have the opportunity to see the optimum performance, the supervisee and client at their best. Supervisees' anxiety about the visit, self-confidence in their preparation, or concern at being evaluated may need to be factored into the information obtained. With prearranged visits, the supervisor and supervisee can plan together to observe specific behaviors and use the same recording systems so that they can compare observations readily at a later conference.

Spontaneous visits, when the supervisor drops

in unannounced or uses closed circuit television for undistracting observation, provide a more accurate picture of a routine session. The risk of not seeing clients or supervisees at their prepared best may be offset by a later prearranged visit. Both types of visits should be included in a systematic observation approach.

Focused

Developing a focus pattern for observing will increase the supervisor's efficiency. Typically such a routine will include scanning, microfocus, and macrofocus in various patterns throughout an observation. Scanning, using both eyes and ears to take in the whole scene quickly, is frequently the first step of a supervisor's routine. Next, the supervisor uses appropriate micro-macro patterns, zooming in and out like the lens of a camera, to obtain the specific kinds of information needed. For a complete picture, both microfocus and macrofocus need to be used, either within one session or over several sessions; the supervisor synthesizes the total picture from a number of different focused samples.

Supervisor trainees benefit from opportunities to practice focusing and to develop their own patterns so that focusing eventually becomes automatic; when trained to use their own system, supervisors need not worry about inadvertently leaving out a crucial focus and can observe efficiently and reliably. Exercises in focusing may include (a) videotaped diagnostic and therapeutic sessions in which students are directed toward certain views; (b) work on identifying personal biases; (c) self-paced lessons to identify specific occurrences and characteristics in ongoing live sessions using macrofocus and microfocus; (d) practice in blocking out extraneous visual and auditory information; (e) practice in concentrating on different behaviors (e.g., nonverbal, verbal), contexts, persons, communication characteristics (syntax, semantics), or directions (left to right, right to left); (f) practice with various patterns or combinations of focusing (e.g., scanning–macrofocus–microfocus–different microfocus–macrofocus, with 2 to 3 minutes per focus); (g) practice in switching focusing patterns to build flexibility; (h) supervisor-to-supervisor discussions and idea exchanges; and (i) use of patterns in supervisory experiences.

Guided versus Solo

Supervisor trainees need both guided and solo observation opportunities. In guided observation, which may occur in a training program classroom or one-to-one while observing a live or videotaped session, the trainee is directed to observe certain aspects. The direction may be oral or written and may consist of goals and objectives, lesson plans, test or history forms, or specific instructions (e.g., "Watch how the clinician keeps the child on task during the naming of colors"). An effective way to demonstrate micro- and macrofocus is to talk about something as it is going on, encouraging the observers to tune in to specifics; an oral commentary from the supervisor on a videotaped session replayed without the sound is highly effective in helping the development of visual focus. Audiotaped sessions with annotated scripts that observers can follow are helpful in developing auditory focusing skills (e.g., "Listen to the audiologist's directions to the woman who is having her hearing tested; are the directions clearly stated?"). Oral or written preparation of observers just before a viewing (e.g., "When I turn on the tape, let's all look at the client's facial expression," or "Read the first objective; now watch this section to see if the objective is met") increases success in learning to focus. Directed focus activities can also center on macrofocus aspects (e.g., "Watch the first 5 minutes of the tape; is the session positive? negative? communicative?"). When observation is guided individually, the supervisor can adapt focusing activities to the specific needs of the supervisor trainee (e.g., "You commented that the clinician does not seem to have good rapport with this client; what nonverbal behaviors do you observe that support your comment?"). Whether in a group or individual situation, the supervisor guides the observer through the observation, providing preparation, clarification, direction for focusing, and immediate information and response; as the supervisee gains proficiency in observing, the supervisor decreases the amount of direct guidance.

In solo observation, the supervisor or supervisor trainee views a live or taped session alone and highlights, records, or responds to the occurrences. The observer independently determines focus based on the purpose of the observation.

By learning and practicing the elements of systematic observation, each supervisor develops a system of observation that (a) allows efficiency and thoroughness; (b) centers on the purpose for the observation; (c) includes frequency, duration, a balanced focus, prearrangement or spontaneity, and guided or solo observation; and (d) yields information that can be synthesized to produce the whole clinical picture. This gathering of detailed observation, however, requires a method or system of recording.

OBSERVATION RECORDING SYSTEMS

The *systematic recording* of intervention (events, occurrences, behaviors, data, interactions, and analyses) is habitual in professional clinicians. Communication Disorders supervision employs two kinds of recording systems: supervisees use one kind in clinical work, and supervisors use another to record supervision occurrences. Observation recording systems, which are organized procedures for written documentation of occurrences and behaviors, are well reported in the literature. Numerous systems have been developed and widely used; Simon and Boyer reported approximately 78 category systems for observation in use prior to 1967, and Schubert reviewed additional observational evaluation systems (Schubert, 1978). Anderson (1988) described the currently used methods for recording and analyzing observational data, including interaction analysis systems; she recommended that supervisors try various systems and pursue research designed to improve present approaches. Clinical training programs tend to use their own formats (their original, favorite standard, or adapted system) based on the needs of the program, the philosophies and biases of the supervisory staff, and the perceived strengths and limitations of the students. Formats specifically for observation in supervision generally take the form of specific ratings, narrative data, checklists, timing, or tallying.

Ratings

Rating scales are groups of symbols used to indicate relationships. The observer rates or assigns a symbol to something in relation to a standard or norm, a preset scale for measurement, or established guidelines. Symbols assigned may be numbers representing percentage or percentile, grades A to F, numbers ranged on a competency grid, and so on. For rating observation information in supervision, any type of symbol that is meaningful to the supervisor and supervisee is appropriate. Supervisor trainees who practice using various symbols to rate observation information learn to use rating techniques flexibly and adaptably.

Rankings, which order information relative to a base, are a type of rating. A rank indicates something in relationship to something else; percentile, percentage, and certain descriptors (e.g., maximum, moderate, or minimum supervision) are examples. A priority ranking from *most important* to *least important* may help organize supervisory feedback. Rankings for which reference points are defined specifically and concretely (e.g., "number of hours per week this supervisor spends in each of the supervisory roles in a full-time employment block of 40 hours") may be more objective than those whose criteria leave more room for judgment (e.g., "the performance of this supervisee in relation to all the other supervisees at this hospital within the past 5 years" or "the supervisee's performance in relation to supervisor's expectations"). Either kind may generate a useful hierarchy. Supervisors may use ranking to evaluate either themselves or supervisees.

Narrative Data

Narrative data are written descriptions (phrases, sentences, paragraphs, and journal entries). Formats include anecdotal descriptions; ecological narratives; specimen records; photographic records; ethnological, sociological, or psychoanalytic descriptions and field notes; audiotape and videotape recordings; and activity logs.

Anecdotal descriptions tell about situations and events in narrative form. They are objective stories relatively devoid of judgments or evaluations. Their purpose is to recreate in writing for someone who was not present an action, situation, or person that the supervisor observed.

Ecological narratives describe environments without describing the interactions of people within the environment. If a supervisee visits the home of a client, a description of the home itself would be an ecological one. In the Administrator role, the supervisor might write an ecological description of a new clinic setting as part of the request for a new facility.

Specimen records are objects that are meaningful parts of the observation, items picked up from the environment, such as children's drawings, homework pages from school, somebody's hearing aid that got chewed by the dog, a letter, or a completed job application form.

Photographic records include cinefluorographic films, pictures of ultrasound studies and spectrographic samples, still photos (commercially developed or polaroid prints), movies and slides, and x-rays. A single photographic record can be used to support or refute a diagnosis, to serve as baseline prior to treatment, or to demonstrate unique features of a disorder. Taken over time, photographic records serve as valuable means for comparison.

Anthropological or ethnological descriptions include the context or setting (e.g., the home, culture, neighborhood, barrio, classroom, hospital), the people in it, and the people-environment interactions. *Sociological descriptions* also include the context and the people in it but may be more confined to the close or immediate group and its interactions. *Psychoanalytic descriptions* are more behaviorally based and interpret or judge people's behaviors in relation to their environment. *Field notes* are descriptions or notes written on the spot (in the classroom or therapy area, during the staff meeting) rather than after the fact.

Audiotape and videotape recordings are electronically recorded, dated tapes of partial or entire evaluation or therapy sessions, conferences, or counseling sessions. They are useful for comparisons to document growth or change in condition; for supporting programs and plans (a videotape of a cross-generational program can help show field readers why a gerontology grant should be renewed); for clinical education using commercial videotapes that demonstrate new tests or materials; or as part of a data base of recorded supervisory interactions for later analysis and teaching.

Activity logs are journals used to keep track of specific events over time. Organized according to a preset plan, logs might include what supervisees are doing with certain materials or strategies, what locations the supervisor has observed, or which units of study are being used in therapeutic situations. In narrative form and kept regularly, logs are especially valuable for reference in long-term planning.

Narrative descriptions of the supervisee's physical condition and appearance (health, extent of physical limitations, professional dress) may be appropriate in tracking change over time. The supervisor should use objective terms and statements when preparing the narrative (e.g., "The supervisee coughed and sneezed approximately every 2 to 3 minutes throughout the therapy session," rather than "The supervisee's allergies interfered with the session.")

Checklists

Checklists are an objective method of recording information according to preset criteria. Efficiency, completeness, and conciseness are the primary advantages of checklists; the predominant disadvantage is lack of flexibility. Checklist responses are easily transferred to a data base or can be quickly scanned visually. Commercially produced checklists and supervisor-prepared, situation-specific checklists fall into similar categories: static descriptors, action descriptors, discrete event records, standardized situation responses, contrived situation responses, and performance records.

A checklist of *static descriptors* records characteristics readily observed, such as height and weight, hair and eye color, use of glasses, hearing aid, or leg brace, and so on. The supervisor quickly progresses through the checklist, checking presence or absence and sometimes adding description, such as type of hearing aid.

A checklist of *action descriptors* includes characteristics of movement, mobility, or behavior, such as gait, ambulatory or nonambulatory mobility, active or passive behavior. The reader may quickly scan the completed checklist to receive information efficiently.

Discrete event records are checklists of small portions of situations or behaviors; they provide a concise way to record the results of a microfocus. For example, if documenting seizure behavior, the supervisee can quickly chart factors associated with the occurrence (e.g., time of day, what was happening before the seizure, how long the seizure lasted, what the client did during the seizure, what happened afterwards). If the supervisee's responses during the client's seizure are being recorded, the supervisor can quickly chart what the supervisee does or says before, during, and after the seizure.

Checklists of *standardized situation responses* give the supervisor an efficient way to note the supervisee's performance in standardized situations (screening hearing, administering a standardized test), or in certain places (in a particular classroom with a variety of clients, in an office).

With *contrived situation responses,* the supervisor sets up specific situations to elicit desired responses and then records the responses on a checklist. Role-playing, using a particular meeting format, or following a script are ways for the supervisor to maximize the chance of producing the desired responses.

Performance records are checklist components used on a number of commercially produced checklists as well as the typical Individual Education Plan (IEP). Test protocols and report cards could also be considered performance records. The supervisor can quickly progress through the checklist, recording whether the supervisee did or did not perform each task (e.g., begin the session on time, explain fee schedule to family, have client sign the medical release form). Performance records kept over a month or semester or year provide even more valuable comparative information.

Timing

Observation timing includes a wide range of possibilities, from the macrofocus of examining an entire process to the microfocus of a few seconds. Timing records kept on a macrofocus plan might document the whole therapeutic intervention program (from referral to discharge for a client), the entire training process of the supervisee (from first course or client to completion of graduate program), or the supervisee's employment record (from initial interview through resignation). Records kept systematically over a significant period of time are valuable resources for supervisors in all supervision roles.

Microfocus observation records might cover a one-time diagnostic or therapy session, a specific part of a session (one activity, occurrence, or short timed segment), or specific responses, such as the client's diadochokinetic rate or length of phoneme prolongations or the supervisee's reaction time latency.

Timing thus includes observing within the confines of time as well as recording the timing of occurrences and behaviors. A watch with a second hand or digital second counter or a stopwatch is needed to time occurrences.

Tallying

Tallying is the marking or counting of categorized occurrences or behaviors. Supervisors choose which behaviors to observe and then mark each time they occur within the set observation period, thus deriving a numerical value for their frequency. Tallying can be used comparatively (e.g., the supervisee talked 17 times, the client talked 4 times during the first 5 minutes of the session). Summaries of tallying may be raw numbers or percentages.

The observation recording systems presented in this section are ways for the supervisor to show the supervisee what is happening in a situation and to document the occurrences. Supervisor trainees should practice using various recording systems so as to develop a repertoire of options for supervision in different circumstances, roles, and employment settings.

SUMMARY Observation competence, the ability to apply observational knowledge and skills to all dimensions of behavior, is an essential basis for the Communication Disorders supervisor. It develops from training and experience. An observation training program includes information and practice of skills in visual literacy, nonverbal and verbal behaviors, modes for observing, systematic observation, and use of recording systems. The supervisor trainee progresses from guided observation to becoming an independent, self-evaluating, competent observer who uses observation competence in all roles of supervision.

APPLICATIONS Discussion Topics
1. Discuss the concept of visual literacy and why a Communication Disorders supervisor must be visually literate.
2. Discuss your personal biases. Identify how your biases might affect your ability to observe.
3. Discuss the differences between CCTV and videotape recordings. When is CCTV more valuable than videotape recording?
4. Discuss why a supervisor should use different observation modes (e.g., videotape, live observation, CCTV, observation window, audiotape).
5. Discuss the advantages and disadvantages of each mode of observation.

Laboratory Experiences
1. Try different kinds of observational recording systems. List the advantages and disadvantages of each to supervisors and supervisees.
2. Develop a proficiency-based training program to teach supervisors and supervisees to use videotaping equipment.

3. Design activities for self-confrontation training of supervisees and supervisors.
4. Develop a video library of supervision conferences for demonstration in training.
5. Develop your personal plan for systematic observation.

Research Projects

1. Compare observation information recorded on a checklist with that recorded in anecdotal, narrative format using a 10-minute videotape of a supervision conference.
2. Study supervisors' macro and microfocus patterns in relation to their personal biases.
3. Compare narrative accounts of the same nonverbal behavior as observed (a) live in the room and (b) through a CCTV system.
4. Compare and contrast the performance of a specific observation skill by two groups of supervisor trainees, one group trained through guided observations and the other through solo observations.
5. Study supervisees' preferred modes for receiving observational feedback (e.g., in writing, supervisory conferences, audiotaped messages).

REFERENCES

American Speech-Language-Hearing Association. (1984). *Accreditation of educational programs in speech-language pathology and audiology.* Rockville, MD: ASHA Educational Standards Board.

American Speech-Language-Hearing Association. (1985). Clinical supervision in speech-language pathology and audiology (position statement). *Asha, 27* (6), 57–60.

Anderson, J. (1981). Training of supervisors in speech-language pathology and audiology. *Asha, 23,* 77–82.

Anderson, J. (1988). *The supervisory process in speech-language pathology and audiology.* San Diego: Little, Brown/College-Hill Press.

Behrmann, M. (Ed.). (1984). *Handbook of microcomputers in special education.* San Diego: College-Hill Press.

Boehm, A., & Weinberg, R. (1977). *The classroom observer: A guide for developing observation skills.* New York: Teachers College Press, Columbia University.

Cartwright, C., & Cartwright, G. (1974). *Developing observation skills.* New York: McGraw-Hill.

Dowling, S. (1981). Observational analysis: Procedures for training coders and data collection. *Journal of the National Student Speech and Hearing Association, 9,* 82–88.

Dowling, S. (1984). Clinical evaluation: A comparison of self, self with videotape, peers, and supervisors. *The Clinical Supervisor, 2*(3), 9–17.

Farmer, S. S. (1981). Providing a visual literacy awareness training program for communicative disorders specialists. Unpublished manuscript.

Farmer, S. S. (1982, March). *Visual literacy: Information and training program for communicative disorders specialists.* Paper presented at the American Speech-Language-Hearing Association South Central Regional Conference, Colorado Springs, CO.

Farmer, S. S. (1987). Visual literacy and the clinical supervisor. *The Clinical Supervisor, 5*(1), 45–71.

Goldberg, S. A. (1976, November). *The effect of nonverbal behaviors upon clinical evaluations.* Paper presented at the annual convention of the American Speech and Hearing Association, Houston, TX.

Golper, L., McMahon, J., & Gordon, M. (1976, November). *The use of interaction analysis for training in observation.* Paper presented at the annual convention of the American Speech and Hearing Association, Houston, TX.

Gonzales, D. (1985). *Critical observation: A training program for beginning communicative disorders students.* Unpublished Master's thesis, New Mexico State University, Las Cruces.

Grijalva, L. (1982). *A training program to develop observation skills in beginning clinicians.* Unpublished Master's thesis, New Mexico State University, Las Cruces.

Guinty, C., & Scudder, R. (1980, November). *Effects of training on observers' ability to count nonverbal behaviors.* Paper presented at the annual convention of the American Speech-Language-Hearing Association, Detroit, MI.

Hagler, P., & Holdgrafer, G. (1987). Effects of supervisory feedback on clinician and client discourse participation. In S. Farmer (Ed.), *Clinical supervision: A coming of age. Proceedings of a national conference on supervision* (pp. 106–111). Las Cruces: New Mexico State University.

Harris, R. A. (1979, November). *A self-teaching, programmed approach to preclinical observation.* Paper presented at the annual convention of the American Speech-Language-Hearing Association, Atlanta, GA.

Harvey, J. (1980). *A program to develop observation skill in graduate student clinical supervisors.* Unpublished Master's thesis, New Mexico State University, Las Cruces.

Irwin, R., & Nickels, A. (1970). The use of audiovisual films in supervised observation. *Asha, 31,* 363–367.

Jaggar, A., & Smith-Burke, M. T. (Eds.). (1985). *Observing the language learner.* Newark, DE: International Reading Association.

Klevans, D., & Volz, H. (1976, November). *The nonverbal behavior system: A procedure for evaluating clinical interactions.* Poster session presented at the annual convention of the American Speech and Hearing Association, Houston, TX.

Klevans, D., Volz, H., & Friedman, R. (1981). A comparison of experiential and observational approaches for enhancing the interpersonal communication skills of speech-language pathology students. *Journal of Speech and Hearing Disorders, 46,* 208–213.

Knapp, M. (1978). *Nonverbal communication in human interaction* (2nd ed.). New York: Holt, Rinehart & Winston.

Kunze, L. H. (1967). Program for training in behavioral observation. In Miner, A. (Ed.). A symposium: Improving supervision of clinical practicum. *Asha, 9,* 471–481.

Lougeay-Mottinger, J., Harris, M., & Stillman, R. (1987). Use of a videotape coding system to change clinician behavior. In S. Farmer (Ed.), *Clinical supervision: A coming of age. Proceedings of a national conference on supervision* (pp. 86–91). Las Cruces: New Mexico State University.

Peaper, R., & Mercaitis, P. (1987). The nature of narrative written feedback provided to student clinicians: A descriptive study. In S. Farmer (Ed.)., *Clinical supervision: A coming of age. Proceedings of a national conference on supervision* (pp. 138–143). Las Cruces: New Mexico State University.

Rassi, J. (1985). Comparing methodologies of clinical instruction and observation: A supervisors' exchange. *SUPERvision, 9*(1), 2–9.

Rassi, J. (1987). The uniqueness of audiology supervision. In M. Crago & M. Pickering (Eds.), *Supervision in human communication disorders: Perspectives on a process* (pp. 31–54). San Diego: Little, Brown/College-Hill Press.

Roberts, J., & McCready, V. (1987). Different clinical perspectives of good and poor therapy sessions. *Journal of Speech and Hearing Research, 30,* 335–342.

Rowen, B. (1973). *The children we see: An observational approach to child study.* New York: Holt, Rinehart & Winston.

Runyan, S., & Seal, B. (1985). A comparison of supervisors' ratings while observing a language remediation session. *The Clinical Supervisor, 3*(2), 61–75.

Schubert, G. (1978). *An introduction to clinical supervision in speech pathology.* St. Louis: Warren H. Green.

Smith, K., & Mawdsley, B. (1987). Analysis in the supervisory process. In S. Farmer (Ed.), *Clinical supervision: A coming of age. Proceedings of a national conference on supervision* (pp. 164–175). Las Cruces: New Mexico State University.

Stallings, J. (1977). *Learning to look: A handbook on classroom observation and teaching models.* Belmont, CA: Wadsworth.

Stubbs, M., & Delamont, S. (Eds.). (1976). *Explorations in classroom observation.* New York: John Wiley.

Thompson, J. (1973). *Beyond words: Nonverbal communication in the classroom.* New York: Citation Press.

Vaughn, G., Kramer, J., Lightfoot, R., Faucett, R., & Tidwell, A. (1982, March). *TEL-Communicology, REMATE Computer and SPACE Devices.* Paper presented at the South Central Regional Conference of the American Speech-Language-Hearing Association, Colorado Springs, CO.

7
Decision Making: The Science

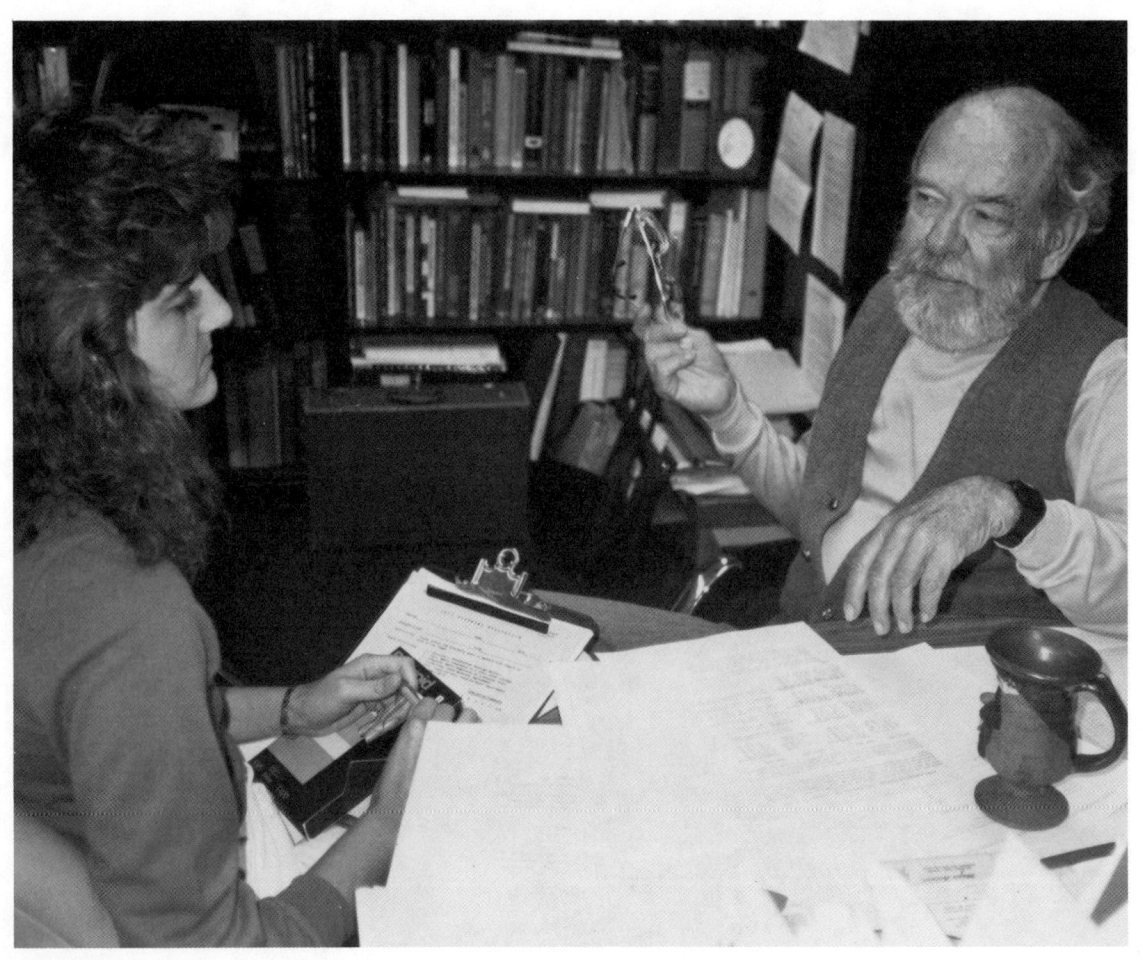

CRITICAL CONCEPTS

Decision making:
- ☐ *incorporates a number of theories and models.*
- ☐ *requires a five-step analysis.*
- ☐ *applies to all five supervision domains and roles.*
- ☐ *reduces the uncertainty associated with outcomes.*
- ☐ *is systematic.*

OUTLINE

INTRODUCTION
THE MODEL
DECISION ANALYSIS
   Probability
   States of Nature
   Utility and Value
   Alternative Actions
   Outcomes
   Restatement
   Information Processing
   The Decision Axis
   Signal Detection Theory
   Optimal Decision
   Risk
DECISION MAKING
SUMMARY
APPLICATIONS

INTRODUCTION

Consider the following scenario: Your clinicians had requested an in-service workshop by the currently popular expert in language disorders. You had made the arrangements and paid the consultant's fee and expenses from your already tight operating budget. The workshop had been a good one; your clinicians' responses had been positive; during the workshop, the consultant had been wise enough to have your clinicians practice the techniques she advocated. All told, it looked like a good investment.

    As you made your routine visits to your clinicians, you found that the therapy in progress showed little or no application of the procedures the consultant had presented. The game boards and spinners were still out. The clients' rates of response weren't being controlled. The reinforcement schedules didn't match the clients' performance levels. What had seemed to be a certain payoff in change of therapy procedures had not taken place.

    In most instances, we can make decisions without an extensive analysis because the best choice is clear to us or the decision isn't important enough to fuss over. In this instance, what had seemed the best choice obviously wasn't. Considering your depleted budget and the lack of change in your clinicians, you realized that a

---

This chapter was contributed by Edgar R. Garrett, New Mexico State University.

thorough analysis of alternative ways to spend your money might have identified another choice that would have affected your clinicians' behavior. You had learned the hard way that desired outcomes are probable rather than certain, that events or conditions you cannot control nor predict with certainty can modify outcomes, and that there is some risk associated with any choice you make. In short, you now had some insight into what the experts in mathematical probability, risk assessment, and decision theory have in mind when they talk about making decisions under conditions of uncertainty.

Decision theorists use a variety of techniques, but they all approach a decision problem by gathering data to calculate the *probability* that the alternative actions they have identified will lead to the outcome they desire. Since a probability is just that, they next figure out the amount of *uncertainty* associated with each probability and calculate the *risk* of taking each of the alternative actions. Finally, they look at the *utility* or *value* associated with the choices available to them. This approach to decision making cannot control the uncertainty that exists in the world, but it can and does reduce the uncertainty associated with the alternative outcomes that have been analyzed.

Supervisors live and make decisions in a world of uncertainty where good workshops do not always change clinicians' behaviors. In this uncertain world we deal with probabilities rather than certainties, try constantly to balance the value of an outcome against its cost, and make decisions on the basis of how much we are willing to risk to achieve the outcome we have selected. Technically, we all practice decision making under uncertainty and its associated risks.

Each of your roles as a supervisor demands that you make decisions. As a Professional you decide to join some organizations and not others, to be actively involved in some and not others. As a Researcher you decide to gather information about the effectiveness of different therapy delivery systems or concentrate on the effects of one system. As an Educator you decide to introduce many diagnostic tools to your clinicians or concentrate on a few. As an Administrator you decide to assign your clinicians under a block or itinerant schedule for individual or group therapy, or under some other therapy delivery model. And as a master Clinician you decide which therapeutic methods to use with your clients.

Good decision making depends on how thoroughly you examine your options before you make your choices. Did you investigate all of the alternatives available to you? Did you gather as much information as you could? Did you evaluate the probability that your choice will actually provide the result you hope for? Did you establish that the cost of your choice is not greater than its benefit to you? The labor of making a thorough analysis is justified; developing your decision making skills will help you reach more good decisions and fewer poor ones.

THE MODEL

This chapter presents a model built of elements from a number of theories. No one knows how humans operate when we make decisions; we probably never will have access to all the details. Researchers have approached the decision making process from a variety of viewpoints and have investigated different but related aspects of the process. When you study information theory, you are also using elements of signal detection theory. When you study decision analysis, you are using elements of information theory. When you study signal detection theory, you necessarily work with probability. The interrelationships and overlaps go on and on. My generalized model will, I hope, provide you with an approach to decision making that you can apply to any of your supervision problems.

DECISION ANALYSIS

If you don't have a problem confronting you, you don't have a decision to make. A demand from your administrator to increase the number of clients served isn't a problem if you have clinicians with light loads and a waiting list. But if your clinicians have full loads, you have a problem.

Similarly, if you do not have at least two possible actions to choose from, you don't have a decision to make. But since your boss's demand was absolute (you couldn't talk him out of it), you do not wish to resign, and your clinicians do have full loads, you have to decide whether to go from individual to group therapy, shorten therapy sessions, combine the two alternatives, or find a solution other than these obvious ones.

Given a problem and at least two alternative actions, your first obligation to yourself is to state the problem as well as you can in objective terms. Then you will start the decision analysis itself.

In any decision analysis you must include five procedures:

1. Identify the *alternative actions* available to you.
2. Identify and gather information about the environmental conditions or *states of nature* that could be in effect when you select an action.
3. Identify the *outcomes* that may result in light of the action you have selected and the state(s) of nature at the time the action is taken.
4. Establish the *utility* or *value* to you of the outcomes of the various alternative actions.
5. Assess the *probability* that each state of nature will be the one that exists when action is taken.

By following this kind of decision analysis, you can reduce the uncertainty associated with the outcome you select, calculate the expected worth of the outcome, establish the cost to achieve the outcome, and increase your confidence that the outcome you want will be the one you get.

The parts of a decision analysis need not be followed in a rigid sequence, but decision makers do have to consider each part and their interrelationships. The italicized terms in the list above are the key to each part, so let's examine the terms separately before we look at the process itself.

Probability

Probability in this context cannot simply be equated with what you learned about probability in your study of statistics. Statistics can help in making decisions, and the more knowledge the better, but our focus is on individual and complex decisions in which statistical probability is only one of many considerations. Decision analysis identifies two kinds of probability, *objective* and *subjective* probability. Unfortunately, the two are frequently confused.

The usual way of establishing *objective probability* is mathematical. The procedure is to take the number of times a particular outcome can occur and divide by the number of times that particular outcome and all other possible outcomes can occur. Think of a die: it has six faces, each with a different number of dots. The outcome you are interested in is rolling the die so that the uppermost face shows one dot. You know there are six possible outcomes, for you could roll any one of the six faces. The probability of rolling the one-dot face is 1/6, or .16666. Take out a coin and flip it. There are two possible outcomes: you could get heads or tails. You want heads. The probability of getting heads is 1/2, or .50.

A mathematical probability is objective and gives you information about the relative frequency of a particular outcome. The probability of getting heads is 1/2 or .50 whether you flip the coin once or a million times. You will never know what will happen on a given flip, but you will know the probability associated with the outcome you are interested in.

The mathematical approach works very well in predicting the probabilities in games of chance where we can identify all possible outcomes. But in many situations we do not have all the information we need and must collect data before we can make an objective estimate of probabilities.

As a supervisor who wants to be able to predict dismissals from therapy, you first go to your records and establish two things: (a) the total number of individuals with certain characteristics (type of disorder, original baseline, current baseline, age, sex, grade level, length of therapy, etc.), and (b) the number of dismissals in a given period of individuals with those characteristics.

Once you have the needed data in hand, you go back to the mathematical approach to figure your dismissal probabilities: the number of occurrences of a given outcome divided by the total number of outcomes that did happen. For example, suppose a total of 50 children were classified as dysfluent, were male, aged 8 to 9, and had received 2 years of therapy. Of this group, 10 were dismissed. The probability of dismissal, for individuals with these characteristics, is 10/50 or 1/5 or .20.

Again, knowing the probability does not tell you which individuals will be dismissed and which retained in therapy, but only how many dismissals will *probably* occur in a group of 50. The information you have only gives you the relative frequency of a given outcome among the total possible outcomes.

Before leaving objective probability, it is worth noting that we have more faith in a probability that has held up over many events than we do in a probability that proved true in a single instance. Technically, there is more validity or truth in a probability that is confirmed repeatedly. This is why you give more weight to an article or convention paper that reports hundreds of instances of the successful use of a therapy technique than to a report of its successful use with one client.

Finally, objective probability is a public probability. Everyone who looks at the data can agree on the relative frequency of a given outcome, and consequently on the probability. Use as much objective probability in your decision analysis as possible.

In contrast, *subjective probability* is a private measurement of degree of belief. Let's go back to coin flipping. Your last four flips came up heads. Objectively you know that each flip is independent of every other flip: getting heads one time has nothing to do with getting heads the next time; the probability of getting heads remained at .50 for each flip. Subjectively, however, you react a different way, for you believe that the string of heads can't continue. You express a high subjective probability when you say that the next flip "just has to" result in tails.

Any time we talk about a single event, we are expressing a subjective probability, our degree of belief in something happening. That holds whether we are betting on a throw of the dice or the outcome of an election or whether our client's next response will be acceptable. The degree of belief expressed in a subjective probability can range from 0.00, an absolute lack of belief that something will happen, to 1.00, an absolute belief that something will happen. When you say, "That's not likely to happen," you are expressing your belief that something has a low probability of happening. When you say, "I'd bet my shirt on that," you are expressing your belief that something has a very high probability of happening.

The numbers we often use to express the degree of our belief can be misleading. If I hear you say, "The probability is .75 that Clara will be late today," I can't know whether you are talking about an objective or subjective probability unless I have more information. If this is the first time Clara is to appear for therapy, the statement tells me about your degree of belief. If you have been keeping a record of Clara's arrival times, the statement tells me about the relative frequency of Clara's arriving late.

Objective probability comes from assembled data and tells us about the relative frequency of something happening. Subjective probability tells us how strongly someone believes that a particular thing will happen. Professionally we use both kinds of probability, but we do not want to confuse them. A systematized, data-based therapy has an objective probability of success that you and others can examine, a public matter. Using or not using a systematized therapy in a given case will depend upon the subjective probability you assign, a private matter.

States of Nature

Decisions are not made in a vacuum. Rational decision making includes attending to and evaluating environmental conditions that could be in effect when you choose an action. Pay attention to the qualifying words "could be in effect." It is relatively simple to draw up a new plan for scheduling therapy so that you can increase services; before you put it into operation, however, you need to be sure there isn't something in the environment that will interfere seriously with your plan.

Weather is a clear example of an environmental condition or state of nature in decision analysis. You can do nothing about the weather, but the kind of weather you will probably encounter on a given day can be very important to the outcome of an action you have selected. When you have planned a trip to the beach all week long and then learn the night before that there is an 80% chance of rain the next day, you may well reconsider your plans.

There are two kinds of environmental conditions. The states of nature we like are those that could support the action when we put it into effect. The states of nature we do not like are those that could be detrimental. It is not simply a matter of what exists in the environment—people, materials, activities, physical facilities, equipment, money, or philosophies. It is a matter of (a) whether what is out there can affect our chosen action, and (b) whether we can control it.

A simple two-question binary-answer sequence helps you identify the attributes of a state of nature. Let's continue our exploration of your plan to modify scheduling to increase services, and specifically the question of whether clinicians and clients can be reassigned to different time slots. You start with the first question:

"Does it matter to my decision?"

If the answer is *no,* then it cannot affect the outcome of the action you have selected; it is not relevant. In our example, being able to reassign clinicians and clients is not essential to the action you have chosen. With this information, you can stop the sequence and go about your business. If the answer is *yes,* then it can affect your decision, it is relevant. In our example, being able to reassign clinicians and clients is essential if your plan is to work. Do not abandon the plan at this point; go to the second question in the sequence:

"Can I do anything about it?"

If the answer is *yes,* then you can control this aspect of the situation. You have identified a state of nature favorable to your plan, since you can reassign your clinicians and clients. Breathe a sigh of relief and keep going through the decision analysis. If the answer is *no,* then you cannot control the situation. You have identified a state of nature that does not support your plan, since you cannot reassign your clinicians and clients. Go back to the beginning of the analysis and start reexamining some old alternative actions and/or developing some new ones.

Having gone through the drill, let's look at some practical shortcuts. Some things in the environment are fixed. Most of us live with fixed budgets, a financial state of nature over which we have no control. In such cases there is no point in fighting the situation; accept the environmental condition and plan within it.

On the other hand, some things within the environment can be changed. Shifting allocations on line items in your budget may be possible. Similarly, most clinicians have favorite therapy techniques that they tend to apply without a careful analysis of individual differences among clients. Given that other techniques are available, the clinicians could be brought to use another technique, particularly when pushed by their supervisor. Here is an environmental condition that could be changed.

In all instances it is important to know the probabilities associated with an environmental condition. The probability of changing the allocated budget is very low if not zero (though it never hurts to ask!). The probability of arranging a shift among line items might be very high. Similarly, the probabilities of getting clinicians to change their therapy techniques can range from low to high depending upon the individual clinicians. Knowing the probability that each state of nature will be in effect when you choose and begin your action can mean the difference between success and failure.

Utility and Value

Utility and value should not be confused. Both utility and value are tied to the question, "What is it worth to me?" but different things are being measured.

Value is based on objective probability that is established by mathematical analysis. The foundations of modern probability theory were laid in the 1600s in the study of gambling (hence the prevalence of examples involving coins and dice in any discussion of probability). The underlying assumption was that a rational person would look at the alternatives on the basis of their expected values as determined by a mathematical probability analysis, and that the payoffs associated with their respective probabilities would be as satisfying to the gambler as a sure payment and its expected values. The justification for this reasoning is that gamblers continue to gamble, and the law of large numbers says repeated independent gambles will, in the long run, give an average payoff equal to the expected value. So value is an assessment of the payoff in money based on mathematical probability (not of the probability itself).

As supervisors, we have to attend to the value of therapy. A monetary payoff comes from correcting or at least alleviating a disorder as early as possible. The cost of the disorder to society increases with each passing month, both in the expenditure of resources to change the disorder and in the loss of the client's contribution to society.

Utility is more personal and more variable; it is how satisfied you would be with a given outcome. The utility you assign to an outcome may not be the utility I would assign; for each of us the utility we assign is the one that matters (Bross, 1953).

Consider this situation: We each have a lottery ticket that gives us equal chances of winning $1,000 or $0. How much would you ask if somebody wanted to buy your ticket? How much would I ask? Mathematical probability says that on the average we would each win $500 (.5 × $1,000 + .5 × $0 = $500) if we kept our tickets, but that information isn't of much use in this one-shot situation. We have to decide whether to sell our tickets or keep them. We both decide that the right offer will be better than the risk of losing and getting nothing. We each get an offer of $250 for our tickets. I am satisfied with the offer and accept. You are not satisfied and refuse. The $250 had utility for me, but did not have utility for you.

Exactly the same kind of reasoning is involved when we look at how we run our therapy programs. We each have the same number of clinicians that we supervise, the same number of clients being served. Utility appears when you accept one degree of change in behavior (or number of dismissals per established criterion) and I accept another. These are purely utility judgments.

In a situation where the event will not be

repeated, individuals may and usually do base their decisions on the utility of, rather than the expected value of, the outcomes available to them. As we shall see later, while we do incorporate both value and utility into our professional decisions, we do not want to confuse them.

Alternative Actions

"I can do anything I want to do!" True or false? False. The alternative actions that matter in a decision analysis are those that are available and acceptable to us, not all those that might exist. Theoretically, anything is possible; practically, only certain things are probable. We decision-making supervisors need to stay with the probable.

Your recent acquisition of a software program that combines word processing, a spread sheet, and a data base has gotten you more and more involved with the Super Clone in your office. For several weekends you have carried the Clone home on Friday and back to the office on Monday. At times you want access to it for an hour or so in the evening, but a daily transporting of the office micro isn't a satisfactory solution. In short, you want a microcomputer and printer of your own.

Getting a computer and printer calls for cash or credit. You add up the monthly payments you are already making and choose the cash route. Only an exact duplication of your office equipment will satisfy you: a Super Clone with a letter-quality printer. Adding the balances in your checking and savings accounts, you identify a state of nature, an environmental condition, that keeps you from what you want: you don't have enough cash.

You start thinking of the different ways you could alter that state of nature. You could marry a rich person. You could rob the local convenience store or even the local bank. You could set up a bogus investment agency. You could break the bank at Monte Carlo, or Atlantic City, or Las Vegas. You could stop eating and live in a tent. You could murder your rich Aunt Sophie.

You could . . . (continue with your own list; not only is it a fun game, but the brainstorming can make you aware of workable alternatives that cold logic would never identify).

Clearly, not all of the alternative actions you can dream up are actually available to you. Some of the actions violate your personal value system; some violate the standards of people who matter to you; some violate the law. You are not willing to accept the unpleasant consequences that would result. Utility, personal preference, will eliminate such alternatives. The alternative actions you ultimately consider will be those that are available and acceptable to you both objectively and subjectively.

If you insist that a Super Clone is the only unit you will consider, and you do not have the needed cash, you can (a) wait until you can assemble the needed dollars, (b) forget about the whole thing, or (c) modify your desired outcome or the conditions that affect it.

The last alternative immediately produces a number of additional alternatives. If you still insist on staying with the new Super Clone option, you can now consider (a) borrowing the money from a friend, (b) taking out a loan at your bank, or (c) signing an installment payment plan with the computer store. And if you stop insisting on a new Super Clone, you can (a) buy a used Super Clone, or (b) buy a Clone Jr.

These new alternatives that appeared when you opened up the constraints on your options point to a very important fact: too often we do not identify all the actions available to us, and unwittingly reduce the number of outcomes that could result. Identifying alternative actions is not simple. You have to keep objective and subjective probabilities separated so as not to confuse what you want with what you might probably get. You may move your top alternative far down the list once you have explored utility (what the outcome means to you), value (what the price tag and payoff will be), and states of nature (that you can and cannot control). You will frequently conclude that some highly probable outcomes are not acceptable.

Outcomes

An outcome is the result of an action. We have no difficulty in accepting that definition. We do find it hard to accept that a given act does not automatically result in a given outcome. Outcomes are uncertain. Our excursion through probability showed us that the act of flipping a coin does not necessarily give us the outcome of heads coming up. In human affairs, we saw that even when we knew the probability associated with dismissals from therapy, we could not predict who would be dismissed.

We can usually identify the "reasonable" outcomes of an action. What makes them reasonable is that we pay attention to uncertainty by evaluating the possible effects of the states of nature that could exist at the time we act.

Restatement

Decision analysis gives us a systematic way to examine our options when we make a choice. By taking care to include each of the five parts in the analysis, we can identify the action that is most likely to result in the outcome that has the greatest utility for us. (Whether we take that action is a different matter.)

Decisions are made every day in our profession, actions are taken, and outcomes result. Most of our decisions are not reached through systematic analysis but are made on the basis of our individual sets of values, derived from experience, judgment, and intuition. We often cannot identify the factors in a given set of values. Decisions based on such sets are not necessarily bad, but they lack quantitative or logical procedures for predicting the possible outcomes. Diedrich (1974) and Garrett (1973) found that both new and experienced school clinicians can predict how long a child will be in articulation therapy before dismissal. But we also found that the clinicians could not identify the factors that led to their predictions.

Such a finding was not surprising. A clinical profession like ours deliberately uses educational and clinical experiences to shape student clinicians in the image of their teachers and supervisors. In one sense, considering that we are selective in what we observe and in what we remember from what we observe, it is amazing that we have such similar maps of the world. In another sense, there should be no amazement; while we may have been selective in observing and remembering all the details, we had to recall and apply the main ideas and many supporting details in class and in clinic or we would not have been given passing grades by our teachers and supervisors and would not be—or be on the way to being—professionals now.

Information Processing

We can better understand the process of observing and remembering by employing an information processing model. Our senses gather information from the environment in the form of physical stimuli (auditory, visual, kinesthetic, etc.); our brain selects some of the information for transfer to short-term memory (which holds it for immediate use), and then transforms and transfers the meaning of that information into long-term memory (the storehouse from which we call information when we want it later). When we make a decision, we retrieve information from long-term memory, compare what we had stored to what we are currently considering, and then act.

It is the content and organization of the information we retrieve from long-term memory that concerns us now. The content is made up of repeated observations of what we attend to in the world; our supervisors directed us as we listened to the sounds that clients produced, their similarities, their differences. The organization is provided by the "boxes" where we stored and grouped the observations: our supervisors told us which observed sounds were to go into the box marked *normal* and which into the box marked *abnormal*. Sometimes it was difficult to decide whether some sounds were normal or not, but we had to make a decision and we did. Because our observing and organizing were guided by people who were generally in agreement, we too are likely to agree more than we disagree. (You can find a good discussion of information processing in Gagne's [1985] *Conditions of Learning*.)

The Decision Axis

Schultz (1972) chose the term *decision axis* to identify this organized long-term information when we retrieve it from memory and use it to make a decision. We will use his simple but effective graphic representation of a decision axis as a horizontal line. We know that a line is a series of points arranged in a particular way. That knowledge helps us remember that an observation set is a series of repeated observations organized into categories. If we are determining normality, our decision axis will look like Figure 7-1.

We also use our stored information to establish criteria. In our example of speech sounds, our observations have included a great variety of normal and abnormal instances. Repeated confirmation of our decisions by our supervisors told us that we were using appropriate criteria to separate the normal and abnormal productions. We were developing a set of *decision criteria* for identifying and separating normal and abnormal sounds. Placing those decision criteria at a point on the decision axis gives us the *criterion cutoff* we use to separate normal and abnormal speech sounds (Schultz, 1972), as shown in Figure 7-2.

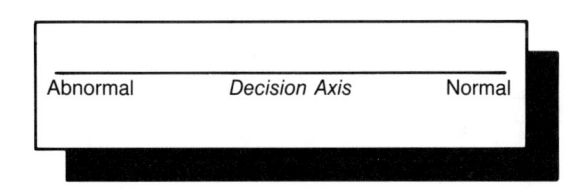

FIGURE 7-1
A decision axis for abnormal to normal

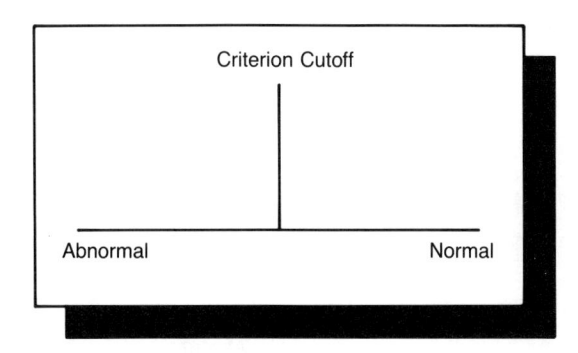

FIGURE 7-2
A decision axis with abnormal speech sounds to the left of and normal speech sounds to the right of a criterion cutoff

Ideally, our decision axes and decision criteria should be exact measures of what exists in the world. Information theory shows that that is impossible; we cannot sense, process, organize, or store all of the information that is available. That explains why we continue to have difficulty in telling whether some sounds are abnormal or normal. Recall from your speech science class that when we compare physical measures of speech sounds as displayed in spectrographs with our perceptions of those sounds, the matches are not perfect. We are not going to resolve the problem here, but we will consider some consequences.

In using the decision axis model, you need to consider not only the axis and the criterion cutoff, but the distribution of your observations on the axis. When you record the frequency of occurrence of scores by marking each score with a dot on a piece of graph paper, you produce a *plot* of the distribution of the scores. For our example, such a plot would show two distributions on our decision axis, one for all the instances we labeled *abnormal* and another for all the instances we labeled *normal*. Included in these distributions are the instances when we were unsure but had to decide and classify anyway. These instances would produce an overlap of the two distributions, and the result would look something like Figure 7-3.

FIGURE 7-3
Distributions of abnormal and normal speech sounds on a decision axis

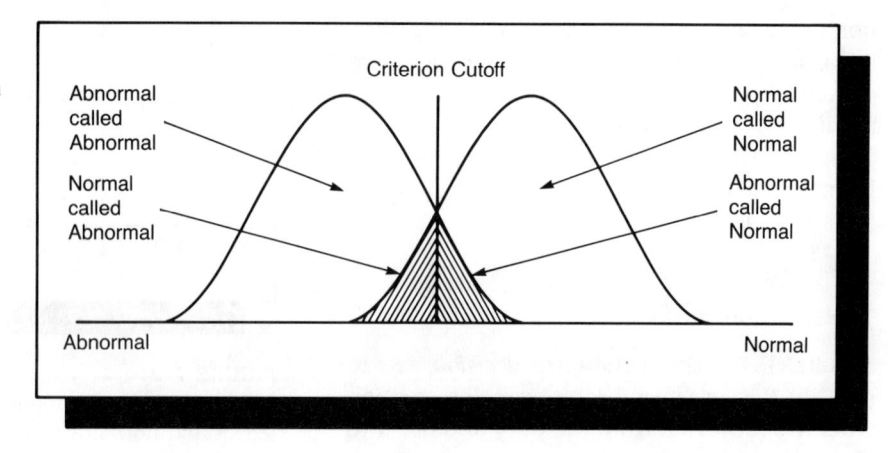

[Figure: Two overlapping bell curves on an axis from "Abnormal" to "Normal" with a "Criterion Cutoff" line in the middle. Labels: "Abnormal called Abnormal", "Normal called Abnormal", "Normal called Normal", "Abnormal called Normal".]

These overlapping distributions are troublesome and can lead to consequences we don't like. Even with the modifications to our decision axis and decision criteria that have come with experience, we will continue to put some abnormals under the normal label and some normals under the abnormal label. We are back to the issue of uncertainty. Since we cannot escape it, we will turn to signal detection theory to help us understand the consequences and how we can modify them.

(Before we continue the abnormal/normal example, notice how pervasive this problem of categorizing people and their performances is. As a teacher you have no problem identifying the A and F students, but separating the B− and C+ or C− and D+ students can be difficult even when your grading criteria are objective. As an administrator you have no difficulty in assigning performance ratings to your clinicians if they are really good or really bad; those who fall in the middle take much more thought.)

Signal Detection Theory

Signal detection theory is the part of information theory that explains how we decide whether a signal is present or not (Egan, 1975). You may have encountered this concept in an acoustics course when you worked with the relationship between signal and noise. For our purposes, think of a signal as "the thing we are looking for," and rather than using the term *signal,* use the term *target.* The conditions involved in any detection problem are:

1. The random occurrence of one of two events—target and nontarget—with each event occurring in a specified interval of time.
2. Varying amounts of information in the form of physical stimuli in the events, which produce a probabilistic condition.
3. The necessity of making a decision after each observation about whether or not the target is present.

To rephrase the conditions, there is a target we are looking for; the target is accompanied by nontargets that we are not looking for but do respond to; the amounts of stimuli from both the target and the nontarget vary; in each case we must apply a criterion measure and say whether the event we are observing is the target or not.

Using the code of *X* for the target and *Y* for a nontarget, we can represent the four possible outcomes of our decision this way:

1. *Hit:* X called X.
   The target was present when we said *yes.*
2. *Miss:* X called Y.
   The target was present when we said *no.*
3. *False alarm:* Y called X.
   The target was not present when we said *yes.*

4. *Correct rejection:* Y called Y.
 The target was not present when we said *no.*

(I chose this rather awkward phrasing to emphasize that we are always looking for the target. The question is always "Is this a target?" The answer is always *yes* or *no.*)

We can show these four possible outcomes in the 2 × 2 *decision matrix* given in Figure 7-4.

We are dealing with probabilities. The presence of a target is a probability that depends on the distribution of targets in the events being observed, that is, how much overlap there is in the populations on the decision axis. Similarly, identifying a target is a probability that is influenced by where we locate our criterion cutoff on the decision axis. Further, we have to accept that we are not perfect observers and that some degree of uncertainty will be associated with our decisions.

We are all familiar with the practical application of this concept. When we conduct screenings for communication disorders, we always follow up with definitive tests. In signal detection terms, screenings produce false alarms (normals called abnormal) as well as hits (abnormals called abnormal). The definitive tests confirm our hits and reduce our false alarms.

Suppose we are screening for voice problems. Assume a total population of 110 individuals, of whom 10 have abnormal voices (our target events) and 100 have normal voices (our nontarget events). Now assume that the location of our criterion cutoff results in 9 hits, 1 miss, 5 false alarms, and 95 correct rejections. Our *rate* or percentage would be:

 Hit Rate:
  X called X = 9/10 = .90 = 90%
 Miss Rate:
  X called Y = 1/10 = .10 = 10%
 False Alarm Rate:
  Y called X = 5/100 = .05 = 5%
Correct Rejection Rate:
  Y called Y = 95/100 = .95 = 95%

Taking these rates and putting them in the appropriate cells of the decision matrix enables us

	Decision Yes	Decision No
Target	HIT	MISS
Non-Target	FALSE ALARM	CORRECT REJECTION

FIGURE 7-4
A signal detection decision matrix

to answer some important questions. Adding across the target or X row confirms that we did look at all the targets (HT 90% + MS 10% = 100% of targets). Adding across the nontarget or Y row confirms that we did look at all the nontargets (FA 5% + CR 95% = 100% of nontargets). We also have confirmation that we did observe all the cases in the total population (100% of targets is 10; 100% of nontargets is 100; and 100% of the total population is 110). The important point is that while the numbers in the cells can change, the sum across each row must always equal 100%, and that all the Xs and Ys must equal 100% of the total population being observed.

Adding down the Yes column tells us that with a HT of 90% (9 Xs) and a FA of 5% (5 Ys) we identified 14 cases as having abnormal voices. Adding down the No column tells us that with a MS of 10% (1 X) and a CR of 95% (95 Ys) we identified 96 cases as having normal voices. Again we have confirmation that all 110 cases were observed. We can't add rates in columns the way we did in rows, but an examination of the decision matrix tells us a great deal about the accuracy of our observations in relation to our criterion cutoff's location. The four cells have an active relationship, so that a change in one cell produces a change in the other three. A basic premise in signal detection theory is that increasing the hit rate (HT+) automatically means increasing the false alarm rate (FA+). Referring to the matrix, you will see the other automatic changes: an increased hit rate (HT+) means a decreased miss rate (MS−), and an increased false alarm rate (FA+) means a decreased correct rejection rate (CR−).

(I deliberately avoided taking a mathematical approach to signal detection theory so that we could focus on the concept and how it fits within this generalized model of decision making. For those of you wanting detailed information about the mathematical base, I recommend Egan (1975) and Raiffa (1970), who provide excellent insights into the techniques for figuring the probability of probabilities within the matrix.)

By now you will have realized that the terms in the four boxes of the decision matrix in Figure 7–4 correspond to the four groups of individuals we identified in Figure 7–3. Given the target *abnormal* and a set of criteria for identifying abnormality, each time we applied our decision criteria we placed an individual either to the left or to the right of the criterion cutoff on our decision axis. We know from information theory that our decision criteria are not perfect and from signal detection theory that our observations are not perfect, so that probably we misclassified some individuals. We need some way to compensate for these inaccurate placements on the decision axis. The answer is to select the criterion cutoff that best serves our purpose.

Consider the implications of our attempting to identify individuals with a communication disorder that is related to an active pathology. Since not identifying such individuals could have very undesirable consequences, ranging from progressive loss of communication to life-threatening physical conditions, we want to identify every case that we possibly can; in other words, we do not want to miss a case. With the decision matrix in mind, we know that to identify more targets, we must increase our hit rate or decrease our miss rate. And with the decision axis in mind, we know that moving the criterion cutoff to the right will give us these desired results.

When we *loosen* our criteria and move the criterion cutoff to the right on the decision axis, we will identify more abnormal events, simultaneously adding to our hit rate (HT+) and reducing our miss rate (MS−), both desirable consequences (HT% + MS% = 100%). Figure 7–5 represents what happens on the decision axis as a result of this procedure.

There are other consequences, however, that we must consider; as we can see in Figure 7–5, loosening our criteria also means that we automatically increase the number of false alarms (HT+ means FA+) and decrease the number of correct rejections (MS− means CR−), both undesirable consequences. Moving our criterion cutoff to the right clearly enabled us to identify more of the individuals we were concerned

FIGURE 7–5
A representation of the effect of loosening the criterion cutoff

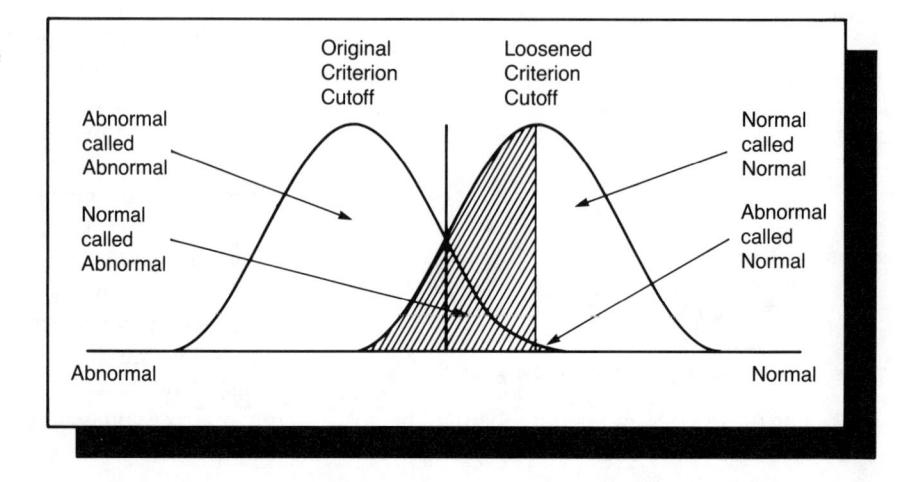

about. At the same time, that outcome was achieved at a high cost; we ended up telling more people who do not have a problem that they do.

Now let's look at another example in which our concern is quite different. Rather than wanting to identify active pathologies, we are worried about a screening procedure that keeps pointing us toward individuals who really don't have a serious problem. With the decision matrix in mind, we know that we must reduce our false alarm rate and increase our correct rejection rate. With the decision axis in mind, we know that moving the criterion cutoff to the left will give us the desired results.

When we *tighten* our criterion cutoff, or move it to the left, we will identify fewer abnormal events, simultaneously increasing our correct rejections (CR+) and reducing our false alarm rate (FA−), both desirable consequences (FA% + CR% = 100%). Figure 7-6 shows us the effect of a tightened criterion cutoff.

Again there are consequences we must attend to, for in increasing the number of correct rejections we will automatically increase the number of misses (CR+ means MS+), and in reducing the number of false alarms we will automatically reduce the number of hits (FA− means HT−), both undesirable consequences. This time the cost comes in eliminating kids from therapy who may well need our help.

These two examples show that when we modify our decision criteria to attain a desirable goal, the new criterion cutoff produces consequences we may not like. To live with this quandary, we have to understand how to select a decision that may not be perfect but serves our purpose best.

Optimal Decision

Signal detection theory does not remove uncertainty from our decisions, but it does enable us to evaluate systematically the outcomes produced by different decision criteria. We must conduct such an examination in order to select the outcome that has the most utility for us. We have seen the interrelation between benefits (identifying more active pathologies in your population) and costs (telling individuals they have a problem when they don't). In each situation the task is to decide how much tightening or loosening will produce the best balance between benefits and costs that has the most utility for you. When you answer that question, you will have identified your *optimal decision*.

Before we look at an example, note that in human affairs benefits and costs may be tangible or intangible. They may consist of dollars, units of time, degree of personal satisfaction, number

FIGURE 7-6
A representation of the effect of tightening the criterion cutoff

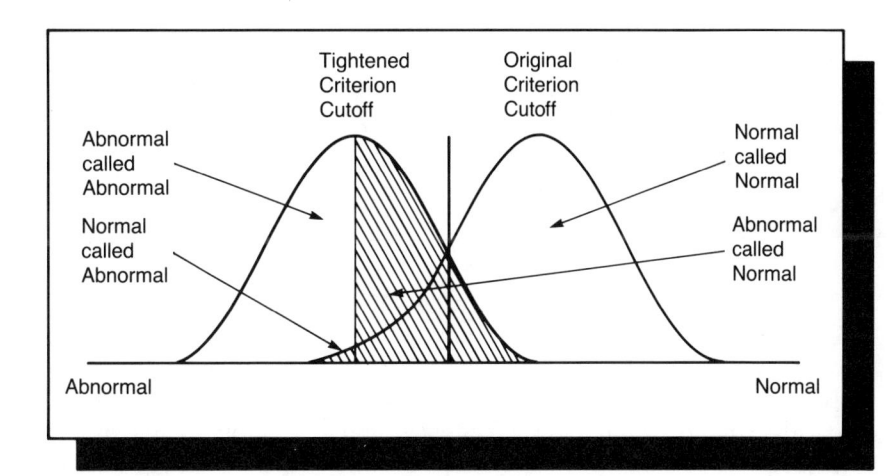

of individuals, degree of behavioral change, or any other measure that concerns you at the time. Tangible things are easy to count. Intangible things, such as personal satisfaction, can also be counted by assigning them to a scale that represents the degree or intensity of your feeling. You may be (1) very satisfied, (2) satisfied, (3) not satisfied, or (4) completely unsatisfied with a particular outcome. When a cost-benefit analysis calls for assigning numbers to intangibles, that is how you do it.

Now an example you can approach either as a clinician or as a supervisor, or both. You have identified 70 kids in your school as having abnormal speech. You cannot serve all of them, because you are expected to stay within the guideline of 35 to 40 active cases and a severe case overload would be detrimental to your performance. You certainly do not want to waste your scarce resources by assigning a kid to therapy who doesn't really need it. You turn to what you know about the decision axis, distributions on it, and the criterion cutoff.

These factors emerge as you look at the problem systematically:

1. The identified population of 70 includes both hits and false alarms.
2. The criterion cutoff's location was determined by:
   a. Your personal "by the ear" criterion.
   b. The scores from a standardized test.
3. You can tighten your criterion by:
   a. Making your listening criterion tougher.
   b. Picking a higher cutoff score from the standardized test.
   c. Adding new information from another evaluation measure.

Setting up a new "by the ear" criterion is possible, but it would take a lot of labor you don't have time for right now, so you eliminate that choice. Either of the other two choices would move the criterion cutoff to the left and give you the needed reduction from 70 to 35 or 40. But there could be a difference in the *quality* of the outcomes in terms of hits and false alarms.

1. Picking the higher number on the standardized test could reduce the total number of cases identified without necessarily altering the ratio of HT to FA, for you do not know the degree of overlap of abnormal and normal distributions that is producing the false alarms.
2. Adding new information would also produce the needed reduction in numbers but would have two accompanying effects. Adding information to the decision criterion could produce a more robust tool that would help you reduce the number of false alarms and increase the number of hits. Second, if the new information were also incorporated in your decision axis, your modified axis would more nearly approximate reality.

I have deliberately built a case in which the addition of new information would be the optimal choice. If we equate HT to benefits, and FA to costs, any choice that promises an increase in HT and a decrease in FA will be the choice with the best cost-benefit payoff.

At the same time, we have not considered all the factors that might be involved. If you have to establish your caseload within the next 3 days, time is a factor you can't ignore. Submitting your list on time is a benefit you would gain at the cost of losing a possible increase in HT. With this additional factor, your optimal choice is to raise the standardized score cutoff, rather than adding new information, and get your list into the office on time.

This discussion of information theory and signal detection was intended to help us understand the process that shapes our decisions. We established that our decision axes and decision criteria come from our educational and clinical experiences. Where we position the criterion cutoff on an axis comes from the same source. And although our decisions are made under uncertainty, we can improve them by approaching them systematically.

Three articles by Turner and others (Turner, Frazer, & Shepard, 1984; Turner & Nielsen, 1984; Turner, Shepard, & Frazer, 1984) describe the application of clinical decision analysis to a problem in audiology. There you will find elaborations and applications of signal detection theory beyond the scope of this chapter.

Risk

We need to look at *risk* before we put the whole process together and make some decisions. The term *risk* has appeared before, and it should be evident to you that any decision made under uncertainty has some element of risk. At first glance, my definition of an optimal decision seems complete: the decision with the best balance of costs and benefits, the one with the most utility. The difficulty is that, as individuals, we do not always see the action with the best cost-benefit ratio as the action with the most utility.

Utility is a personal thing. "Wheel of Fortune," the TV game show, provides an excellent example. You are one of three contestants. You have escaped the "Bankrupt" and "Lose a Turn" spaces on the wheel, and your correct calls for letters to complete the phrase have resulted in your earning $3,000. From the viewpoint of utility, the important fact is that you have identified the phrase, even though a number of letters are still missing. You can spin again or give the answer now.

These two alternative actions lead to different outcomes. You know there is no risk in giving the answer now, for that action can lead to only one outcome: you get $3,000. There is a risk in spinning the wheel again, for that action can lead to any of three outcomes: (a) adding to what you have already earned; (b) losing your turn, having someone else provide the answer, and losing everything; or (c) going bankrupt and losing everything. How you view the utility and risk of these outcomes will determine whether you spin again or give the answer now.

Risk-taking is an element in the utility we assign to an outcome. Depending on the possible outcomes, we are sometimes willing to take a risk and sometimes not. Technically, a number of strategies exist for handling the element of risk in making a decision. We need to consider only two strategies: minimax and maximax (Bross, 1953).

The *minimax* strategy says, "Minimize maximum risk." If you used that strategy, you would give the answer now to avoid the maximum risk of losing everything on the next spin of the wheel. Generally, low risks produce low gains.

The *maximax* strategy says, "Maximize maximum gain." If you used that strategy, you would spin the wheel again knowing you might add a sizable amount to your earnings. Generally, high gains involve high risks.

Don't be misled by the $3,000 figure in the "Wheel of Fortune" example. The decision has to do with the alternative actions available and the factors that go into your selection of an action. Remember the lottery example earlier in the chapter? I decided to sell my ticket, a minimax strategy. You decided to keep your ticket, a maximax strategy. What about all of those computer generated mailings you receive about winning $10,000,000? You invest the needed postage to return the entry form because you are using a maximax strategy. If you saved the money for all the postage stamps, you could buy a new tape for your cassette player, a minimax strategy.

Going back to the matter of optimal decisions that led us into this examination of risk, you can now see that we are influenced as much by the subjective element of utility as by the relatively objective element of the ratio between costs and benefits. When we select an alternative that promises a greater gain, we have decided that alternative has more utility for us even if it has more risk. When we select an alternative that has a lower risk, we have decided that alternative has more utility for us even if it promises less gain.

DECISION MAKING

Supervisors are professionals filling a variety of roles, individuals facing decisions in every role. We've been through a number of brief examples up to this point; now let's tackle a more complex problem that asks us to look at the effects of a series of decisions. I will not specify any particular setting; while some of the details would change, the considerations would not. Regardless of setting, too, the five parts of the decision analysis remain the same:

1. You must identify the *alternative actions* available to you.
2. You must identify and gather information about the environmental conditions or *states of nature* that could be in effect when you select an action.
3. You must identify the *outcomes* that may result in light of the action you have selected and the state(s) of nature at the time the action is taken.
4. You must establish the *utility* or *value* to you of the outcomes of the various alternative actions.
5. You must assess the *probability* that each state of nature will be the one that exists when action is taken.

The problem you face is this: your boss has directed you to increase the number of clients served during the year without modifying your dismissal criteria. In other words, the same level of service is to be delivered to more individuals in the same period of time. Having concluded that ignoring the edict would result in a loss of income that you couldn't tolerate, you also realize that what the boss wants does merit consideration. You have a waiting list of individuals needing service, and your evaluation procedure is not part of the problem. You know that your boss is being pressured by those funding your program to demonstrate that the money is being well spent.

There is no possibility that more resources in the form of salary will be available. This state of nature eliminates the alternative of adding more clinicians to the program. Since all salaries come from the same pot, you cannot add aides, either. Reducing the salaries of your clinicians enough to add another clinician or several aides is an alternative that passes through your mind. But since salaries have been established for the year and contracts signed, you eliminate that alternative, too.

The operating budget for your program carries a 5% limit on the amount that can be shifted from one line item to another. Your experience with paperwork tells you that juggling $400 will be more trouble than it is worth. But wait. Last year you reached the goal of a microcomputer for each clinician, and your group selected a batch of software for language therapy. Most of the clinicians have used some of the programs, and the research you've seen indicates that computer-based therapy is effective. If the $400 went for some new programs that had received good reviews in the journals, and if use of the micros increased...

What you are looking at is your therapy delivery system. If you can reduce the amount of time your clients spend in individual face-to-face therapy by using more microcomputer-delivered and/or group therapy, then you can serve more clients. Given the right software and appropriate assignment of your clinicians and clients, one group could receive micro-delivered therapy while another group received clinician-delivered therapy, and the clients who most needed individual help could still receive it.

This mental bouncing around is how many of us approach decision making. We bounce from alternative actions to possible outcomes, back to states of nature and their probabilities, to utility, to risk, and this method is fine as long as all the elements in the decision analysis are included. In our example, you have examined a number of alternative actions and rejected them in quite a reasonable manner. But now that you realize that modifying your therapy delivery system can help you achieve the goal your boss set, you can reduce the bouncing by systematically following the sequence in the decision analysis and know that you are covering all the bases.

First, you identify the alternative actions available to you as

1. requiring an increased use of micro-delivered therapy.
2. requiring an increased use of group clinician-delivered therapy.

Second, you cannot identify any states of nature affecting your outcomes that are beyond your control. Several of your clinicians are set in their ways and resist change, but you can probably get their cooperation by approaching them the right way and showing them the seriousness of the situation, or you can keep them doing individual therapy.

Third, you identify the outcomes that may result from your requiring an increased use of micro-delivered therapy as

1. the addition of at least two new clients to each clinician's active caseload.
2. the addition of at least 30 minutes of therapy daily for at least 60% of each clinician's caseload.

You identify an outcome that may result from your requiring an increased use of clinician-delivered group therapy as

1. the addition of at least four new clients to each clinician's active caseload.

Unfortunately, no research exists to allow you to predict a more rapid change of behavior with either of your actions. But there is also no research that says not to take the actions.

Fourth, you establish that the outcomes of your two actions would have a high utility for you. You would have the personal satisfaction of having achieved a difficult goal. You would work diligently to ensure that your clinicians also found utility in implementing the program. We will not consider value here because it would involve introducing a whole set of numbers. But the numbers would support your claims of increased cost efficiency and financial benefit.

Fifth, since the states of nature appear to be ones you can control, your only concern is to assign a probability that represents how your individual clinicians will most likely react and how those reactions will average out in the whole delivery system.

If you had sat down in your office with paper and pen to think through that decision, you might well have ended up drawing a series of simple decision trees to help you check your analysis of the outcome(s) of each possible action (Raiffa, 1970). The structure of a decision tree is shown in Figure 7–7. Remember that each outcome is accompanied by a state of nature. Thus you could have two branches, three branches in Figure 7–7, or more, each with its accompanying state of nature.

Your first thought was to reject your boss's demand. That act could have led to O1, having him retract the demand, or O2, having him reassert it. The states of nature in the form of the waiting list and the pressure for accountability produced an extremely high probability that O1 would be rejected and O2 would occur. You projected the decision tree your boss would use if

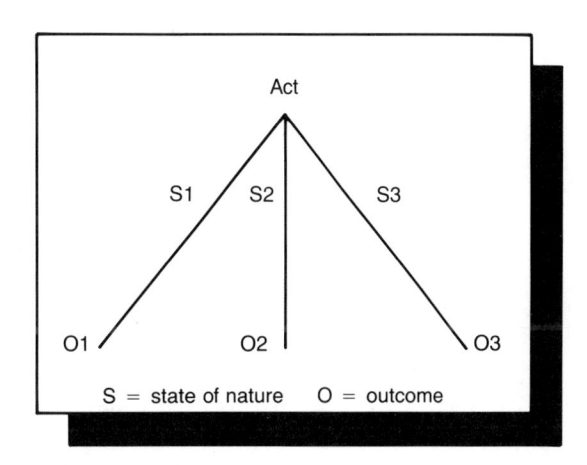

FIGURE 7–7

A decision tree showing the act, with different states of nature leading to different possible outcomes

you still refused to tackle the problem, and the probable outcome was that he would fire you and select another supervisor. There was far more utility for you in staying employed than in defending your clinical philosophy, so you started looking at the problem.

The problem was to serve more people without lowering dismissal criteria. How to do it? Act: Ask for more money. Possible states of nature: S1, you get the money; S2, you don't get the money. Possible outcomes: 01, if S1, you add more clinical personnel; 02, if S2, you don't add personnel. The probability that the money will be available when you ask is 0.00. You discard that action. The possibility of pulling money out of your clinicians' salaries is also rejected because of the 0.00 probability that you can do it.

In our example, this was the moment when you started focusing on the therapy delivery system and being systematic. You were touching all the bases and assuring yourself that your conclusions were justified, even though my narrative could have been interpreted as showing how disorganized your thought processes were. The important point is that when we act professionally, we examine many alternative actions and their possible outcomes, even those we may not like.

Keep the concepts of uncertainty and risk in mind as you go about your decision making. None of us is infallible; we all struggle in selecting the optimal decision and in deciding how much we are willing to risk. Approaching your problems systematically can help you be sure you are exploring all the probabilities and identifying all your options.

SUMMARY

Supervisors continually make decisions; some are easy, some are difficult. Good decision making depends on how thoroughly you examine your options before you make your choices and act. Decision analysis enables you to look at problems as objectively as possible, to identify the alternative actions available to you, and to predict the likely outcomes of the different actions so that you can make the decision that has the greatest utility. Decision analysis is a five-step process: identifying alternative actions, identifying states of nature that could affect the actions, identifying the resultant outcomes, establishing the utility of the outcomes, and assessing the probability that the states of nature will be present when we act.

Good decision making depends on your understanding that any choice you make has an element of uncertainty in it, that you are acting on a probability rather than a certainty. The models from information processing and signal detection theory combine with those from mathematical probability and risk assessment to help you identify the strategy that has the most utility, that will lead to the outcome that best serves your purpose.

You use decision making strategies every day as you fulfill the multiple roles of supervision. Applying decision analysis techniques efficiently and systematically can give you a high degree of confidence that you have considered all the options, that the outcome you selected is optimal and highly probable, that you are a good decision maker.

APPLICATIONS

Discussion Topics

1. Discuss the similarities and differences between the decision axis model and the decision analysis model.
2. The term *risk* is used in many ways. Identify at least 10 examples of different uses of the term. Which ones fit the concept of risk as it is presented in this chapter?
3. Discuss how you can apply signal detection theory to therapy in speech-language pathology. Are there ways you could improve your signal detection ability? What are some possible outcomes of such a change in your clinical behavior?
4. Discuss the application of information processing to the supervisor's role as a clinical educator.
5. Discuss the concept of the *optimal decision* as it was presented in this chapter, paying particular attention to the effect of utility and risk on the basic cost-benefit notion of what is optimal.

Laboratory Experiences

1. Using the "more clients, same dismissal criteria" example from this chapter,
    a. identify at least one additional alternative action that could have been available to you.
    b. identify at least two additional states of nature that could have led you to reject the option of adding personnel.
2. Using the decision axis model, identify three instances where a tightened criterion cutoff would be preferable to a loosened cutoff. Justify your argument on the basis of risk.
3. Develop a case supporting the active involvement of supervisors in professional organizations using
    a. a cost-benefit argument involving dollars and cents.
    b. a utility argument based on personal satisfaction.
4. Now refute the arguments you presented in exercise 3.

Research Projects

1. Using elements of decision making theory, design and execute a research project to study how best to establish an electronic bulletin board for CUSPSPA on SpecialNet, BitNet, or a comparable national telecommunication system to which supervisors in all settings could have access.
2. Survey existing Communication Disorders training programs and establish a data base describing the education and training that each provides in formal decision making for speech-language pathology, audiology, and/or supervisor trainees.

3. Design and execute a study that uses the decision axis model to evaluate the competencies of speech-language pathology and audiology trainees. How does training in the use of the decision axis model affect the reliability of supervisors' evaluations of supervisees' clinical competence?

4. Design and execute a study to redistribute the funds in an existing budget for a specific service delivery site. Compare the minimax risk strategy of allocation with the maximax strategy.

5. Survey the procedures clinicians use to determine dismissal from therapy. Are the procedures effective and efficient? With what aspects of decision making theory are they most compatible?

REFERENCES

Bross, I. D. J. (1953). *Design for decision.* New York: Free Press.

Diedrich, W. S. (1974, November). *Analyses and management of articulation learning.* A short course presented at the annual convention of the American Speech and Hearing Association, Las Vegas.

Egan, J. P. (1975). *Signal detection theory and ROC analysis.* New York: Academic Press.

Gagne, R. M. (1985). *The conditions of learning* (4th ed). New York: Holt, Rinehart & Winston.

Garrett, E. R. (1973). *A systems approach to the optimization of speech therapy services in the schools: Quarterly report.* U.S. Office of Education, Project No. 412498.

Raiffa, H. (1970). *Decision analysis.* Reading, MA: Addison-Wesley.

Schultz, M. C. (1972). *An analysis of clinical behavior in speech and hearing.* Englewood Cliffs, NJ: Prentice-Hall.

Turner, R. G., Frazer, G. J., & Shepard, N. T. (1984). Formulating and evaluating audiological test protocols. *Ear and Hearing,* 5, 321-330.

Turner, R. G., & Nielsen, D. W. (1984). Application of clinical decision analysis to audiological tests. *Ear and Hearing,* 5, 125-133.

Turner, R. G., Shepard, N. T., & Frazer, G. J. (1984). Clinical performance of audiological and related diagnostic tests. *Ear and Hearing,* 5, 187-194.

8
Creative Problem Managing: The Art

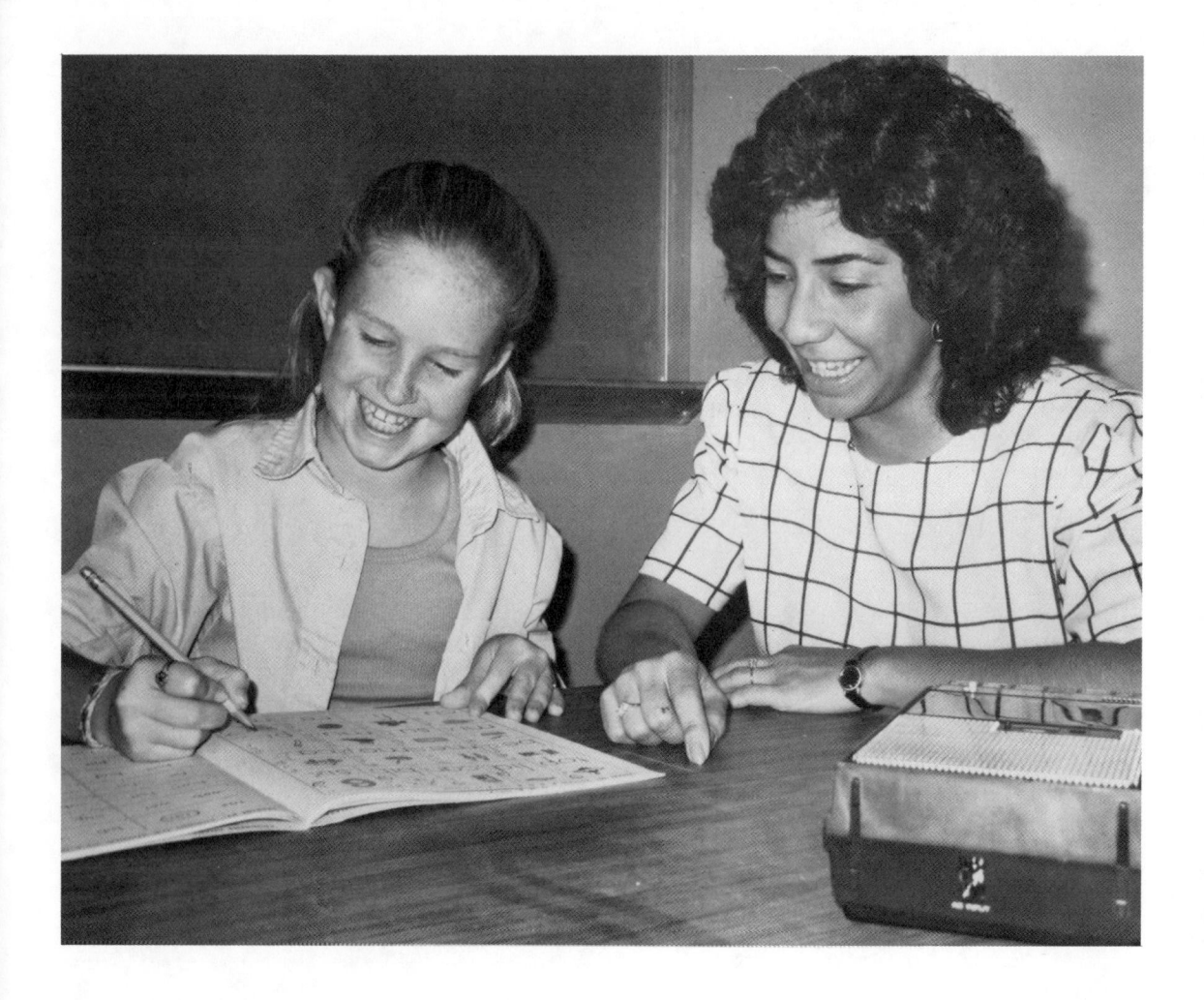

CRITICAL CONCEPTS

- *Problems can be dealt with using different approaches.*
- *Problem managing and problem solving are different concepts.*
- *Algorithms, vertical thinking, and convergent thinking are systematic, high-probability approaches to problems and are associated with problem solving.*
- *Heuristics, lateral thinking, and divergent thinking are planned, low-probability approaches to problems and are associated with problem managing.*
- *Programs for creative problem managing are available and have been used in Communication Disorders supervision.*

OUTLINE

INTRODUCTION
PROBLEMS
PROBLEM MANAGING
THEORIES OF PROBLEM MANAGING
    Behaviorist/Associationist Theory
    Gestalt Theory
    Information Processing Theory
    Schema Theory
OBSTACLES TO PRODUCTIVE PROBLEM MANAGEMENT
PROBLEM MANAGING PROGRAMS
    Specific Problem Managing Strategies
    Applications to Communication Disorders Supervision
SUSTAINING PRODUCTIVE PROBLEM MANAGING
SUMMARY
APPLICATIONS

INTRODUCTION

Supervisors encounter problems daily and need a variety of strategies to manage many different kinds of problems. Chapter 7 presented scientific techniques of decision making to help supervisors manage problems that require a systematic, sequential, logical approach. Not all problems need that kind of management, however, and supervisors should develop alternative strategies as part of their supervisory competence. This chapter, therefore, presents information about problems and how to manage them in creative, nonsystematic, nonlogical ways.

What is creative problem management, and how does it differ from the systematic decision making described in chapter 7? To answer these questions, this chapter addresses the nature of problems, the process of problem managing, and theories of problem management. It identifies obstacles to productive problem management, describes programs for overcoming the obstacles, and suggests methods of sustaining productive problem management.

People need decision making or creative problem managing strategies only when a problem is present. Just what constitutes a problem?

This chapter was contributed by Stephen S. Farmer, New Mexico State University.

PROBLEMS

Problems can be described by examining their components. Miller (1984) states that a problem "involves decision making or choice making without all the necessary information available" (pp. 199–200). Mayer (1977) and Winkelgren (1979) suggest that problems consist of four components: (a) *givens,* the items of knowledge a person uses when managing a problem; (b) *operations,* the procedures or process used when managing a problem; (c) a *goal,* the outcome or end point of the management process; and (d) *obstacles,* the cognitive operations and states of nature that interfere with, rather than facilitate, the outcome. Two types of problems exist: those that require logical, inferential, sequential strategies, and those that require holistic, simultaneous, pattern-seeking strategies. Problems arise because of some type of functional fixedness, a rigidity or constraint present in an entity because of either linguistics or perception. For example, when something is given a label, it absorbs all the semantic qualities associated with the label and at the same time restricts most people from thinking beyond the semantic constraints; the label thus may prove to be beneficial in that it provides some focus, or it may be detrimental because it is too restrictive. Historically, the term *supervision* in the Communication Disorders profession has carried the semantic constraint of being equated with clinical education, thereby restricting the idea of what a Communication Disorders supervisor is and does. The problem is a linguistic one of identity and definition.

The other common source of problems is perceptual; these problems, too, have a linguistic component. Consider the following scenario: As a supervisor, a student clinician, and a parent observe a child in therapy, the three observers make these comments about the tears that begin coming from the child's eyes:

STUDENT: Oh-oh, Amanda is upset. She's beginning to cry. I'd better go in and help my co-clinician.

SUPERVISOR: No, I think she got some of the flour from their cooking project in her eyes. See how she's rubbing them? She'll be OK after she blinks a few times. You stay out here and let your colleague handle it.

PARENT: Actually, she has allergies, and today there is such a high count that she's tearing because of overactive histamines. I need to go in and give her her allergy medicine.

Various perceptions of the same event may be labeled differently by different people and, as a result of the semantic label, will be managed differently. Reacting to a child's tearing by assuming that the child is sad (the student clinician's tack) would produce a management approach very different from the physical irritant approach (the supervisor's). The allergy viewpoint (the parent's) provides even another approach. In short, problems may arise from the way a situation is perceived or from the way it is labeled when described. Managing problems, then, involves altering perceptions or redefining what is being observed.

PROBLEM MANAGING

The literature that is relevant to managing problems generally uses the term *problem solving,* which reflects the logical, systematic, scientific approach to dealing with problems. The word *solve* implies a finality to the problem: that it will not occur again once a solution is found. Most problems in Communication Disorders supervision, because they involve people, are ongoing; they appear over and over but in different forms. Supervision interactants involved in dealing with a problem often suppose that once the problem has been attended to and a solution reached, it should not appear again. When it does, they may feel a consternation detrimental to their approach to problems. Why solve problems when in fact nothing has been solved? Supervision participants might more realistically think in terms of *managing* problems: working to find meaningful outcomes for the present state of the problem, but acknowledging that the problem will likely emerge again in a different form and will need renewed management efforts. This approach requires that supervision participants accept problems as continuous rather than episodic, so that, when the problem does re-emerge, participant energies can be channelled toward productive management of the problem.

The concept of problem management is related to two concepts already presented: systems and change (see chapter 3). In the context of general systems theory (Bertalanffy, 1968) and general systems thinking (Coulter, 1986), it is clear that (a) problems will occur in open and closed systems; (b) all parts of a problem are related, and change in one part causes change in others; (c) similar initial conditions can yield different outcomes, and similar outcomes can result from different initial conditions (*equifinality*); (d) feedback can maintain (*morphostasis*) or change (*morphogenesis*) a problem; (e) problems are ongoing (rather than episodic), have movement and form, and have both relationship and content levels; and (f) problems can be managed using metacognitive operations. Further, management of problems in Communication Disorders supervision requires preparation for change. (See chapter 3 for a discussion of systems and change.)

Various philosophical and psychological approaches to learning were discussed in chapter 3. Inherent in each of those theories is a basic approach to managing problems.

THEORIES OF PROBLEM MANAGING

Behaviorist/Associationist Theory

Much of what is known about problem managing has been learned by observing people involved in the process. Before the late 1950s the predominant theory used to study problem management was behaviorism, or functional analysis (Miller, 1984). This school emphasizes stimuli, responses, and the associations between them. Behaviorists (also referred to as associationists) argue that responses previously used in a problem situation are most likely to be tried when the situation arises again. According to this theory, when a problem re-emerges an individual will probably do what was done before; a corollary is that behaviors that have not helped in managing a given problem will lose strength, whereas those that do facilitate productive management will move up the hierarchy of strategies. The major limitation of the behaviorist/associationist theory is that it fails to explain the problem management process in new situations; it does not account for the rapid processing that occurs. Instead, the theory predicts that an individual in a new situation will engage in a trial-and-error application of past habits, an inefficient and time-consuming procedure. This deficiency in the theory led to a broader perspective on learning: the Gestalt theory.

Gestalt Theory

Identifying the influence of perceptual organization in problem management was a major achievement of Gestalt psychologists. The Gestalt theory of problem management is considered a diametric opposite to the behaviorist/associationist theory; it is a structural analysis approach to problem management. Gestaltists view problem managing as resulting in the ability to comprehend how the parts of a problem fit together to satisfy the requirements of the goal (Bourne & Ekstrand, 1982). They describe a creative process at a high cognitive level that uses perceptual organization (the categorizing of stimuli) to give form to the problem. The process is believed to consist of a series of stages or steps through which the participants progress. However, the theory gives little or no consideration to the mental processes of attention, memory, cognitive style, or motivation. Information processing theory supplies those components.

Information Processing Theory

The dominant means of studying problem managing now is the information processing approach. In this model, problem management is seen as a process of evaluating a problem, selecting one of a number of possible steps toward the preferred outcome, evaluating the resulting situation, then selecting and applying the next most appropriate step and so on. This process continues until the desired outcome is reached. The process can be reactivated as needed to manage a changed form of the problem.

Bourne and Ekstrand (1982) present a classic description of the information processing approach to problem managing as represented in their computer program *General Problem Solver (GPS)*. In this model, the authors characterize a person's internal memory representation of a problem as *problem space*. All management activity (thinking) is conducted within the problem space. This space includes a number of components: the *initial state* (givens) of the problem, the *goal state* (the outcome to be achieved), possible *intermediate states* (subgoals), and *operators* (procedures) that can be applied to move from one state to another and finally to the goal state. These components of the problem space can be identified in nearly every type of problem researchers have studied.

The concept of a problem space within which people work toward a desired outcome implies constraints on the steps or moves that are possible or that a manager is willing to make in the process. The problem space defines a limited set of possibilities, and occasionally problem managers need to move beyond the boundaries of that set. The boundary setting can become functional fixedness if the manager has defined the problem space in a way that restricts possible uses of a key element.

A phenomenon known as *incubation* is relevant to the discussion of problem space. Incubation occurs when a problem manager leaves the process temporarily and, upon returning to it, immediately discovers a new productive outcome that seems obvious. Incubation is considered by some to be a kind of unconscious management process. Others suggest that incubation creates a new and more effective problem space. Whatever the explanation, incubation shows the advisability of trying completely different approaches when working on difficult problems.

A critical aspect of problem managing is selecting and applying operators, the information organizing methods that facilitate movement in the process. Two types of operators are discussed in the problem solving literature: algorithms and heuristics.

Algorithms. An *algorithm* is a guaranteed path to a productive outcome. The scientific decision making process described in chapter 7 is algorithmic. While algorithms offer guaranteed solutions, they have a number of disadvantages. One is that they can be inefficient and time-consuming; if applied automatically step by step, they may obscure the easiest paths and solutions. Also, not all problems can be managed by the logical, sequential, vertical thinking approach.

Vertical thinking is described by deBono (1970) as an analytical, sequential, high-probability, finite process. Vertical thinkers take the most reasonable view of a situation and then proceed logically and carefully to work it out. According to deBono (1968), vertical thinking has always been the only respectable type of thinking, and our educational system urges all minds to strive for its ultimate form, logic. Computers are the best example of vertical thinking. The programmer defines both the problem and the logical step-by-step procedure for solving it. The computer then employs the procedure unvaryingly and efficiently to work out the problem.

An alternative to using algorithms when managing problems is to use heuristics.

Heuristics. A *heuristic* is a method of deriving and evaluating potential productive outcomes.

Lateral thinking, planning, goal revision, semantic mediation, and creativity are heuristics that supervisors can use to manage many Communication Disorders supervision problems.

Lateral thinking. Lateral thinking, or low-probability thinking, was developed by deBono (1968) as a way to explore many alternative views of a problem rather than accepting what is apparently the most promising and proceeding from there. Lateral thinking is not only used in problem managing but also for looking at new ideas and situations of every sort. It is a productive strategy for enlarging one's problem space or world of knowledge. To use deBono's metaphor, if the goal is to dig a bigger and deeper hole, even though the hole may be in an inadequate location, then vertical thinking is the way to work. However, if the goal is to dig the best hole in the best location, then lateral thinking must be used. Vertical thinking is the tool used to dig holes bigger and deeper; lateral thinking means trying again somewhere else.

Many people find it difficult to abandon a half-dug hole, so to speak, because they are reluctant to give up an investment of time and effort without seeing some return. Besides, it is easier to go on doing the same thing than to explore other possibilities.

It is impossible to look in a different direction while looking harder in the same direction. When two thoughts are strung together they create a direction; it is easier to add further thoughts along the same line than to ignore the line. It is difficult work to ignore an idea, especially without an alternative.

Historically the greatest amount of scientific effort is focused on the logical enlargement of some accepted hole; this holds true for Communication Disorders supervision also. However, new ideas and scientific advancements have usually come when someone either ignored a hole that was in progress, was dissatisfied with or ignorant of the old one, had a temperamental need to be different, or acted on a whim. Such hole-hopping is rare because the current educational system stresses appreciation of existing holes. It would be difficult to build competence by encouraging general dissatisfaction with an existing array of holes. Also, education is not always concerned with progress; often its purpose is to make useful knowledge available on a wide scale, to disseminate rather than to create.

To conclude this hole-digging analogy, an incomplete hole offers a direction in which to expend energy. Energy needs direction, and few situations are more frustrating than eager energy looking for a direction. Most often, efforts require reward by some tangible result; the more immediate the result, the more energy goes into the effort. Enlarging the hole being dug offers visible progress and assurance of future achievement. Finally, a well-dug hole has a comfortable, secure familiarity. Because Communication Disorders supervision is a young discipline, we must consider the consequences of enlarging and deepening the various supervision holes and of finding new holes to explore. Table 8-1 compares vertical and lateral thinking.

The second heuristic to be discussed is planning

Planning. Rather than pursuing a problem one step at a time, it can be profitable to plan ahead and develop a sequence of moves. The planning operator can help identify intermediate problem states that could be obstacles to a productive outcome. Planning, however, is only one of a number of metacognitive operations, and Communication Disorders supervisors must use it as such. To be able to plan effectively and efficiently, you need to understand metacognition.

Metacognition is knowledge about cognition. It includes conscious access to one's own cognitive operations and reflection about those of others. Metacognition involves analyzing, planning, regulating, controlling, monitoring, evaluating, and revising thoughts and actions through operations including (a) analyzing and characterizing the problem; (b) reflecting on what one already knows or needs to know to manage the

TABLE 8-1 Comparison of vertical and lateral thinking

Vertical Thinking	Lateral Thinking
1. Selective; rightness matters	1. Generative; richness matters
2. Moves only if there is a direction in which to move	2. Moves in order to generate a direction
3. Analytical	3. Provocative
4. Sequential	4. Can make jumps
5. Each step must be correct	5. Each step does not need to be correct
6. Negative aspects are used to block off certain pathways	6. There is no negative
7. Concentration and focus exclude what is irrelevant	7. Chance intrusions are welcome
8. Categories, classifications, and labels are fixed	8. Categories, classifications, and labels are negotiable and transactive
9. Follows the most likely paths; logical	9. Explores the least likely paths; not logical
10. A finite process	10. A probabilistic process
11. Digs a hole deeper	11. Changes the site of the hole
12. High-probability outcomes	12. Low-probability outcomes

Source. *Lateral Thinking: Creativity Step by Step* by E. deBono, 1970, New York: Harper & Row.

problem; (c) devising a plan for attacking the problem (thinking ahead about what to do in the future); (d) monitoring progress; and (e) evaluating the process separate from the outcome.

Planning means designing a way to change some current state, the *status quo,* into some other desired state, the *goal* state (Patterson & Roberts, 1982). The process of planning includes understanding its purpose and knowing when to plan. Planning is used to decide or schedule actions or to make decisions about how to do an activity. Many activities will not work if they aren't planned, and become problems that must be managed. Planning must be done in adequate time before an activity, should not be done by someone who does not have major responsibility for executing the plan, and need not be done for activities where the procedures are already known. Planning, as a metacognitive operation, is important in all five domains of Communication Disorders supervision: Professional, Research, Educational, Administrative, and Clinical.

Planning includes selecting both the content and the order of activities undertaken to achieve a goal. Planning requires some knowledge of what actions are to be undertaken and the conditions under which they will be performed. Planning involves hierarchical organization of goals and subgoals. Plans must include criteria for assessing planning efforts and their outcomes. For example, criteria for a good plan might include safety, fairness, how it makes the participants feel, and whether it manages the problem without creating other problems (Camp & Bash, 1981). Good plans are not easy to develop. Planning, according to Pea (1982), is most problematic if difficult decisions must be made, concentrated thinking is required, many things need to be planned, changes need to be made, something must be planned for the first time, the plan repeatedly is not carried out, or the action being planned is disliked. Planning is also difficult if efficient and effective plan execution is desired, the planning context is noisy, the plan execution is rapid, the plan is complicated and difficult to remember, or the plan is not important to the planner(s).

Throughout a problem managing process, a Communication Disorders supervisor needs to monitor self-progress. Self-monitoring requires recognition of the plans of others: acknowledging that other people plan, perspective taking (imagining what others are seeing), person perception (knowing traits or attributes of others), and role taking (imagining the intentions, thoughts, and feelings of others, which requires perspective taking and person perception).

Planning should also involve evaluating the planning process itself, separate from evaluating the outcome of the problem managing process: were the criteria of good planning met?

Planning is an important prerequisite to problem management, and Communication Disorders preparation programs must ensure that trainees develop competence in planning.

Planning, especially the evaluation component, may lead to the use of a third heuristic, this one for revising goals.

Goal revision. Goal revision is used to revise unattainable goals and subgoals into more attainable ones. The process may include subdividing the goals into objectives, clarifying the wording, doing further research or study, and changing the specified time frame. Once a subgoal is reached, more subgoals may be developed or the goal state may be attained.

Heuristics require good background knowledge, what Larkin (1980) terms *domain-specific* or *content-related* knowledge. This knowledge is an aggregate of concepts. Concepts are mediated by semantics.

Semantic mediators. The fourth heuristic to be discussed is the use of *semantic mediators,* or concepts. According to Bourne and Ekstrand (1982), a concept is commonly thought of as an idea or as the meaning of something. Concepts may be concrete (such as *audiogram*) or abstract (such as *sincerity*). A concept is a basic unit of knowledge. It can be present in active awareness or can be held in inactive memory until needed.

Concepts may be thought of in two ways: as building blocks or as bundles or packets of information. As building blocks, concepts can be used variously to create simple or complex knowledge systems. Concepts can also be considered packets or bundles of information that mediate a knowledge system.

Concepts are mediated by *semantic networks.* Single words have meanings; those meanings may be altered when the words are combined with others. Semantic networks are the interrelationships of words that help develop meaning.

Concepts are classified as logical or natural. *Logical* concepts are defined according to certain relevant features and rules about those features. A logical concept is used to categorize, unambiguously, all instances or sets of objects as either having or not having membership in a concept. *Natural* concepts, on the other hand, have "fuzzy" boundaries and better and worse examples, with some items or instances belonging more or less fully to a category. Some theorists define natural concepts in relation to a category prototype, or best example, that serves as a reference point for the category and allows for flexibility of interpretation (Rosch & Mervis, 1975). Logical concepts are most often associated with vertical and convergent thinking, natural concepts with lateral and divergent thinking. It also can be said that logical concepts align with the science aspect of Communication Disorders supervision whereas natural concepts are associated with the art of the process. Combining logical concepts with natural concepts is the science and art of Communication Disorders supervision.

Manipulating concepts in unique ways is called creativity, the fifth heuristic.

Creativity. Some problems involve a clearly defined goal state, clearly identified subgoals, and known operations that can be followed to reach an outcome. But if the management of a problem is less clear-cut, then *creative* problem management is required.

Creative problem managing cannot be defined by any single procedure. Creative outcomes are novel and useful, meet the objectives of the problem, and ideally transform one's concept of what is produced (goal state) or of the source of the problem (initial state) (Jackson & Messick, 1965). Creative problem managers seek a variety of potential outcomes to a problem and continually restructure or redefine the problem as each outcome is found. Creativity encompasses both fluency and flexibility. Fluency means smoothly and rapidly producing a large number of ideas about a problem. Flexibility means finding divergent, unusual ideas. These criteria help to identify whether an outcome is a product of creative thought. They do not, however, tell what abilities or techniques a person must use to reach creative outcomes. Guilford's (1967) Structure-of-Intellect model is a three-dimensional (4 cells × 5 cells × 6 cells) model of intellectual functioning composed of *context* (figural, symbolic, semantic, and behavioral), *operations* (evaluation, convergent production, divergent production, memory, and cognition), and *products* (units, classes, relations, systems, transformations, and implications).

People differ in their ability to use the various mental operations as they are associated with various contents and products. Some mental operations are particularly important in creative thought. Among the most important are those involving divergent production. Like other forms of mental function, creative thought is a joint product of divergent and convergent thinking using various contents and outputting various products. Some individuals are particularly capable of combining divergent and convergent thinking creatively in working with certain content to produce certain outcomes. DeBono (1968) distinguishes between lateral thinking and creativity. He views lateral thinking as a larger concept of which creativity is one part. Creative thinking, according to deBono, often requires a talent for expression, whereas lateral thinking is open to anyone interested in new ideas.

Divergent thinking is associated with creativity. Divergent thinking is being able to overcome the limitations of functional fixedness and mental set, or the dominance of certain ideas. Dominant ideas need not always be obvious to exert a powerful structural influence on how a person or organization thinks and approaches problems. Therefore, divergent thinking, creativity, and lateral thinking must be used to identify dominant, restrictive ideas and to combat them with new thoughts, ideas, concepts, and actions.

Because of the diverse nature of problems, creativity may also require that a person apply convergent thinking to select the most appropriate of the possible outcomes. In short, creative problem managing in Communication Disorders supervision requires a wide range of skills and dispositions and the flexibility to use them productively.

Benefits of Creative Problem Managing. Creative problem managing has a number of benefits for Communication Disorders supervisors. According to Olson (1980) and deBono (1985), creativity in problem managing has been shown to

1. help focus the thoughts of a group for productive management of a problem.
2. pull members of a group together to work for a common goal.
3. improve morale.
4. increase leadership ability.
5. increase persistence.
6. help people develop new interests in work, leisure, and life in general.
7. facilitate open-mindedness toward self and others.
8. help people learn to delay judgment.
9. help people recognize problems earlier so as to manage them more effectively and efficiently.
10. reduce procrastination.
11. increase self-acceptance, confidence, and risk taking.

12. facilitate more enthusiastic acceptance of responsibility.
13. facilitate the generation of new and useful ideas that can lead to effective and efficient management of problems.
14. increase enthusiasm for work and for problem management.

Reasoning. Logic and creativity combine into the process of reasoning. Two kinds of reasoning are recognized: formal logic and natural reasoning. These correspond to logical concepts and natural concepts as discussed earlier in this chapter. *Formal logic* consists of a set of rules for analyzing a situation, position, or statement and deciding whether it is internally consistent. Training in formal logic gives people a set of intellectual skills and dispositions (competence) that they can use to analyze their own and others' situations, positions, or statements. Communication Disorders supervisors who do not have this competence may make reasoning errors that are predictable and understandable as simple deviations from logic. Knowing more about logic can help us understand how people usually reason (see chapter 7).

Most discourse, whether it is conversation, discussion, formal speaking, or text, follows a set of conventions described by Grice (1975) as Cooperative Principles (see also pp. 107 and 114). In essence, the principles state that a competent communicator (speaker or writer) produces language in such a way as to maximize the effectiveness of the communication for a recipient (listener or reader). The four principles are these: (a) the structure of the communication is no more or less informative than required; (b) the sender both believes and has adequate evidence for what is said; (c) the communication is relevant; and (d) the communication is structured so as to be easily understood by the receiver. Although most Communication Disorders personnel follow these principles without much awareness, it must be recognized that they have important consequences. In particular, much information is left for the receiver to infer rather than being explicitly stated. Thus, natural reasoning, based on both the sender's and the receiver's communication competence, is done partly in the process of comprehending, or making meaning.

The last theory of problem managing is the schema theory, which integrates concepts from previous theories.

Schema Theory

A recent theory of problem managing that adopts some ideas about perception from the Gestalt theory and combines them with a refined information processing theory is the *schema theory*. Schema theory describes how knowledge is packaged, or represented in units called *schemata* (Rumelhart, 1980). According to Rumelhart, schemata are data structures used to store concepts; every kind of concept a person stores requires schemata for representing it. In addition, each schema contains "the network of interrelations that is believed to normally hold among the constituents of the concept in question" (p. 34). In this theory, schemata are constructed interpretations of events, objects, or situations, brought by semantic manipulation into comprehensible units that constitute a person's view of the nature of reality. In addition to constructing comprehension, schemata provide a source for predictions about unexperienced events. Schemata allow people to fill in the cracks of their knowledge constructs when only part of the information surrounding an object, event, or situation is received. This is possible because semantic networks are often predictable. In short, schemata allow people to manage problems by moving from known to unknown territory through interpretation and prediction.

Schemata are activated and used in two types of processing: conceptually driven (top-down) and data-driven (bottom-up) processing (Dodd & White, 1980; Norman & Bobrow, 1976).

Top-down processing involves activating a schema and all its subcomponents (sub-schemata). For example, a supervisor is asked by a supervisee to imagine a client's drawing of a person. The supervisor's schema for drawings of human figures is activated, and its sub-schemata are common ways of representing the various body parts, their size, proportions, and relationships. This is conceptually driven processing, based on past experiences stored in memory and on the predictability of the semantic concept *person*. It may or may not produce an accurate representation of the actual drawing.

On the other hand, if the supervisee shows the supervisor the actual drawing, no matter how distorted the drawing may be, viewing the discrete and separate elements will contribute to the supervisor's interpretation of the drawing as representing a person (bottom-up). In this instance, individual data provided as separate components work together to form a generalized concept of *person*. When faced with one type of problem, the Communication Disorders supervisor must use one type of processing (top-down); a different strategy (bottom-up) must be used to manage the second situation. Thus, schema theory explains how different strategies are used for managing different types of problems.

One major factor distinguishes the Gestalt and the information processing approaches to problem management. Gestalt theory views problem managing as an intuitive and sometimes automatic process. The outcome is simple and obvious if the problem is analyzed in the right way. Processing theory, in contrast, describes problem managing as primarily a conscious, planned, and logical activity and considers somewhat more complicated and more natural problems (see p. 208). Like all higher mental processes, problem managing probably involves both intuition and logic. Intuition works best when the outcome is simple and can be attained immediately; logic may be required when many steps are needed to reach an outcome.

What has been said about problem managing theories can be summarized as follows. First, problem managing can be defined as (a) the discovery of relationships or connections between the known and the unknown; (b) the creation or discovery of something new; or (c) the validation of something thought to be true. Second, problems can be defined relatively easily according to component parts, but the *process* of managing problems is not understood by those doing research in the area. Third, the processes one uses to attain outcomes are described in a variety of ways, with the general consensus that problem managing involves knowing about and using different strategies and having a reservoir of background knowledge on which to draw.

Productive problem managing should be the goal of supervisors. However, they may encounter obstacles to that goal.

OBSTACLES TO PRODUCTIVE PROBLEM MANAGEMENT

According to Olson (1980), Mussen, Conger, and Kagan (1974), and Smith (1981), a number of obstacles can interfere with productive problem managing:

1. *Attention:* The ability to select and concentrate on the relevant aspects of a problem is important in every step of the problem managing process. For complex problems, the inability to focus attention may contribute to the random, impulsive strategies sometimes used in problem management.
2. *Failure to comprehend the problem:* Problems may not be managed efficiently and effectively, not because the managers are incapable of doing so but because they do not understand what is to be done.
3. *Forgetting elements of the problem:* Another common cause of failure to generate good outcomes is forgetting basic elements of the problem. The more complex the problem is, the higher the probability of forgetting basic elements.

4. *Cognitive style:* The problem managing process may be affected by cognitive tempo (reflective or impulsive), an aspect of cognitive style. People may respond to a problem quickly with a high rate of inappropriate responses (impulsive) or respond more slowly and make more appropriate responses (reflective).

McKenny and Keen (1976) identified a variety of cognitive styles, the main ones being *systematic–preceptive* and *intuitive–receptive*. Their research showed that about three-fourths of their subjects used only one style, while the remainder favored one style but did not use it exclusively. McKenny and Keen also reported that most people use their preferred style for all problems rather than switching back and forth between cognitive styles. Since many problems lend themselves to one problem managing style more than to others, it is important, when possible, to have people with contrasting styles work together. (Refer to the discussion of cognitive styles and personality types in chapter 2.)

Erhardt and Corvey (1980) suggest that individuals have several styles of thinking and use them for different kinds of problems. They have identified five styles of reasoning used in problem managing:

a. *Rule-governed reasoning.* Problems are managed best when the underlying policies that govern them are known; definitions are important.

SUPERVISOR: We will deal with your excessive absenteeism by referring to our attendance policies on page 15 of the Clinicians' Handbook.

b. *Differences-focused reasoning.* Problems are managed by looking for differences among components; asking "What if . . ." is typical of people with this style.

SUPERVISOR: Let's look at the different ways we are focusing on this problem. You are asking to take the exam on another day because you have two exams scheduled on the same day. Your focus is on rearranging the exam to meet your individual needs. My focus is on meeting the demands of a curriculum and its instructor. What would happen if I allowed all the students in the class to take the exam at another time just because they had more than one exam scheduled per day?

c. *Similarities-focused reasoning.* Problems are managed by grouping similar ideas and developing an outcome based on those commonalities.

SUPERVISOR: We have too many clients to schedule individually, so we're going to try grouping clients as Judi suggested. I think Juan, Sigrid, Troy, and Anna would make a workable articulation group.

d. *Synthesized reasoning.* This is a combination of the three previous styles. Synthesized reasoning generally takes more time.

SUPERVISOR: Each of you has gathered some information about how to work with the marginal students in our program. Let's synthesize your information into supervision guidelines that our entire department can follow.

e. *Deductive reasoning.* Deductive reasoning is logical reasoning, such as is used in mathematics and syllogisms.

SUPERVISOR: If language is symbols and learning occurs by the manipulation of symbols,

then all learning-disabled people must be language disabled, because they have difficulty manipulating symbols, or learning.
5. *Insufficient knowledge:* The lack of appropriate rules or information to manage the problem productively. Life experiences help determine whether an individual will have the knowledge needed to manage a problem.
6. *Motivation:* Beliefs about what causes one's own behavior serve as *cognitive mediators* and thus influence subsequent behavior, such as one's willingness to deal with a new or difficult problem, persistence, effort, and expectations for productive management of problems. Most people attribute the success or failure of their problem managing to effort, ability, problem difficulty, or luck. If they believe that their success is a result of effort, problem managers are likely to expend effort on similar problems in the future. Conversely, if they believe that productive outcomes were due to luck, expense of effort in the future will seem unlikely to increase the chances for productive problem managing.
7. *Firm belief in rules inconsistent with the correct hypothesis:* The "My mind is made up, don't confuse me with the facts" syndrome can be a strong block to creativity.
8. *Fear of error or failure:* Most people are not only afraid of criticism from others if they fail, but want to avoid self-generated shame or humiliation from violating personal standards of competence. Communication Disorders supervisors who are prepared to supervise will recognize the supervisees who are inhibited. Cautious supervisees often know more than they are willing to say. They censor good ideas because they would rather forego the possibility of success than risk failure.
9. *Habit:* This is generally considered to be an uncreative, stereotyped form of response that may prevent the supervisor and interactants from using divergent or lateral thinking.
10. *Time:* Time pressures may force a person to act before thinking. People who have time to be more creative take it out of the same 24 hours per day allocated to everyone else; however, they think (or plan) before acting.
11. *Too many problems:* Problems must sometimes be identified and prioritized to keep Communication Disorders supervisors from becoming overwhelmed.
12. *No problems:* Humans are problem-managing animals, constantly facing problems. If problems are managed automatically, habitually, or by another person, they may never be recognized as problems. Supervisors, supervisees, and others may feel that they have no problems and, consequently, no need to practice creative problem managing.
13. *Need for one answer now:* People often become anxious when they have problems and no immediate answer. Therefore, unsatisfactory outcomes are often chosen to alleviate the anxiety.
14. *Difficulty of directed mental activity:* Supervisors must consider that people may find physical exertion easy but mental exertion difficult, or vice versa.
15. *Fear of fun:* Part of the process of creative problem managing involves intermixing fun, relaxation, and playfulness with serious deliberations.
16. *Recognizing good outcomes:* Some people are unable, or perhaps unmotivated, to find greater value in creative activities than in habitual ones.
17. *Criticism by others:* Creative problem managing may be stifled by untimely or unconstructive critical remarks by others.

Communication Disorders supervisors, to increase their creative problem managing competence, may first need to decrease obstacles to creativity. Until they do this, they will have difficulty interacting effectively with others in problematic situations. Fortunately, several approaches to creative problem managing exist.

PROBLEM MANAGING PROGRAMS

Problem managing training programs have certain necessary components. Good preparation programs should

1. be comprehensive by involving instructors as well as supervisors, supervisees, clients, and ancillary personnel; by addressing social, academic, personal, and professional problems; by acknowledging that change is inherent in problem managing and that change is a difficult process; by emphasizing ways to understand and meet other people's values and expectations and to communicate acceptance to persons being helped.
2. use a variety of procedures, such as modeling (e.g., demonstrating a positive attitude, approaching problems with confidence, applying both inhibition and rational risk-taking in dealing with problems), self-verbalization, self-instruction, role-playing, and individual and group methods. Dyer (1972) suggests that people in today's society need the ability to determine when to be independent from others and when to collaborate with others.
3. last long enough to ensure that strategies have been learned as well as skills and have begun to be employed as dispositions.
4. emphasize the importance of being able to ask productive questions. Good questioning strategies can enhance thinking and problem managing abilities. By employing the questioning strategies outlined in chapter 5, supervisors can learn to develop questions about procedures, tasks, information, and understanding, areas integral to the Professional, Research, Educational, Administrative, and Clinical domains.

Although many paradigms exist for teaching problem management, Feldhusen's (1973) model is the most detailed. It includes 10 steps that can be implemented in three stages:

Stage I: Obtaining the information
  1. Sensing that a problem exists
  2. Defining the problem

Stage II: Understanding the problem
  3. Clarifying the problem
  4. Guessing causes (generating and evaluating hypotheses)
  5. Judging whether more information is needed
  6. Noting relevant details

Stage III: Managing the problem
  7. Viewing familiar situations in unfamiliar ways
  8. Seeing implications
  9. Choosing outcomes
  10. Verifying outcomes

Specific Problem Managing Strategies

Many problem managing strategies have been developed. Some are broad and include all three stages of problem managing mentioned previously, such as Reflective Thinking (Whitman & Boase, 1983); others pinpoint a specific step within a stage, like Synectics for step 7 (Gordon, 1961). Some of the strategies emphasize the logical, sequential methods of vertical thinking; others present creative ways to break through rigid verticality. Communication Disorders supervisors need to be aware of the many tools available to help them manage problems in the most productive manner. Six approaches to problem managing are presented here.

Simulations and Role-Playing. Wasinger and Ortman (1984) discussed the importance of problem managing in the 13 tasks and 81 competencies of supervision and presented a simulation program to improve students' clinical problem managing skills. Role-playing is another technique used to teach problem management. Books that are particularly relevant to super-

TABLE 8-2
Samples of specific problem managing strategies and purposes

I Whole-Brain Thinking Model (Wonder & Donovan, 1984)

Strategy	Purpose
Internal Brainstorming	To discover solutions or concepts by using both left- and right-brain strategies. The open-ended, non-judgmental stage is a freewheeling, right-brain experience; analysis and evaluation are left-brain activities.

II Lateral Thinking Model (deBono, 1985)

Strategy	Purpose
4M (Me-Values; Mates-Values; Moral-Values; Mankind-Values)	To direct attention to four value systems that link events with personal emotions.
TEC Framework (Target/Task, Expand/Explore, Contrast/Conclude)	To focus thinking and make it a deliberate task.
The 5-Minute Think	To focus thinking for a brief, intense period. 1 minute: T/T; 2 minutes: E/E; 2 minutes: C/C.
PISCO (Purpose, Input, Solutions, Choice, Operation)	To focus thinking by separating the stages.

III Conceptual Blockbusting Model (Adams, 1979)

Strategy	Purpose
Bug List	To develop a list of specific small-scale needs: a fluent, flexible, specific, and personal list of things that are personal irritants ("bugs").
Brainstorming (Osborn, 1953)	To develop conceptualization in groups by suspending judgment: to create

---

vision include *Values Clarification* (Simon, Howe, & Kirschenbaum, 1972), *Skill-Streaming the Adolescent* (Goldstein, Sprafkin, Gershaw, & Klein, 1980), and *Special Children in Regular Classrooms* (Epstein, 1984).

Whole-Brain Thinking. Table 8-2 presents two of the six strategies based on the concept of whole-brain thinking (Wonder & Donovan, 1984). The whole-brain strategies attempt to engage both right (creative) and left (logical) hemispheres of the brain in the problem managing process.

deBono's Thinking Course. Three of 30 strategies from deBono's Thinking Course (1985) are presented in Table 8-2. Several of the lessons in deBono's course are derived from the *CoRT (Cognitive Research Trust) Thinking Program,* the most widely used curriculum for the direct teaching of thinking skills. The strategies illustrate lateral thinking.

Conceptual Blockbusting. Table 8-2 describes three of six Conceptual Blockbusting strategies (Adams, 1979) and their purposes. These strategies emphasize creativity as taught in the

TABLE 8-2 continued

III Conceptual Blockbusting Model (Adams, 1979)

Strategy	Purpose
	ideas rapidly without judgment or evaluation.
Synectics (Gordon, 1961)	To develop conceptualization in groups by suspending judgment through the use of metaphor: Personal Analogy, Direct Analogy, Symbolic Analogy, Fantasy Analogy.

IV Communication Dynamics Model (Whitman & Boase, 1983)

Strategy	Purpose
Reflective Thinking (Dewey, 1910)	To encourage an orderly and thorough discussion of problems using Dewey's five-step agenda (define the problem; define the causes; specify the criteria for outcomes; consider more than one outcome; choose the best outcome).
Lecture Forum	To present in-depth information from opposing viewpoints for thorough understanding of the various facets of a problem; low audience discussion.
Panel Discussion	Similar to Lecture Forum but using a panel of experts rather than single experts at different times; panel discusses, audience may participate.
Buzz Sessions	To stimulate widespread participation and prolific ideas.

Design Division of the Stanford School of Engineering.

Communication Dynamics. Four problem managing strategies based on concepts of communication are presented in Table 8-2. They exemplify both vertical and lateral thinking.

DO IT. The DO IT model (Olson, 1980) is the most complete creative thinking program in that it touches on all three stages of the process as represented in Feldhusen's (1973) model. The DO IT Model is an acronym for the process:

D = Define the problem
O = Open self to consider many diverse ideas
I = Identify best ideas
T = Transform best idea into action

Applications to Communication Disorders Supervision

A number of creative problem managing strategies have been applied directly to Communication Disorders supervision.

Farmer and Farmer (1986) presented a short

TABLE 8-3
Problems, management strategies, and supervision types

Problem	Problem Managing Strategy	Model	Supervision Type
Taking a case history	4-M	Lateral Thinking (deBono, 1985)	1 (STYLE I/dyad)
Using productive questioning strategies	5-Minute Think	Lateral Thinking (deBono, 1985)	1 (STYLE I/dyad)
	Internal Brainstorming	Conceptual Blockbusting (Adams, 1979)	
Writing goals and objectives	Lecture Forum	Communication Dynamics (Whitman & Boase, 1983)	4 (STYLE II/group)
Writing reports	Panel Discussion	Communication Dynamics (Whitman & Boase, 1983)	4 (STYLE II/group)
Masking	PISCO	Lateral Thinking (deBono, 1985)	5 (STYLE III/dyad)
Using critical observation skills	Bug List	Conceptual Blockbusting (Adams, 1979)	5 (STYLE III/dyad)
Counseling	Dewey's Reflective Thinking Pattern	Communication Dynamics (Whitman & Boase, 1983)	8 (STYLE IV/group)
Using therapy materials creatively	Buzz Sessions	Communication Dynamics (Whitman & Boase, 1983)	8 (STYLE IV/group)
	Brainstorming	Conceptual Blockbusting (Adams, 1979)	

Source. Unilateral and Bilateral Styles of Dyadic and Group Clinical Education/Supervision, a short course presented at the annual convention of the American Speech-Language-Hearing Association, Detroit, MI, 1986, by S. Farmer and J. Farmer.

course at the ASHA convention using videotaped segments of conferences to illustrate the use of specific problem managing strategies with four of the eight types of supervision (STYLES + forms). The problems, strategies, theoretical models, and types of supervision are shown in Table 8-3.

In a miniseminar at the ASHA convention, Farmer, Farmer, Dimmer, Lyon, Nesbit, Thompson, and Wertzberger (1987), through small-group interactions, implemented five strategies to manage problems associated with each of the Communication Disorders domains. The domain-related problems and the strategies used to generate outcomes are shown in Table 8-4.

An added benefit to both ASHA presentations

was that graduate students took part as presenters. Providing opportunities for graduate students to apply knowledge and skills they have acquired through supervision training is one way to facilitate the growth and development of Communication Disorders supervision.

SUSTAINING PRODUCTIVE PROBLEM MANAGING

Like all the areas of competence discussed in this textbook, creative problem managing competence needs to be sustained. However, before sustaining competence in problem managing, supervisors must develop that competence by implementing appropriately-developed goals and objectives in Communication Disorders supervision preparation programs, continuing education, or self-development. After that, the following methods can be employed to ensure that competence in problem managing is sustained: (a) change environments and elements within environments; (b) exercise physically (being and feeling healthy can aid problem managing); (c) exercise mentally (problem managing takes practice); (d) help others to manage problems.

TABLE 8-4
Roles, problems, and management strategies

Role	Problem	Goal	Problem Managing Strategy
Professional	Of the approximately 1,700 speech-language pathologists and audiologists involved in supervision, approximately 350 (18%) are members of CUSPSPA; a majority of CUSPSPA members are not active participants in the organization.	To increase the number of active participants in CUSPSPA.	DO IT (Define the problem; Open self to consider many ideas; Identify the best ideas; Transform best idea into action) (Olson, 1980).
Researcher	Limited research is being done in the supervision process.	To increase the opportunities for Speech-Language Pathology and Audiology students to do research in supervision.	PISCO (Purpose; Input; Solutions; Choice; Operation) (deBono, 1985).
Educator	Supervisors do not have high intra- or inter-judge reliability when evaluating supervisee competence.	To establish a minimum of one procedure for developing supervisors' reliability competence.	Synectics (Gordon, 1961; Adams, 1979)
Administrator	Supervisors are not competent in developing Communication Disorders programs to	To facilitate the development of supervisors' competence in program development for	TEC Framework using the 5-Minute Think: Target/Task, 1 minute; Expand/Explore, 2

TABLE 8-4
continued

Role	Problem	Goal	Problem Managing Strategy
Administrator	meet the needs of a given context (e.g., worksite, community).	(1) a college or university speech and hearing center; (2) a school program; (3) a community speech and hearing center; (4) a medical setting; (5) a business (e.g., hearing aid dispensing).	minutes; Contrast/Conclude, 2 minutes (deBono, 1985).
Clinician	Supervisors do not carry their own caseloads to maintain personal clinical development.	To develop a means by which supervisors will be actively involved in the clinical process on a regular basis.	Reflective Thinking. Orderly and thorough discussion of problems using Dewey's five-step agenda: Define the problem; define the causes; specify the criteria for outcomes; consider more than one outcome; choose the best outcome (Dewey, 1910; Whitman & Boase, 1983)

Source. Preparation for Supervision Roles: Meta-Cognitive Strategies, a miniseminar presented at the annual convention of the American Speech-Language-Hearing Association, New Orleans, LA, 1987, by S. Farmer, J. Farmer, J. Dimmer, M. Lyon, E. Nesbit, C. Thompson, and D. Wertzberger.

SUMMARY

Mental activities are referred to as cognitive processes. These processes include selecting information from the environment, modifying that information in light of pre-existing knowledge (memory), and using it to meet the demands of a task at hand. Learning, remembering, reasoning, and problem managing are examples of cognitive processes that supervisors use in each supervision role: Professional, Researcher, Educator, Administrator, and Clinician. Problem managing may involve convergent, vertical thinking and algorithms (guaranteed routes to an outcome) or divergent, lateral thinking and heuristics (methods of deriving and evaluating potential outcomes). Planning and creativity are two of the most beneficial heuristics for supervisors, but need to be developed through experience.

This chapter summarized a variety of problem managing strategies that can be included in Communication Disorders preparation programs and then used by trained supervisors in their roles within any worksite. The scientific decision making strategies discussed in chapter 7, combined with the artful creative problem managing strategies presented in this chapter, provide an ample repertoire of methods for managing supervision-related problems productively.

APPLICATIONS

Discussion Topics

1. Discuss several Communication Disorders supervision techniques that could be considered creative and others that are uncreative.
2. Discuss five habits associated with Communication Disorders supervision that most restrict creativity.
3. Name 10 Communication Disorders supervision uses for each of the following items:
   a. toothpick   c. pencil   e. piece of paper
   b. paper clip   d. coffee mug   f. handkerchief
4. Discuss ways that supervisors and supervisees can use the models of problem managing in Communication Disorders supervision.
5. State a supervision problem. Have all members of your group privately rewrite the problem in what they consider to be a clear statement form. Discuss the restatements. Are they the same problem? Would they have similar solutions?

Laboratory Experiences

1. Define a Communication Disorders supervision problem. Ask supervisees from three different levels of supervision (first-time, experienced, advanced) to develop outcomes for the problem. Compare the outcomes with your own.
2. Select five problem managing strategies and apply them to the following domain problems:
   a. Professional: No CUSPSPA organization exists in your state.
   b. Research: You need a Real-Time analyzer to examine the acoustic properties of supervisors' voice qualities associated with the psychological perception of sincerity.
   c. Educational: You are concerned about doing any more demonstration therapy because all your supervisees do only what they see you do and use the same materials.
   d. Administrative: You need to plan activities to get your worksite involved in Better Hearing and Speech Month.
   e. Clinical: You are the only staff member with expertise in dysphagia. The local hospital wants to contract with you to provide diagnostic and treatment services, but you have a full caseload at your university speech and hearing center.

3. Identify a supervision problem associated with each of the five roles of supervision: Professional, Researcher, Educator, Administrator, Clinician. Choose one problem managing strategy to manage all five problems.

4. Use dice to combine the following items randomly to stimulate possible Communication Disorders supervision ideas:

   1. paper
   2. desk
   3. clock
   4. microcomputer
   5. clipboard
   6. videorecorder

   1. pencil
   2. swivel chair
   3. restaurant
   4. audiotape recorder
   5. telephone
   6. food

   For example, if the rolled dice indicated 4–2 (microcomputer–swivel chair), perhaps a swivel chair could be used with the microcomputer during conferences so that the supervisor could attend to the supervisee as they talk and then swivel to the computer to write notes for further supervisor/supervisee reference.

5. Make a list of 10 problems associated with supervision. Decide whether they could be managed best with an algorithmic approach or a heuristic approach.

Research Projects

1. Develop and test a method for expanding visual perceptual constructs (i.e., multiple ways of perceiving the same event) and apply the method to critical observation training in Communication Disorders supervision preparation programs.

2. Select one of deBono's (1985) thinking lessons to incorporate into a Communication Disorders training program and evaluate its effectiveness in problem managing.

3. Select a Communication Disorders supervision problem. Have one group of supervisees manage the problem using vertical thinking strategies and another group using lateral thinking strategies. Compare the outcomes using predetermined criteria of effectiveness.

4. Design a research project to test the hypothesis that problems are ongoing rather than episodic.

5. Conduct a survey of Communication Disorders supervisors to document (a) knowledge of problem managing, (b) preparation in problem managing, and (c) use of problem managing strategies (e.g., types, frequency, duration).

REFERENCES

Adams, J. (1979). *Conceptual blockbusting* (2nd ed.). New York: Norton.

Bertalanffy, L. von. (1968). *General systems theory: Foundations, development, application.* New York: Braziller.

Bourne, L., & Ekstrand, B. (1982). *Psychology* (4th ed.). New York: CBS College Publishing.

Camp, B., & Bash, M. (1981). *Think aloud: Increasing social and cognitive skills. A problem-solving program for children*. Champaign, IL: Research Press.

Coulter, D. (1986). *General systems thinking*. Unpublished materials from 1986 INREAL Trainers Institute, Boulder, CO.

deBono, E. (1968). *New think*. New York: Avon.

deBono, E. (1970). *Lateral thinking: Creativity step by step*. New York: Harper & Row.

deBono, E. (1985). *deBono's thinking course*. New York: Facts on File.

Dewey, J. (1910). *How we think*. Boston: Heath.

Dodd, D., & White, R. (1980). *Cognition*. Boston: Allyn & Bacon.

Dyer, W. (1972). *The sensitive manipulator: The change agents who build with others*. Provo, UT: Brigham Young University Press.

Epstein, C. (1984). *Special children in regular classrooms*. Reston, VA: Reston.

Erhardt, H., & Corvey, S. (1980). *Cognitive style: In search of buried treasure*. Dallas, TX: Mountain View College.

Farmer, S., & Farmer, J. (1986, November). *Unilateral and bilateral styles of dyadic and group clinical education/supervision*. A short course presented at the annual convention of the American Speech-Language-Hearing Association, Detroit, MI.

Farmer, S., Farmer, J., Dimmer, J., Lyon, M., Nesbit, E., Thompson, C., & Wertzberger, D. (1987, November). *Preparation for supervision roles: Metacognitive strategies*. A miniseminar presented at the annual convention of the American Speech-Language-Hearing Association, New Orleans.

Feldhusen, J. (1973). *Teaching problem solving skills: Development of an instructional model based on human abilities related to efficient problem solving* (Final Report, Project 2E051, Grant No. OEG 5720042 —509—). Lafayette, IN: Purdue University.

Goldman, L., & Goldman, N. (1974). Problem solving in the classroom: A model for sharing learning responsibility. *Educational Technology, 9,* 54.

Goldstein, A., Sprafkin, R., Gershaw, N., & Klein, P. (1980). *Skill-streaming the adolescent*. Champaign, IL: Research Press.

Gordon, W. (1961). *Synectics*. New York: Harper & Row.

Grice, H. (1975). Logic and conversation. In P. Cole & J. Morgan (Eds.), *Syntax and semantics: Vol. 3. Speech acts* (pp. 41–58). New York: Academic Press.

Guilford, J. (1967). *The Nature of human intelligence*. New York: McGraw-Hill.

Jackson, P., & Messick, S. (1965). The person, the product, and the response: Conceptual problems in the assessment of creativity. *Journal of Personality, 35,* 309–329.

Koberg, D., & Bagnall, J. (1974). *The universal traveler: A soft-systems guidebook to creativity, problem-solving, and the process of design*. Los Altos, CA: William Kaufmann.

Larkin, J. (1980). Teaching problem solving in physics: the psychological laboratory and the practical classroom. In D. Tuma & F. Reif (Eds.), *Problem solving and education: Issues in teaching and research* (pp. 111–124). Hillsdale, NJ: Lawrence Erlbaum.

Maltz, M. (1960). *Psychocybernetics.* New York: Essendess.

Mayer, R. (1977). *Thinking and problem solving: An introduction to human communication and learning.* Glenview, IL: Scott, Foresman.

McKenny, J., & Keen, P. (1976). How managers' minds work. *Harvard Business Review, 52,* 14–21.

Miller, L. (1984). Problem solving and language disorders. In G. Wallach & K. Butler (Eds.), *Language learning disabilities in school-age children* (pp. 199–229). Baltimore, MD: Williams & Wilkins.

Mussen, P., Conger, J., & Kagan, J. (1974). *Child development and personality* (4th ed.). New York: Harper & Row.

Norman, D., & Bobrow, D. (1976). On the role of active memory processes in perception and cognition. In C. N. Cofer (Ed.), *The structure of human memory* (pp. 35–46). San Francisco: Freeman.

Olson, R. (1980). *The art of creative thinking.* New York: Harper & Row.

Osborn, A. (1953). *Applied imagination.* New York: Scribner's.

Patterson, C., & Roberts, R. (1982). Planning and the development of communication skills. In D. L. Forbes & M. T. Greenberg (Eds.), *Children's planning strategies* (pp. 22–38). San Francisco: Jossey-Bass.

Pea, R. (1982). What is planning development the developing of? In D. L. Forbes & M. T. Greenberg (Eds.), *Children's planning strategies* (pp. 15–27). San Francisco: Jossey-Bass.

Rosch, E., & Mervis, C. B. (1975). Family resemblances: Studies in the internal structure of categories. *Cognitive Psychology, 7,* 573–605.

Rumelhart, D. (1980). Schemata: The building blocks of cognition. In R. Spiro, B. Bruce, & W. Brewer (Eds.), *Theoretical issues in reading comprehension* (pp. 33–58). Hillsdale, NJ: Lawrence Erlbaum.

Simon, S., Howe, L., & Kirschenbaum, H. (1972). *Values clarification.* New York: Hart.

Smith, D. (1981). *Teaching the learning disabled.* Englewood Cliffs, NJ: Prentice-Hall.

Wasinger, J., & Ortman, K. (1984, November). *Simulation: A method of increasing students' clinical problem-solving skills.* Paper presented at the annual convention of the American Speech-Language-Hearing Association, San Francisco.

Winkelgren, W. (1979). *Cognitive psychology.* Englewood Cliffs, NJ: Prentice-Hall.

Whitman, R., & Boase, P. (1983). *Speech communication.* New York: Macmillan.

Wonder, J., & Donovan, P. (1984). *Whole-brain thinking.* New York: Random House/Ballantine.

9
Clinical Literacy

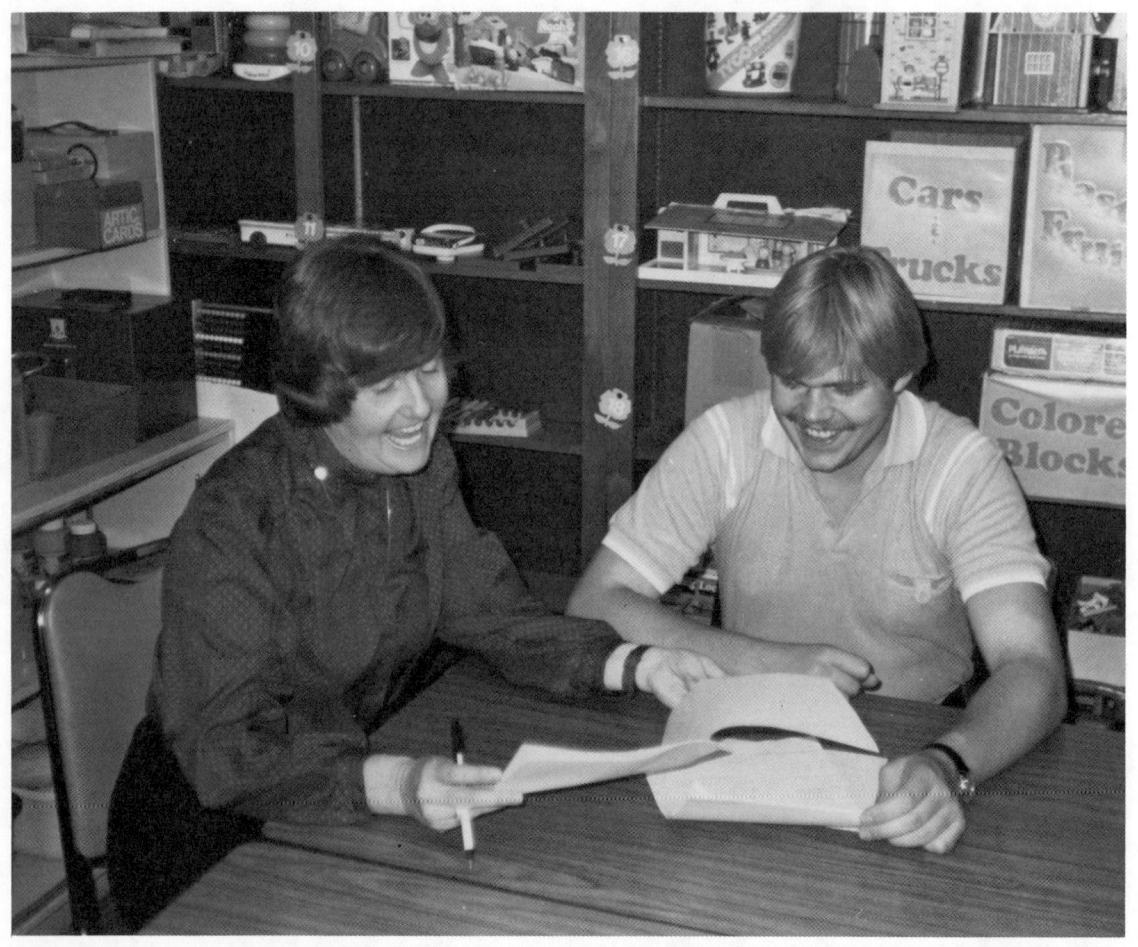

CRITICAL CONCEPTS

- *Supervisors need competency in clinical literacy in order to effectively function in all supervision roles, but especially to guide supervisees as they develop clinical reporting competency.*
- *Clinical report writing skills may be acquired through specialized training, learning to analyze one's own writing, and supervised practice.*
- *Supervisors direct supervisees toward becoming independent in editing what they write.*

OUTLINE

INTRODUCTION
    Dimensions and Importance
    Developing Clinical Literacy
    Professional, Legal, and Ethical Considerations

DEVELOPING COMPETENCE IN CLINICAL REPORTING
    Oral Reporting
    Clinical Report Reading
    Clinical Report Writing
    Forms of Clinical Reporting
    Developing Clinical Writing

DEVELOPING COMPETENCE IN WRITING GOALS AND OBJECTIVES
    Goals and Objectives for the Client
    Goals and Objectives for the Supervisee
    Goals and Objectives for the Supervisor

EDITING
    Editing Competence for the Supervisor
    Editing Competence for the Supervisee

SUMMARY

APPLICATIONS

INTRODUCTION

Communication Disorders supervisors have surely received more than their fair share of clinical reports fraught with errors, and they have always struggled with the mysteries of helping their supervisees develop clinical literacy. *Clinical literacy* (having the knowledge, skills, and dispositions to read, interpret, and write clinical material) is a competence necessary for all supervisors. This chapter provides the supervisor with information about the dimensions and importance of clinical literacy, including ways to develop supervisees' competence in writing goals and objectives, clinical reporting, and independent editing.

Dimensions and Importance

Of all the supervisor's activities, those involving written communication are the most frequently performed, most visible to peers and public, and most often used as indicators of competency or success in all supervisory roles. In the Professional role, the supervisor may prepare a conference brochure or presentation or serve on the ASHA Professional Affairs II Committee, reading and selecting proposals for the annual conven-

This chapter was contributed by Judith L. Farmer, New Mexico State University.

tion. The Researcher must understand and produce written material in papers, articles, reports, theses, dissertations, and professional journals. As an Educator in an academic setting, the supervisor writes course materials, handouts, and examinations, reviews literature in preparation for lectures, and directs and critiques students' writing; as a clinical educator, the supervisor writes procedural manuals and test protocols, reviews supervisees' written plans and progress notes, completes evaluation forms and provides narrative feedback, and guides supervisees in developing clinical report writing skills. The supervisor in the Administrator role may read and write annual reports, grant proposals, contracts, program descriptions, and administrative policies in addition to managing routine correspondence and monitoring employees' clinical reports. The Clinician role includes numerous reading and writing activities, from reading test administration manuals to charting notations on the hospital record to writing notes to the client's parent or teacher.

The importance of clinical literacy in Speech-Language Pathology and Audiology is well documented. Researchers have addressed report writing skills using various approaches (Carnell, 1976; English & Lillywhite, 1963; Moore, 1969; Wing, 1975). Educational preparation programs have emphasized reading and writing of clinical material through academic coursework and clinical practica; many textbooks devote significant space to the development of clinical literacy (Battin & Fox, 1978; Billings & Schmitz, 1980; Cornett & Chabon, 1988; Emerick & Haynes, 1986; Flower, 1984; Hutchinson, Hanson, & Mecham, 1979; Meitus & Weinberg, 1983; Neidecker, 1987; Rassi, 1978). Knepflar's (1976) handbook of report writing has guided many a clinical report writer, supervisor and supervisee alike. Literature in supervision further supports the importance of clinical literacy, with the added expectation that supervisors will assume responsibility for guiding supervisees in developing clinical reporting skills (Anderson, 1988; Broffman, Wiener, & Lawrence, 1985; Hargrave, 1984, 1985; Pannbacker, 1975; Sanders, Middleton, Puett, & Pannbacker, 1985–1986; Schubert, 1978). The ASHA Committee on Supervision has directed further attention to the importance of clinical literacy by identifying 3 of the 13 tasks of supervision as directly pertaining to clinical literacy ("2.0 Task: Assisting the supervisee in developing clinical goals and objectives"; "7.0 Task: Assisting the supervisee in development and maintenance of clinical and supervisory records"; and "10.0 Task: Assisting the supervisee in developing skills of verbal reporting, writing, and editing") (ASHA, 1985, pp. 58–59). That clinical literacy needs to be a part of every supervisor's competence is obvious; that clinical literacy is learned through skill development and practice justifies the inclusion of a clinical literacy module, unit, or emphasis in every supervision preparation program.

Developing Clinical Literacy

As dimensions of communication competence, clinical reading and writing warrant special attention in supervisor preparation programs. Supervisors are expected to be clinically literate, reading and writing clinical materials at a professional level. Supervisors whose clinical literacy is shaky, however, need training before they can help their supervisees develop clinical literacy. Some supervisors may demonstrate clinical literacy and yet not be able to guide supervisees in acquiring similar skills; training and practice in using and presenting the tools of clinical literacy will help these supervisors. Supervisors may facilitate skill development by offering specific instruction, directing practice, guiding self-analysis of the supervisee's writing, delivering oral and written feedback, providing reinforcement, and encouraging independence in clinical reporting. In addition, supervisors should present clinical literacy activities with a positive attitude and emphasize the professional, legal, and ethical aspects of clinical reporting.

Professional, Legal, and Ethical Considerations

As professional speech-language pathologists and audiologists, supervisors are well aware of the ethical principles stated in the ASHA Code of Ethics (1988) and respect those principles in service delivery. They may tend to assume that supervisees are operating with the same code, an assumption that has serious ramifications if incorrect. Supervisors are responsible for (a) sharing information about ethical aspects of the profession with each supervisee; (b) encouraging accountability in the management of oral and written clinical products; (c) expecting high-quality, accurate, objective clinical reporting; and (d) modeling ethical behavior. Supervisees need to learn about the legalities of clinical reporting, the concept of accountability through written forms, and the implications of regulatory and legal documents.

Underlying all professional activity and the resulting clinical management and materials is *confidentiality,* an understanding that what transpires in the clinical process will not be disclosed in oral or written form without the permission of the individuals involved. Supervisors are responsible for guiding supervisees to maintain professional confidences and for maintaining the confidentiality of their own professional interactions with supervisees. In the Clinical role, supervisors model confidentiality in clinical interactions and reporting. Breaches of confidentiality by supervisor trainees are usually unintentional: a misplaced report or chart, a casual remark to a friend, a careless action (e.g., leaving the rough draft of a report visible on the seat of the car parked next to that of the client's mother, who happens to notice the report). Supervisors can guide their supervisees to become aware of actions or situations that can lead to breach of confidence, demonstrate the appropriate use of release-of-information forms, hold conferences in privacy, shred rough drafts of reports, and discuss the consequences of unintentional and intentional breach of confidentiality. All of these steps will contribute to supervisees' understanding of their responsibility to maintain clinical confidentiality.

DEVELOPING COMPETENCE IN CLINICAL REPORTING

Clinical information is transmitted orally or in writing between a sender/talker/writer and a receiver/listener/reader. *Clinical reporting* is the use of clinical literacy to interpret and convey written clinical information and the use of communication competence to comprehend, interpret, and express orally-relayed clinical information. Clinical reporting includes oral reporting (speaking and listening), clinical report reading, and clinical report writing.

Oral Reporting

Communication Disorders professionals have traditionally depended on writing for reporting information, although, with the increasing cost of producing written communication, the use of oral communication is becoming more frequent. The brief telephone call from a physician's office to an audiologist's office to refer a patient and the postevaluation telephone call from the audiologist's office back to the physician's office are time and cost efficient, though not always as accurate or detailed as written referrals and reports. Sometimes an oral report to the client's family, teacher, social worker, or other professional will precede the written report for the sake of immediacy, whereas at other times an oral report follows the written report to provide further information or opportunity for discussion or consultation (Knepflar, 1976). Clinical reporting often carries more weight in person than over the telephone. If the situation warrants a person-to-person conference, a brief visit with a principal, surgeon, or other professional to convey clinical information is an encouragement to two-way communication.

Listening. Oral reporting requires skill in listening as well as in speaking. Supervisor trainees will benefit from practice in accurate listening, in simultaneous recording or charting of information received orally, and in training employees (particularly those who answer the telephone and take messages) to develop listening skills. Supervisors should encourage supervisees to develop listening strengths, to remember information accurately, and to ask questions that facilitate effective oral reporting. (See chapter 5 for an extended discussion of listening.)

Speaking. Giving clinical information orally requires competence in oral communication, organization, and accuracy. Supervisors can help supervisees develop oral reporting skills by reviewing the information to be conveyed before the contact, encouraging peer practice, suggesting that supervisees speak from a brief outline, having supervisees audiotape their side of telephone exchanges for analysis, and modeling oral reporting. (See chapter 5 for additional information on speaking.)

Clinical Report Reading

A supervisee's skill and efficiency in reading clinical reports increases with experience in writing reports and thus is not usually given significant emphasis in the clinical reporting literature. However, supervisors can encourage supervisees to develop clinical report reading skills by directing them to various types of reports to read, encouraging them to critique reports, pointing out strengths and limitations of particular reports, helping them anticipate what kind of information can be obtained from each report, explaining criteria for judging reports, and demonstrating adaptation to different report forms. In modeling clinical report reading skills, supervisors can demonstrate a routine for the efficient reading of clinical reports; the routine depends on each supervisor's biases and experiences and on the information needed from each report.

Clinical Report Writing

Clinical report writing is used to document baseline, occurrences, or change; to maintain an ongoing official record; to relay information; to assure quality services; to establish a data base for research; to provide evidence of service; to complete forms for reimbursement; to acknowledge a referral, service, or courtesy; to request information or services; to substantiate accountability; to demonstrate legal responsibility; and to show the quality of service being provided (Flower, 1984; Meitus & Weinberg, 1983; Neidecker, 1987; Oyer, 1987). The professional competence of the report writer is judged by the quality of the report. Supervisors must be able to guide supervisees as they develop competence in clinical report writing.

Of all the clinical competencies, students express the most concern about report writing, declaring it difficult to learn and extremely time-consuming. Although some Communication Disorders clinical preparation programs provide coursework in report writing, the teaching of this skill usually becomes the responsibility of the supervisor in the clinical setting, because written products are a major part of client management, service delivery, and accountability. Thus, supervisor trainees need to learn techniques for teaching clinical report writing skills.

Writing style in Communication Disorders can be creative/imaginative or professional/technical. Creative/imaginative writing is not encouraged in clinical reporting (although it may be an important strategy in therapeutic intervention). Professional/technical style is the formal tone, vocabulary, and structure used in research literature, policies and procedures, and standard administrative communication. Clinical report writing is professional/technical writing that uses language and format specific to Communication

Disorders reports. Several different forms or types of reports are possible.

Forms of Clinical Reporting

Various clinical reporting forms or types exist to meet the wide range of clinical reporting needs. Clinical reporting format is usually standardized within an employment setting, with different models for different clinical functions and clients. The following kinds of reports are used in many clinical reporting situations:

- *Diagnostic or initial evaluation reports:* Comprehensive, usually detailed reports of results of an audiological, speech, and/or language examination, including pertinent history information, test administration, and clinical impressions. Diagnostic reports are used to determine need for treatment, record present-status data, communicate information to other professionals, the client, or the family, document services being provided, direct intervention programming, and fulfill requirements for reimbursement for services.
- *Intervention plans (therapy plans, IEPs, service delivery plans, care plans, therapeutic records, unit records, problem-oriented charts, operational management data):* Records, reports, or chart entries describing goals and objectives, requirements for implementing them, and time or financial considerations. Intervention plans are used to direct intervention programs systematically and to satisfy government, school, institution, or third-party payment requirements.
- *Session plans (lesson plans, progress notes, daily entries, flow charts):* Specific session-by-session plans. They are often detailed when a clinician is inexperienced and needs to plan on paper but become less detailed with increased clinical experience. Clinicians often devise their own formats. Session plans focus on objectives for the client and may include strategies and materials, postsession evaluation, and recommendations for the next session. Session plans are used to guide planning and evaluation. They may be submitted (either before or after use) to the supervisor, who can respond with questions or comments about specific strategies, activities, or materials, can suggest procedures or tests, and can provide reinforcement.
- *Progress reports (end-of-term reports, interim summaries):* Periodic summaries of a client's therapy program and progress or change. Progress reports include original goals and objectives, therapy procedures, and recommendations for the future direction of the program. They are used to document services, refer for additional services, recommend maintenance or change of the therapy direction, satisfy reimbursement source requirements, and maintain an ongoing record of intervention.
- *Discharge summaries (disposition or transfer statements, end-of-therapy reports):* Summaries that are prepared when a client is being dismissed from therapy because of no further need for intervention, referral to another program, moving from the area, or loss of financial eligibility. Discharge summaries contain information about the client's communication, services received, progress made, and recommendations. They provide a concise record of the client's communication disorder and intervention program and are used to document services and meet financial reimbursement requirements.
- *Third-party payment reports (insurance forms, federal and state government agency forms):* Regulation forms that require specific information, often coded numerically, about service and diagnosis. They are used to determine eligibility for reimbursement.
- *Charts (notations, unit notes):* Records of condition and treatment containing evaluation

or therapy information, written either on a single contact or every day. Charting must be brief because of limited space for reporting. It is most often used in hospital, rehabilitation, nursing home, or other medical settings; if charting is dictated verbally (e.g., over the phone to members of the typing pool), the clinician must carefully monitor the written product, both for content and proofreading. Charting is used to document services, to request referrals or additional services, and to communicate with other professionals.

- *Anecdotal records (logs and journals):* Narrative entries to describe services delivered. These are more detailed than charting and are usually used by multiple professionals (such as the members of a transdisciplinary team). Anecdotal records are used to share treatment information about the client among professionals, providing a variety of perspectives about the intervention program. They are also used to maintain records, document services, facilitate an effective team approach, and foster professional exchange.
- *Checklists (graphs, audiograms, profiles, test forms, diagrams):* Described in chapter 6. Checklists present information about a client's condition, status, strengths, and limitations in a quickly readable form. They are used to supplement narrative data, but can be subject to misinterpretation if the reader is not familiar with the format or source.
- *Professional letters:* Letters written in the traditional business format on professional letterhead. They include the date, a formal salutation, a reference (to the topic or client), a message or messages written in paragraphs, a closing statement, and professional signature. Letters are used to make and acknowledge referrals; request information, services, or consultation; relate intervention protocol or follow up on an oral report; accompany and summarize a detailed narrative (cover letters); recommend individuals for employment, scholarships, honors, or graduate education; thank individuals or organizations for services, donations, or professional courtesies; solicit support for services from businesses, individuals, and organizations; make employment inquiries and submit resignations; introduce self and services to members of the professional community; and commend colleagues for their accomplishments.

Supervisor trainees will also benefit from exposure to and experience with other written products often relevant to supervision: grants, proposals, contracts (Lefferts, 1978), annual and semiannual reports, fiscal year reports/budgets/plans, job descriptions, applications for promotion, position announcements, minutes of meetings, academic and clinical manuals, brochures, newsletters, academic course plans and handouts, quizzes and examinations, in-house notes and memoranda, press releases, and manuscripts of textbooks and professional papers.

Developing Clinical Writing

Developing competence in clinical report writing is an ongoing professional activity; the more one writes, the more skilled one becomes. First, however, clinical writing skills demand concentrated development at the preservice level; the faculty and professional staff in academic and clinical settings, particularly the supervisor, have significant responsibility for teaching report writing. At the service level, supervisors are expected to continue to guide the development of supervisees' report writing in the employment setting.

Supervisors often have trouble differentiating between supervisees who are relatively good writers but need help with the specific vocabulary, mechanics, and style of clinical report writing and those whose report writing suggests a significant written language problem. In general, the former respond rapidly when they are exposed to formula writing and self-analysis, described below, whereas the latter require formal, remedial instruction in writing. A supervisee's style of clinical report writing often differs significantly from the style of the supervisor or the expectations of the site; such stylistic differences may be managed in supervision conferences that include report sampling and comparison, discussion of the rationale for various styles, and appreciation of both styles.

A further challenge for supervisors in clinical settings is the dual responsibility of ensuring that a professional-level report is being produced and of seeing that the supervisee learns and becomes independent in clinical report writing. If a supervisee is having serious difficulties with report writing, should the supervisor become the primary report author, or sacrifice the quality of the report to give the supervisee the writing experience? When time is short, should the supervisee be allowed several weeks of rewriting, analyzing, receiving feedback, and rewriting again, particularly when clinical management depends on or is influenced by the written report? Each supervisor strives to balance the quality of the report with the supervisee's learning experience. Decision making considerations could include the following: How is the quality of service being affected by the supervisee's difficulties in report writing? Is this supervisee academically prepared for report writing? Can the supervisor commit the time to educating, conferencing, and editing when a supervisee demonstrates repeated problems in report writing? Should the supervisor prepare the real report and have the supervisee practice with hypothetical client information? What specific approaches to teaching report writing skills would be appropriate for this supervisee?

Of the numerous approaches that exist for teaching or encouraging the development of report writing skills, formula writing and self-analysis are particularly appropriate for use by Communication Disorders supervisors.

Formula Writing. Formula writing is an approach to clinical reporting that starts from a standard format (organization, sequence, vocabulary, style) and uses a skeletal form containing slots (syntactic positions) for fillers (semantic data). Report formulas range from the *element formula,* prescribing only the sequence of the information, to the *slot filler formula,* containing complete sentences with blanks for filling in data. Formula writing can be a time efficient, cost effective, and self-directed method for developing skills in clinical reporting. Because of the semantic predictability of the fillers (only certain kinds of fillers can fit semantically into specific slots), supervisees progress quickly in organizing and sequencing report information. Supervisors should use care, however, in preparing the formula; a too-tight formula produces stilted, sometimes inaccurate reports and can discourage independent thinking and progress in clinical writing. In supervisor preparation programs, using a number of different formulas (e.g., one for university clinic reports, another for hospital charting, another to design an IEP) can be a good way to teach reporting skills. Supervisors can vary the formulas according to how much report writing practice the supervisee has had, giving less experienced writers more detailed formulas. In employment settings, supervisors determine the formulas according to the priorities, needs, and traditions of each setting; supervisors' biases and experiences significantly affect the nature of the formula.

Formula writing can be used for classroom learning, on a supervisor-to-supervisee basis, or in a self-paced program; content may come from clinical observation, diagnostic and therapeutic intervention, research data, or correspondence. The process of developing clinical reporting skills through formula writing may include these steps:

1. Supervisor describes the expected product, the goal, the whole picture.
2. Supervisees read sample reports, identify the elements and the slot fillers, and outline the formula; supervisor gives written feedback.
3. Supervisees select reports from the clinical files and independently identify the elements

and slot fillers and describe the formula; supervisor gives feedback in a conference.
4. Supervisees are given the written formula and data with which to fill the slots.
5. Supervisees are given the written formula and a videotape to observe; on the basis of the observation, they fill the slots. Supervisor provides feedback.
6. Supervisees observe and report on selected videotapes, moving gradually from slot filler to element formulas as they progress in writing. Considerable practice at this stage helps prepare supervisees for more independent report preparation. Supervisor provides feedback.
7. Supervisees prepare reports, independently selecting their formulas, using data from live or videotaped observations, diagnostic or therapy sessions, or research. Supervisor gives feedback in conferences.
8. Supervisees become less dependent on slot filler and element formulas and develop their own schema as they gain experience in report writing; when confronted with unfamiliar settings or clients, supervisees will return to dependence on formulas until they become comfortable writing about the new subject.
9. Supervisees independently apply formula writing principles to clinical reporting; they use their own formulas to prepare reports and can devise and adapt formulas for various settings, clients, and situations.

Thus, supervisees develop from formula dependence to independence, gaining clinical reporting skills that can be applied to computer use, goals and objectives, and all aspects of clinical and supervisory reporting.

Formula writing is the basis for computer-generated reports. Beyond word processing, in which the computer or word processor reproduces text in much the same way as a typewriter, computers can store whole report formulas, both element and slot filler types, and can systematically process correspondence or the products of data processing and analysis (Neidecker, 1987; see also chapter 10). In word processing, supervisors can make templates for the various formulas and writing skill levels of supervisees, as appropriate for the preparation program or employment setting. Report generating programs are used more often in employment settings than in clinical preparation programs, where students require considerable practice in clinical report writing.

Self-Analysis. A second method for guiding supervisees in the development of report writing is self-analysis, a system of examining one's own writing, identifying strengths and limitations, and determining steps needed for improvement. The supervisor helps by targeting specific problems in the supervisee's reports, encouraging self-discovery of weaknesses, and allowing the supervisee to devise corrective measures aimed at the identified problems. (Table 9-1 shows strategies for supervisees to use in response to the problems identified by the supervisor; the accompanying Analysis Forms A, B, C, and D are found in Tables 9-2, 9-3, 9-4, and 9-5.)

To summarize, clinical reporting, spoken and written, requires competence in oral reporting, report reading, and report writing. Communication Disorders supervisors must demonstrate competence in their own clinical reporting functions and guide supervisees as they develop clinical reporting skills and dispositions.

DEVELOPING COMPETENCE IN WRITING GOALS AND OBJECTIVES

The use of goals and objectives has long been recognized as instrumental in changing behavior (Mager, 1962, 1972). Goals state intentions for change over a long term; they include a description of the planned outcome, criteria for measuring the change, and a time frame. Objectives state short-term plans that contribute to the accomplishment of the goal; like goals, objectives

TABLE 9-1
Strategies for supervisees' problems in report writing

Problem	Strategies for Supervisees
A. Content	
Accuracy of information	Apply Analysis Form A; use column 1 for raw data (from history form, audiogram, test forms, etc.) and column 2 for the corresponding information in the report; compare columns for accuracy.

Completeness of information
  Detail: too detailed
        not detailed enough
	Apply Analysis Form A; use column 1 to list information from the raw data and column 2 for corresponding information in the report; compare columns for details and completeness.

Objectivity/subjectivity Facts versus assumptions or inferences	Apply Analysis Form D with target of *objectivity;* comment "objective," "subjective," "fact," "assumption," or "inference" for each sentence.
Terminology correct and professional; use of accepted nomenclature and classification	Apply Analysis Form A in one of two ways: 1) Use column 1 for listing terms identified in the report and column 2 for listing the definition from Nicolosi, Harryman, & Kresheck (1983); compare the columns; comment. 2) Use column 1 for listing words or phrases used instead of professional terminology and column 2 for the professional terms that could be used instead.
Integration or synthesis of information	Apply Analysis Form D with target of *synthesis of information;* instead of selecting a paragraph, write the topic sentences throughout the report; comment on whether the topic sentence information is reflected in the summary, impressions, or recommendation areas. Schedule a supervision conference to talk about "understanding the whole."
Focus: directed misdirected	Apply Analysis Form D with target of *focus;* comment on whether focus is or is not directed toward the purpose of the report.
Perspective: positive tone negative tone	Apply Analysis Form D with target of *perspective: positive/negative;* comment on the tone of each sentence (be aware of negatives such as *cannot* or *did not* as well as semantic intent of sentences).
Criticism of client, family, other professionals/programs	Apply Analysis Form D with target of *criticism statements;* record all sentences containing criticism; schedule supervision conference to discuss personal biases, semantic constructs.
Intimate information	Apply Analysis Form D with target of *intimate information;* record all sentences containing information you perceive as private or intimate; schedule supervision conference to discuss personal biases, importance in including the information, semantic constructs.
Ethical aspects	Apply Analysis Form D with target of *ethics;* record all sentences containing information relating to professional ethics, law, and state/federal regulations; schedule supervision conference to discuss their ramifications.
B. Written Language	
Style differs from the traditions of the employment setting	Read sample written products from the setting; apply Analysis Form A; use column 1 for listing the characteristics of the style of the setting's reports and column 2 for listing the corresponding characteristics of the supervisee's style; comment on similarities and differences. (Refer to Strunk & White, 1979, for basics in written language.)

TABLE 9-1
continued

Problem	Strategies for Supervisees
Organization; categorization	Apply Analysis Form D with target of either *organization within paragraphs* or *organization of entire report;* record headings or sentences that are markers of the paragraph's or report's structure; comment on the organization of each section and of the report as a whole; examine form of presentation of information (e.g., a table that might convey complicated information more readily than detailed narrative).
Sequencing: chronological / by importance	Apply Analysis Form D with target of either *sequence: chronological* or *sequence: importance;* record sentences in the order written in the report; comment if order is or is not appropriate for the target given.

Vocabulary
  Unnecessary jargon
  Nonspecific, precise
  Qualifiers
	Apply Analysis Form B with target of listing vocabulary according to problem identified by supervisor (e.g., needless professional jargon, nonspecific words used when more precise or concrete words are needed, use of "fancy" words, incorrect use of words from other professions, use of qualifiers such as *appeared, seemed, very, rather*); if frequency-of-occurrence information is needed, count occurrences of words listed.

Redundancies	Apply Analysis Form B with target of listing either vocabulary or information that occurs more than once in the report; in righthand column, record number of times the word or information appears.
Wordiness	Apply Analysis Form C to examine sentence structure and length; rewrite sentences with attention to use of terminology, focus, completeness/detail, style, organization, vocabulary, sequencing, redundancy, length, and sentence structure.
Tone: too formal / too informal	Apply Analysis Form D with target of *tone;* select paragraph and write each sentence, underlining words that influence the tone; comment on whether the tone is too formal, too informal, or appropriate (watch for words that sound professional, casual, serious, flippant, humorous, sincere, careless).

Sentences: complete
  too short
  too long
  length not varied
	Apply Analysis Form C, selecting a paragraph typical of the report. Rewrite sentences with attention to completeness and length.

Verbs: correct tense
  consistent tense
  subject-agreement
	Apply Analysis Form B, targeting use of verb tense, consistency of tense, or subject-verb agreement. List verbs in one column with target information in the other. Examine for correctness or frequency of occurrence.

Length of report	Examine report for length in relation to purpose, setting, content, and destination. Consult with supervisor for specific length guidelines.
C. Mechanics Proofreading	Use different methods of proofreading: read slowly, read aloud, follow along with finger while reading, read text in reverse order, have someone else read it. Make a list of errors you typically miss when proofreading and consult it before the final reading.

TABLE 9-1
continued

Problem	Strategies for Supervisees
Identifying information	Compare identifying information given in the report with that from data (history form, intake sheet, administrative chart); if problems continue, apply Analysis Form A, comparing the information from two sources.
Spelling	List words frequently misspelled (Analysis Form B may be used with target *spelling*). Refer to list whenever writing.
Punctuation	Apply Analysis Form C to examine which punctuation is being used regularly; if errors are occurring, consult standard grammar text (e.g., Baugh, 1987); list repeated errors and use list as a reference when proofreading.
Pronoun: use of personal reference	Apply Analysis Form D with target of *pronoun use;* note the referent for each pronoun and comment whether correct or incorrect; consult standard grammar text if having pronoun-referent problems; consult supervisor for tradition or policy regarding use of personal pronouns.
Abbreviations	Apply Analysis Form B, listing abbreviations used in the report; on the corresponding line, indicate whether or not the use is appropriate (typically, abbreviations reduce clarity of a report); consult supervisor for setting's traditions regarding use of abbreviations.
Contractions	Apply Analysis Form B, listing all contractions used in the report; on the corresponding line, write the full form and compare the influence each has on the tone of the report; consult supervisor for setting's traditions regarding use of contractions in report writing.
D. Time	
Report writing taking too much time	Analyze how long report writing is taking by keeping track of time spent on preparation, writing, proofreading, editing, consultation; schedule specific time for report writing; make a time line; practice dictating a report into a tape recorder before actually writing; consult with supervisor and other colleagues for shortcuts; set specific goals to become more efficient in report writing.
Difficulty meeting deadlines	Set a time line for report writing, planning writing activities within a specific time frame.
E. Format	Use formula writing techniques; follow format of setting or requirements of destination.
F. Word Processing	
Typographical errors; proofreading	Use software designed to identify spelling or grammatical errors; proofread hard copy as well as the screen image.
Spelling; grammar	Use spelling checker programs; use grammatical checker programs.
Formatting	Use template for report format.
Disk problems	Always make a backup disk and keep it current; be sure to make editorial changes on the backup disk as well as on the original; treat disks with care.

TABLE 9-2
Analysis Form A: Comparison format

Column 1:	Column 2:	Comparison

Summary of Analysis:

Personal Goal:

_____   _____
Supervisee's Signature   Date

_____   _____
Supervisor's Signature   Date

1. At column headings, enter sources or type of information to be listed.
2. From the two sources or types of information given, enter data on corresponding lines.
3. Compare each column 1 entry with the column 2 entry; comment on the comparison. Summarize your analysis.
4. On the basis of your comparisons, revise report.
5. Write a personal goal to facilitate development in this area of report writing; include how and when goal will be accomplished.
6. Sign and date this form; give to supervisor, who will sign, copy, and return.

TABLE 9-3
Analysis Form B: Listing format

Target:

_____   _____
_____   _____
_____   _____
_____   _____
_____   _____
_____   _____
_____   _____
_____   _____
_____   _____
_____   _____
_____   _____

Summary of Analysis:

Personal Goal:

_____   _____
Supervisee's Signature   Date

_____   _____
Supervisor's Signature   Date

1. At "Target," enter type of information to be listed in either or both columns.
2. In the columns, list information; if frequency-of-occurrence information is desired, give it on corresponding line of opposite column. Summarize your analysis.
3. On the basis of your lists or frequency information, revise report.
4. Write a personal goal to facilitate development in this area of report writing; include how and when goal will be accomplished.
5. Sign and date this form; give to supervisor, who will sign, copy, and return.

TABLE 9-4
Analysis Form C: Sentence format

Sentence Number	Number of Words	Complete/ Incomplete	Simple	Com- pound	Com- plex	Compound- Complex	Punctuation
1							
2							
3							
4							
5							
6							
7							
8							
9							
10							

Summary of Analysis:

Personal Goal:

_____   _____
Supervisee's Signature   Date

_____   _____
Supervisor's Signature   Date

1. Select a paragraph from the report.
2. Number each sentence in the paragraph; for each, record number of words per sentence, whether the sentence is complete or a fragment (incomplete), type of sentence (simple, compound, complex, compound-complex), and the punctuation used.
3. Note completeness, length, variety of type, variety of punctuation. Summarize your analysis.
4. On the basis of your analysis, revise report.
5. Write a personal goal to facilitate development in this area of report writing; include how and when goal will be accomplished.
6. Sign and date this form; give to supervisor, who will sign, copy, and return.

TABLE 9-5
Analysis Form D: Written language analysis format

Target:	
Sentence	Comments

Summary of Analysis:

Personal Goal:

_____   _____
Supervisee's Signature   Date

_____   _____
Supervisor's Signature   Date

1. Select a paragraph or portion of the report to examine; write the target feature selected for analysis.
2. Copy each sentence in the order given in the paragraph.
3. Circle or highlight the target feature in each sentence; record comments. Summarize your analysis.
4. On the basis of your analysis, revise report.
5. Write a personal goal to facilitate development in this area of report writing; include how and when goal will be accomplished.
6. Sign and date this form; give to supervisor, who will sign, copy, and return.

specify the planned outcome, measurability, and a target time. Communication Disorders supervisors use goals and objectives in all supervision roles, particularly in planning personal development (see chapters 2 and 5) and in guiding supervisees to set goals and objectives for clients and for themselves. How supervisors can best help supervisees establish goals and objectives depends on the level of the supervisees' clinical experience, the client's therapeutic status, the clinical management plan, and the clinical setting.

Goals and Objectives for the Client

The process of writing goals and objectives has been approached from various different directions, and many models are available (Jones & Healey, 1973; Mager, 1962, 1972; Neidecker, 1987). For purposes of supervision, the supervisor selects one such model and guides the supervisee in creating goals and objectives for the client. During the initial evaluation, the supervisee is encouraged to consult previous reports, to obtain baseline data, and to confer with the client and/or family. In determining the intended outcome, the supervisee examines the evaluation information, consults academic references, discusses client and/or family considerations, and explores remediation strategies. When the purpose of the intervention program has been determined, the supervisee can begin to specify long-range plans (listed as goals) and short-range plans (listed as objectives). Time limits and methods of judging results are set. A format is selected for writing goals (in a school setting, the IEP format could be appropriate; in a hospital setting, a problem-oriented charting system might be used). A formula writing approach may help the supervisee ensure that all the necessary parts are included:

Element formula:

1. What (the intended outcome)
2. When (time frame)
3. How (plans to effect the change; criteria that will measure change or indicate accomplishment; evaluation process)

Slot filler formula:

By the end of (month) (year) ,   (client)   will be able to   (intended outcome)   (criteria)   as judged by   (evaluation process) .

Although the process of setting goals and objectives becomes easier with clinical experience, many supervisees have difficulty determining the purpose of an intervention program, understanding the importance of accountability, and choosing a realistic intended outcome. Supervisors can assist supervisees by using conferences to discuss purposes, accountability, and expectations for client change. After supervisees have established goals and objectives for clients, they can use the same process to set goals and objectives for self-development.

Goals and Objectives for the Supervisee

When program direction and strategies have been set for a client, the supervisee can determine what clinical competencies can be developed given the client's disorder, the intervention program, and the level of clinical development. Appropriate self-development goals and objectives seem to be considerably more difficult for supervisees to generate than those for the client, and the supervisor's guidance may need to be strong. Evaluating what the supervisee can do and assessing what knowledge and skills need developing next is the typical procedure.

One way to help the supervisee select goals is to refer to the previous term's competency evaluation form, having the supervisee list areas that require further development and target those that could be worked on with this particular client. The supervisor can also encourage self-analysis that relates the supervisee's present level of skill development with the clinical competencies required by the clinical preparation program or by ASHA. (See Table 11-3, p. 281-282 for specific guidelines.) A supervision conference often uncovers a skill the supervisee does not feel competent in but may not have considered appropriate for a goal. Comparing the supervisee's past and present academic courses with the disorder and needs of the client may reveal academic areas that need to be reinforced by specific clinical goals or objectives. After self-development goals and objectives are written (in the same form as those for the client), a supervision conference will help determine how the supervisor can support the supervisee's development; the parties should set type and frequency of evaluation, feedback, and supervisor demonstrations. (See chapter 11 for a discussion of evaluation and feedback.)

Goals and Objectives for the Supervisor

Involving the supervisee in the supervisor's own goals and objectives for the supervision process allows the supervisor to model self-evaluative behavior and to gain the supervisee's assistance. If, for example, the supervisor wants to work on interacting with the supervisee in planning, executing, and analyzing supervisory conferences, the supervisee may be willing to participate in additional or differently conducted conferences, be videotaped during conferences, or provide feedback on specific conference behaviors displayed by the supervisor.

EDITING

Competence in clinical literacy includes editing: the revising, refining, altering, assembling, and adapting of written material for clarity, accuracy, completeness, correctness, and meeting publication standards. The importance of producing high-quality written materials has been a theme of this chapter. This section discusses editing as a process (knowledge), techniques to use in editing (skills), and ways to develop "an eye for editing" (dispositions).

Editing Competence for the Supervisor

Supervisors need the knowledge, skills, and dispositions of editing to function effectively in all roles of supervision (a) as editors of their own written products and those of colleagues or employees, and (b) as developers of editing competence in supervisees. Each supervisor develops a system of steps to ensure careful reading and review of written material. Steps may include (a) initial reading for content, (b) review of format, (c) reading for mechanics (e.g., punctuation, typographical errors), (d) reading for language proficiency (e.g., style, organization, vocabulary), and (e) final reading for content (e.g., accuracy, completeness, perspective, focus). A coding system (traditional proofreader's marks or the setting's or supervisor's own system) increases efficiency in marking and deciphering needed changes. Typical symbols used to edit clinical reports are

ɣ	delete
⌢	combine
¶	begin new paragraph
O	error, especially in punctuation
*	see extended notation on page
∧	insert here
∽	reverse word order
ⓢⓟ	spelling
T	typographical error
cap	capitals

Supervisors may find it helpful to prepare checklists of typical errors in their writing for reference during editing. Practice in accurate proofreading leads to more efficient editing; techniques such as reading aloud or following along with a finger are helpful. Feedback from colleagues will also assist supervisors in editing their own work. Supervisors should specify the areas in which they would like feedback (e.g., content, logical sequencing, use of pronouns). A supervisor-to-supervisor exchange of written material will benefit both parties. Planning time to edit is also essential; editing time should be built into the entire clinical reporting process.

Thus, the editing process for supervisors includes systematic review of the material, efficient and accurate proofreading, use of a coding system, colleague input, and time allotted for editing. Supervisors should aim for competent self-editing, independence in editing one's own writing.

Editing Competence for the Supervisee

In addition to editing their own material, supervisors guide supervisees in developing editing skills. Supervisees, too, should work toward competent self-editing. Many supervisees find independence in editing a difficult-to-reach goal. They learn to revise a particular clinical report according to the supervisor's feedback but have difficulty generalizing those editorial changes to subsequent reports. Supervisors can encourage supervisees to develop a system for editing and can direct them toward self-analysis of report writing using the strategies given in sections B and C of Table 9–1.

SUMMARY Clinical literacy—having the knowledge, skills, and dispositions to interpret and produce written clinical material—is required of all Communication Disorders professionals and thus demands a significant role in academic and clinical preparation programs for clinicians and supervisors. By becoming competent in reporting clinical information orally and in writing, in preparing goals and objectives, and in self-editing written clinical materials, supervisors can function effectively throughout the supervision roles of Professional, Researcher, Educator, Administrator, and Clinician.

APPLICATIONS Discussion Topics

1. Discuss what should be done to help supervisees who do not possess adequate written language skills. Is it the supervisor's responsibility to provide remediation? If not, who should?
2. Discuss the advantages and disadvantages of storing lesson plans for future use and reference.
3. Discuss what role a supervisor should take in improving the clinical report writing skills of the supervisee.
4. Discuss strategies that help with editing and proofreading.
5. Discuss why supervisors should have various models of report styles in their professional repertoire.

Laboratory Experiences

1. Write goals and objectives for yourself as a supervisor, following a specific format.

2. Develop a personal portfolio of good examples of diagnostic reports, lesson plans, end-of-term reports, anecdotal records, chart notations, and professional letters.
3. Develop a symbol system for editing that would be time efficient in providing feedback to supervisees.
4. Develop a model for formula writing of diagnostic reports, lesson plans, end-of-term reports, anecdotal records, chart notations, professional letters.
5. Develop a matrix of common writing errors and some solutions to those errors.

Research Projects

1. Compare the development of report writing skills in a group of students who use formula writing with the development in a group of students who do not use formula writing.
2. Survey graduate students' attitudes toward clinical report writing; compare their attitudes with those of Communication Disorders professionals.
3. Explore the understanding of terminology typically used in Audiology and Speech-Language Pathology reports among groups of physicians, psychologists, social workers, teachers, and occupational or physical therapists.
4. Study the number of actual preparation hours and the total length of time undergraduate and graduate students require to produce clinical reports, including rewrites and turn-around time.
5. Design and evaluate a computer program for proofreading clinical reports, including punctuation, sentence completeness and structure, pronoun reference, and format.

REFERENCES

American Speech-Language-Hearing Association. (1985). Clinical supervision in speech-language pathology and audiology (position statement). *Asha, 27*(6), 57–60.

American Speech-Language-Hearing Association. (1988). *Code of ethics of the American Speech-Language-Hearing Association, 1988. Asha, 30*(3), 47–48.

Anderson, J. (1988). *The supervisory process in speech-language pathology and audiology.* San Diego: Little, Brown/College-Hill Press.

Battin, R. R., & Fox, D. R. (Eds.). (1978). *Private practice in audiology and speech pathology.* New York: Grune & Stratton.

Baugh, L. (1987). *Essentials of English grammar: A practical guide to the mastery of English.* Lincolnwood, IL: Passport Books/National Textbook Co.

Billings, B. L., & Schmitz, H. D. (1980). *Report writing in audiology.* Danville, IL: Interstate.

Broffman, S., Wiener, F. D., & Lawrence, J. B. (1985). Improving writing skills in college students through speech/listening activities. *SUPERvision, 9*(1), 10–17.

Carnell, C. M., Jr. (1976). *Development, management and evaluation of community speech and hearing centers.* Springfield, IL: Charles C. Thomas.

Cornett, B., & Chabon, S. (1988). *The clinical practice of speech-language pathology.* Columbus, OH: Charles E. Merrill.

Emerick, L., & Haynes, W. (1986). *Diagnosis and evaluation in speech pathology* (3rd ed.). Englewood Cliffs, NJ: Prentice-Hall.

English, R. H., & Lillywhite, H. S. (1963). A semantic approach to clinical reporting in speech pathology. *Asha, 5,* 647–650.

Flower, R. M. (1984). *Delivery of speech-language pathology and audiology services.* Baltimore: Williams & Wilkins.

Hargrave, J. K. (1984, November). *Developing report writing skills.* Paper presented at the annual convention of the American Speech-Language-Hearing Association, San Francisco.

Hargrave, J. K. (1985, November). *Developing report-writing skills.* Paper presented at the annual convention of the American Speech-Language-Hearing Association, Washington, DC.

Hutchinson, B. B., Hanson, M. L., & Mecham, M. J. (1979). *Diagnostic handbook of speech pathology.* Baltimore: Williams & Wilkins.

Jones, S., & Healey, W. (1973). *Essentials of program planning, development, management, evaluation: A manual for school speech, hearing and language programs.* Washington, DC: American Speech and Hearing Association.

Knepflar, K. J. (1976). *Report writing in the field of communication disorders.* Danville, IL: Interstate.

Lefferts, R. (1978). *Getting a grant: How to write successful grant proposals.* Englewood Cliffs, NJ: Prentice-Hall.

Mager, R. F. (1962). *Preparing instructional objectives.* Palo Alto, CA: Fearon.

Mager, R. F. (1972). *Goal analysis.* Belmont, CA: Fearon.

Meitus, I. J., & Weinberg, B. (Eds.). (1983). *Diagnosis in speech-language pathology.* Baltimore: University Park Press.

Moore, M. V. (1969). Pathological writing. *Asha, 11,* 535–538.

Neidecker, E. A. (1987). *School programs in speech-language: Organization and management* (2nd ed.). Englewood Cliffs, NJ: Prentice-Hall.

Nicolosi, L., Harryman, E., & Kresheck, J. (1983). *Terminology of communication disorders: Speech—language—hearing* (2nd ed.). Baltimore: Williams & Wilkins.

Oyer, H. (Ed.). (1987). *Administration of programs in speech-language pathology and audiology.* Englewood Cliffs, NJ: Prentice-Hall.

Pannbacker, M. (1975). Diagnostic report writing. *Journal of Speech and Hearing Disorders, 40,* 367–379.

Rassi, J. (1978). *Supervision in audiology.* Baltimore: University Park Press.

Sanders, K., Middleton, G. F., Puett, V., & Pannbacker, M. (1985–1986, Winter). Report writing: Current issues and proposed directions (summary). *SUPERvision, 9*(4), 23–32.

Schubert, G. W. (1978). *Introduction to clinical supervision in speech pathology.* St. Louis: Warren H. Green.

Strunk, W., Jr., & White, E. B. (1979). *The elements of style* (3rd ed.). New York: Macmillan.

Wing, D. (1975). A data recording form for case management and accountability. *Language, Speech, and Hearing Services in Schools, 6,* 38–40.

10
Supervision Applications of Microcomputer Technology

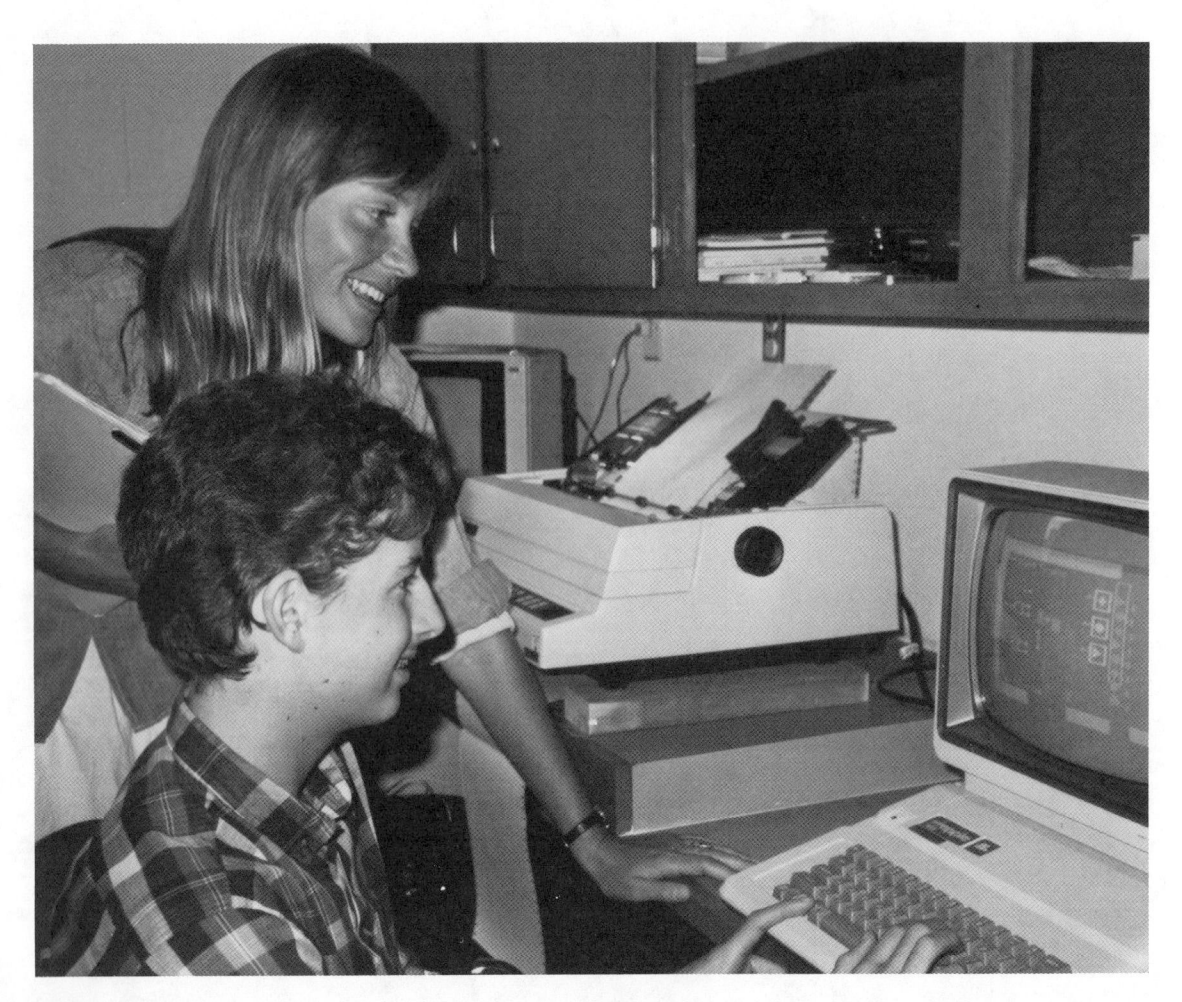

CRITICAL CONCEPTS

☐ *Supervisors need to know about microcomputers for personal development, to help students learn about and use them, and to judge the competency of clinicians who are using them clinically.*

☐ *Microcomputers can be used by supervisees, supervisors, and clients.*

☐ *Microcomputers are applied in four general ways in supervision: word processing, data bases, spreadsheets, and telecommunications.*

☐ *Microcomputer application in supervision requires education and training.*

OUTLINE

INTRODUCTION
RECORD KEEPING
    Supervisee Record Keeping
    Supervisor Record Keeping
    Client Record Keeping
    Equipment Needed
    Understanding Data Base Programs
    Setting up a Client Records Data Base
TELECOMMUNICATIONS
    File Transfers
    Bulletin Boards
    Data Bases
OTHER APPLICATIONS
    Computerized Library Card Catalogs
    Research and Creative Activity
    Networking
    Graphics
    Education/Training
CONCERNS
    High Tech/High Touch
    Practical Use
    Confidentiality and Security of Records
    Expense
    Preparation
SUMMARY
APPLICATIONS

INTRODUCTION

Supervisors are responsible for exploring new tools that make their jobs and clinicians' jobs more efficient, thus producing higher quality services. Tools used in the Communication Disorders profession include typewriters, telephones, standardized assessments, pictures, and so on. Microcomputers have also proven valuable to supervisors, student clinicians, and in-service personnel. Microcomputer knowledge, skills, and dispositions are important to supervisors on two levels. First, competent supervisors must know about and be able to use microcomputers themselves. Second, they must be able to instruct clinicians about clinical applications of microcomputers and then evaluate clinicians' competence in using them.

Most college and university training programs, as well as continuing education programs, now

---

This chapter was contributed by Gary E. Rushakoff and Stephen S. Farmer, New Mexico State University.

offer (a) specific courses in microcomputer applications, (b) exposure to microcomputer applications in several courses, and/or (c) exposure to microcomputer applications in clinical work. This chapter explores applications that may be of value to Communication Disorders supervisors and supervisees, including word processing, data bases, spreadsheets, and telecommunications.

The first application of microcomputers to supervision is record keeping.

RECORD KEEPING

Supervisee Record Keeping

Clock Hours. Students in Communication Disorders programs are required by ASHA to clock their clinical hours to obtain certification. Depending on the number of clinicians in a university program, this can be an onerous and time-consuming task. The use of microcomputers can not only save time, but also probably reduce mathematical errors. Early efforts to keep track of student practicum hours (Mahaffey, 1973; Peterson, 1977) used a university main frame computer. Each student's records had to be prepared on punch cards (hardly ever seen any more). Even one typing error in preparing one of these cards meant retyping the entire card.

Hood and Miller (1984) described a computer program to maintain information on students, including clock hours. Technological advancement allowed them to use a terminal connected to the university main frame computer. Because a terminal was used, entry errors could be corrected easily.

While several universities have reported computer programs for maintaining clock hours, few programs are commercially available as yet. *The Clock Hours Program* (Schwartz & Rushakoff, 1985) is a template for use with the spreadsheet of the *Appleworks* program (Lissner, 1983), an integrated program commonly used in educational settings. Clock hours are entered for each semester by disorder category. The resulting table automatically lists the number of hours required, the number of hours accrued, and the number of hours remaining in the various categories (see Table 10-1). Individuals with moderate experience in developing spreadsheets can develop clock hours templates in a few hours.

Grades. The microcomputer can be used to maintain grades in student practicum. Grade maintenance can be boring and inefficient if letter grades are used, but the microcomputer can show its power when point systems are used for grading. For example, most clinical competency forms can be adapted to spreadsheet format for electronic computation of competency grades. Such a program not only maintains the scores but can instantly compute the mean score for a given student and even quickly highlight deficit areas. It can determine the progress of any one student or compare the scores of several students.

Word Processing. A survey conducted in 1981 (Rushakoff & Lombardino, 1984) reported word processing to be the primary application for microcomputers in university speech and hearing programs. This is likely still to be true. In 1982, when microcomputers were first made available to student clinicians in the Communication Disorders program at New Mexico State University, all therapy and diagnostic reports were prepared with typewriters. Since diagnostic reports were often sent to various agencies, they had to be completely retyped by the secretarial staff. Within 2 years, virtually 100% of clinical reports were created using word processing programs; the secretarial staff no longer needed to retype reports. Indeed, reports were completed more quickly because the entire report never needed to be retyped.

In general, supervisors believe that reports achieve a higher standard of quality when word processing is used. Under the old system, some supervisors felt guilty having students retype a

TABLE 10-1
Clinical clock hours form

Clinical Hours for Certification
(Speech-Language Pathology)

STUDENT: Mills, J.   SEMESTER: Fall, 1988

	Hours Needed	Previous UG Hours	Previous GR Hours	Total Hours	Hours Remaining
Articulation	25				(−20)
Diagnostics		4	0	4	
Therapy		41	0	41	
Language	75				38
Diagnostics		0	0	0	
Therapy		37	0	37	
Voice	25				25
Diagnostics		0	0	0	
Therapy		0	0	0	
Fluency	25				25
Diagnostics		0	0	0	
Therapy		0	0	0	
Diagnostics	50			4	46
Audiology	35	4	0	4	31
Diagnostics	15	4	0	4	
Therapy	15	0	0	0	
	300	86	0	86	214

(Minus sign indicates excess hours.)

Director   Date

whole report when only small changes were needed. Now that supervisors know that changes can be made in seconds, they feel no compunction about correcting just a few errors in an otherwise acceptable report.

Silbar and Konarska (1984) described a data base system of formula writing for reports and letters. The program uses an assembly form to select variables to be included in the document. Speech-language pathologists can complete the assembly form and then operate the program, or they can complete the assembly form and then have the secretarial staff run the program to complete the document.

One attendant problem of word-processed reports was what to do with all the trial printouts and drafts. Few college and university Communication Disorders training programs have shredding machines, so students are instructed to tear up all documents before discarding them. While not guaranteeing complete confidentiality to clients, the policy prevents the casual breaches that the presence of early drafts could cause.

Useful accessory word processing programs are now available. One category is spelling checkers. These programs will check for typographical errors in a report and give the writer a chance to correct them. They will not help with errors like *for* instead of *four* or *boy* instead of *boys,* where the word is a mistake only in the context. However, they will find those spelling errors that are usually the most embarrassing when found months later. One attractive feature of these programs is that the user can add new words to the program's dictionary. A spelling check program does not assume that a word is misspelled; it may just not be in the program's dictionary. If the word is not found in the speller dictionary but is spelled correctly, then it can be added to the dictionary so that the program will know how to spell it the next time. One might think that spelling checker programs could produce lazy report writers who know the computer will do most of their proofreading. They may in fact produce better spellers by highlighting recurring errors.

Also available are grammatical and thesaurus programs that point out common grammatical errors and suggest alternatives to overused words and expressions. However, the efficacy of these programs in professional report writing has yet to be documented.

Career opportunities presented in data base programs offer students the opportunity for career planning.

Career Data Bases. Students who have been enrolled in Communication Disorders programs but have decided against Speech-Language Pathology and Audiology as majors, marginal students who are not suited for the profession, or students who have never heard of Communication Disorders all might benefit from career data base programs. Some of these programs are computerized interest or preference profiles. Some are computerized catalogues of career or profession descriptions. Many yield printouts that can be kept as supervisee records.

Supervisors, too, can keep records more easily by using microcomputers.

Supervisor Record Keeping

Word Processing. Word processing can be applied across the five roles of Communication Disorders supervision: Professional, Researcher, Educator, Administrator, and Clinician. It can be used to write professional papers, letters, recommendations, and clinic reports, to produce tests, and to develop brochures. It can also be used to produce typescripts of clinical sessions and supervision conferences for later analysis.

Analysis of Session Interactions. In the Educator and Clinician roles, supervisors often want client/clinician interaction patterns analyzed. Holloway (1984) computerized the Conover Analysis System (Conover, 1974). The program (*CONAN*) requires the user to take a 5-minute representative sample of a therapy session, enter the utterances into the program, and then categorize them according to the Conover system. *CONAN* then summarizes the client/clinician interaction. Although other computerized programs can analyze language, they do not provide interactional data (data about the effect of one speaker's communication act on another speaker's utterances).

The program *Systematic Analysis of Language Transcripts (SALT)* (Miller & Chapman, 1982) examines the communication of one or two speakers (not interactional communication, however) by performing grammatic, semantic, or discourse analyses selected by the examiner. *SALT* uses 31 symbols for coding each utterance. These symbols enable the examiner to (a) code key features of the utterances, (b) mark particular structures for subsequent analysis, (c) add background information or comments about nonverbal behavior, and (d) indicate unintelligible, incomplete, or omitted entries. Both qualitative and quantitative profiles can be generated from the language samples. The utterance-coding process is complicated but not difficult.

Other available programs include the *Computerized Language Sample Analysis (CLSA)* (Weiner, 1984), *Lingquest 1: Language Sample Analysis* (Fitch, 1986; Mordecai, Palin, & Palmer,

1982), and *Word Class Inventory (WCI)* (Bennet & Alter, 1985). These provide data about such elements as the number and percentage of complete and incomplete utterances, the type-token ratio (TTR), and the mean length of utterance (MLU). Programs such as these can now be developed as templates for a spreadsheet.

Supervisor-supervisee conferences can also provide material for interaction analysis.

Analysis of Supervision Conferences. In the Researcher, Educator, and Administrator roles, supervisors may analyze supervisee-supervisor conferences. (See chapters 4 and 11 for discussions of supervision conferences and interaction analysis tools.) Word processing facilitates the production of a typescript (hard copy) of the data to be analyzed by a computerized interaction analysis (IA) program. Three such programs are the *Multi-dimensional Observational System for the Analysis of Interactions in Clinical Supervision* (M.O.S.A.I.C.S.) (Weller, 1971) and *Pattern Recognition* (Oratio, 1979) for dyadic interactions, and the Proana 5 (Lashbrook & Lashbrook, 1975) for group interactions. All three of these interaction analysis tools have been computerized, although not for microcomputers. The CONAN (Holloway, 1984), which does operate on a microcomputer, can be adapted to supervisee-supervisor interactions.

The *Computer Language Sample Analysis* (Weiner, 1984), *Lingquest 1* (Mordecai et al., 1982), and the *Word Class Inventory* (Bennet & Alter, 1985) lend themselves to analysis of supervisors' metalinguistic behavior from conferences or from written responses, such as those produced by supervisor subjects in a study by Farmer (1985).

Spreadsheets. Spreadsheets can also be useful for supervisors' record keeping. A spreadsheet is a computer program in which a user can enter, modify, and manipulate data organized in rectangular arrays of rows and columns (tables).

The Supervision Hours Summary Form (Table 11-5, p. 293-294) lends itself to a spreadsheet format. Data about how much time supervisors devote to specific aspects of their jobs can be entered regularly. Row and column tallies are automatically totaled after each entry and at the end of the recording period. Total work hours and specific duties within roles are documented in this way.

Billing. Commercial billing programs are available, but a spreadsheet format can be developed within the setting, so it would be a waste of money to purchase a special billing program or even have one programmed. Figure 10-1 shows a spreadsheet billing template using the *Appleworks* (Lissner, 1983) spreadsheet and gives an example of the formulas. Not only does the spreadsheet perform the arithmetic, thereby eliminating possible errors, but it reduces the paperwork that can clutter any speech-language and hearing worksite.

FIGURE 10-1
A spreadsheet with formula of billing in a speech-language and hearing center

	A	B	C	D	E	F
1						
2		Speech and Hearing Center				
3		Statement of Services				
4						
5	Date	Descript	Charge	Credits	Balance	
6						
7	2/23/88	Therapy	$200		(C7-D7)	
8	3/2/88	Payment		$100	(copy it relative)	
9						
10						

FIGURE 10-2
Maintaining therapy data on a spreadsheet

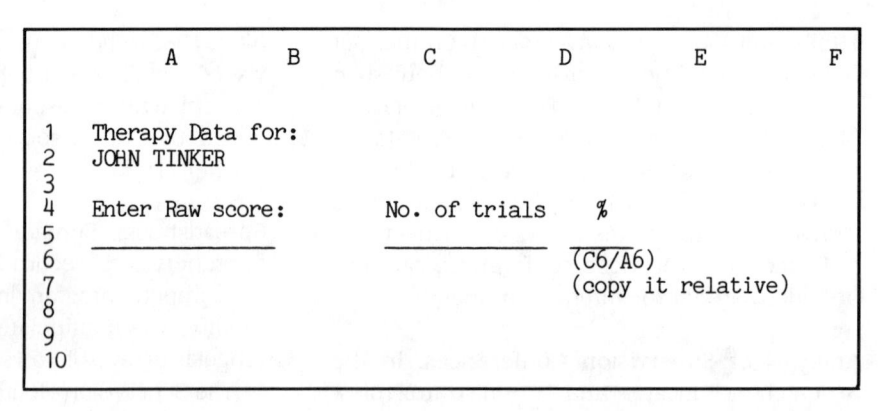

```
            A           B           C           D           E           F

1      Therapy Data for:
2      JOHN TINKER
3
4      Enter Raw score:              No. of trials    %
5      ──────────                    ──────────
6                                                    (C6/A6)
7                                                    (copy it relative)
8
9
10
```

The third use for microcomputer record keeping involves clients or patients.

Client Record Keeping

Numeric Therapy Data. Therapy data, especially numeric data, can be kept and analyzed on the microcomputer; when the clinician enters raw data, the program can produce percentage scores, mean scores, ranges, and so on (see Figure 10-2). Some programs, for example *Clinical Data Manager* (Katz, 1984), are interactive in that they ask the clinician to enter the data.

Some spreadsheet programs come with a graphics program, or have a graphics program that can be purchased separately. These programs can take the data described above and put it into pictorial forms such as line graphs, bar graphs, or pie charts (see Figures 10-3 and 10-4). Graphic presentation may help clients, clinicians, or supervisors to visualize progress.

Maintaining client records on a microcomputer system may prove the most interesting of current applications of technology in supervision.

Client Information. Traditionally, in speech-language pathology and audiology programs, client

FIGURE 10-3
A line graph of therapy data

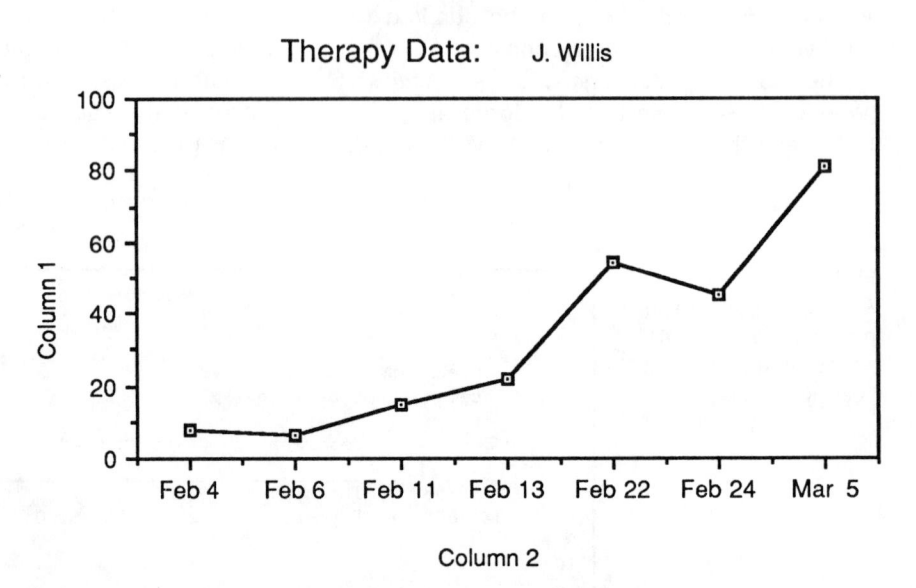

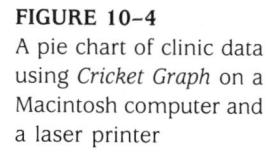

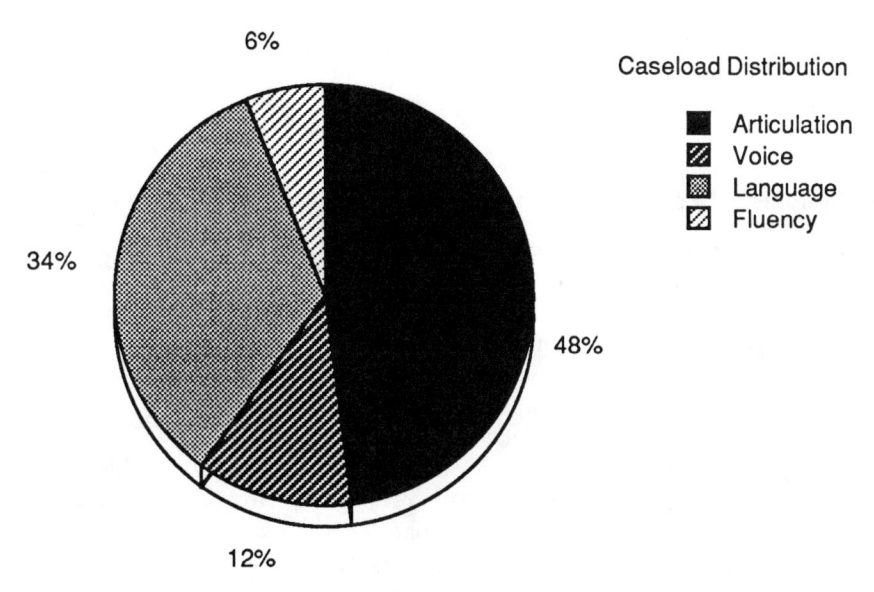

FIGURE 10-4
A pie chart of clinic data using *Cricket Graph* on a Macintosh computer and a laser printer

Caseload Distribution
- Articulation
- Voice
- Language
- Fluency

6%
34%
48%
12%

information has been kept on paper that is then stored. This archival information can rarely be used to compare and process information between people or to generate summary information about the types of services provided by a clinical program, a specific clinician, or a supervisor.

Drawing information from the archival storage system manually is laborious, time-consuming, and occasionally impossible. Once client records are stored on the microcomputer, however, supervisors have quick access to information for (a) administrative reports; (b) grants for program development; (c) budget justification for personnel, equipment, materials, and training; and (d) research projects of many kinds. Not only can more specific information on clinical program needs be available, but supervisors are more likely to notice changes in the distribution of clients being served. Awareness of demographics may allow clinical programs to plan and justify projected service needs. For example, if a hospital utilizes an electronic high-risk registry, then the local or regional school systems, rehabilitation centers, and speech-language-hearing clinics can network with the hospital system to plan appropriate home or school special education programs. Such a system benefits not only the high-risk population but also the administrators (often supervisors) of the service-providing agencies.

Several studies have documented the development and benefits of record keeping in speech and hearing facilities using main frame computers (Elliott, Vegely, & Falvey, 1971; Harden, Harden, & Norris, 1977; Kamara & Kamara, 1976; Mueller & Peters, 1976; Rushakoff, Vinson, Penner, & Messal, 1979). Some researchers have worked on developing microcomputer-based client record systems (Jackson, 1983).

Computer-generated client data may show trends in needs and services that are so subtle as not to be noticed by supervisors using archival systems. For example, after computerizing 50 pieces of speech, language, and hearing information on 1,200 individuals at a residential facility for mentally retarded individuals, Rushakoff et al. (1979) found that 67% of the residents did not or could not communicate through speech. This figure provided a strong budget and grant justification for more communication devices, materials on Blissymbols and sign language, in-service training funds, and focus on specific skills for new speech-language and hearing personnel.

Equipment Needed

Most of the widely used microcomputer systems allow client record keeping through data base software. However, other equipment is also necessary. To maintain as much information as possible in the computer file system and to have it operate at its fastest, it is advisable to get the maximum RAM (random access memory) available.

Clinical programs that wish to maintain large records on many people may need a hard disk drive, hardware that has become more economical in recent years. If a clinical program has a hard disk drive and several microcomputers, users can hook all of the systems to the hard disk drive. The result is known as a local area network (LAN) and means that computer client records can be accessed by any microcomputer system in the building. (See p. 268-269 for a discussion of confidentiality and computer record keeping.) The network is expensive because it means wiring all of the microcomputers to the hard disk drive and also purchasing a controller device that allows only one microcomputer to access the hard disk at any one moment.

A *modem* allows transfer of full or partial client record data to another microcomputer over the telephone. This method can be used to transfer information about clients to funding and referral agencies. A modem may also be of value for clinicians who work in several locations. For example, a microcomputer with a data base program and client record disk may be located at one facility. The clinicians may operate that microcomputer and the data base program using the microcomputer in another building, via a modem, if the main system is near a telephone. Clinicians could call the secretary and ask to have the telephone hooked to the microcomputer. If the clinical program can afford an extra telephone line, the main system can even be kept on line to bypass the secretary. The clinician need only have the computer dial the telephone number of the main microcomputer system, which will automatically respond. Obviously such a setup would require a data base program that allows the use of a password. This LAN system of client records can be useful to supervisors in the Researcher, Educator, Administrator, and Clinician roles.

Understanding Data Base Programs

To decide which software to purchase and how to set up and use a client records data base, it is necessary to understand some common terminology.

A *data base* is a collection of information (data) that may or may not be related. The most common data base known is the library, which has information on thousands of topics, available in books, newspapers, periodicals, records, films, and so on. The encyclopedia is also a data base, a collection of information.

A *file* is a collection of information that is related. The telephone book is a collection of information about almost everyone who owns a telephone in a community. A data base is, therefore, made up of many files. For example, the telephone book (file) can usually be found at the library (data base). For clinical record keeping, the file could have information about all clients who have received or are currently receiving services.

A *record* is a single cluster of information stored in a file. In a clinical record keeping system, each record could be for a different client. If the clinic were providing services to 80 people, 80 records would be in the file. This terminology is different from what is commonly used in archival storage systems. Supervisors may be used to saying, "Pull David's file from the file cabinet." If a computer based system is used, the request will be to "pull David's record from the file."

TABLE 10-2
Examples of data base file structures

File:	Client records	
	Record: Person	
	Fields:	1. Name
		2. Address
		3. Phone
		4. Date of evaluation

File:	Standardized assessments in clinic	
	Record: Test	
	Fields:	1. Name of test
		2. Age range
		3. How long to administer
		4. Author
		5. Year of publication
		6. Publisher

File:	Clinic inventory	
	Record: Item	
	Fields:	1. Item
		2. Location
		3. Condition of item
		4. Tag number
		5. Cost of item

Each record is made up of specific pieces of information. Each piece is called a *field*. In a client record keeping system, the name, address, telephone number, date of birth, and so on are each called fields.

To summarize, a file is made up of a number of records and a record is made up of a number of fields (see Table 10-2). Virtually all data base software is designed from these three building blocks, and understanding them helps to understand the differences in the capabilities of various programs.

Setting up a Client Records Data Base

In some clinical programs it may be a difficult process to decide what information should be collected on each client. Unlike the paper record system, which allows supervisors to collect any information they would like included, computerized record systems must be specific (Elliott et al., 1971; Kamara & Kamara, 1976; Rushakoff et al., 1979). Some information lends itself to computer filing and other information does not. For example, it is easy to record whether a client presents a semantic language problem (1 = *yes*, 2 = *no*); it is not easy to record a long description of that problem in a computer data base.

Supervisors should determine their current information needs. For example, many clinical programs need to produce data on the number of clients evaluated or the number of clients in various age groups or disorder categories. Even though supervisors may not find a current need for knowing hearing level in each ear, this information might prove useful later. For example, is the facility seeing only one degree of hearing impairment, or impairments at all levels? Information about the specific needs of a clinical program could provide focus and justification for equipment, personnel, and materials. Most current data base programs allow users to change the file structure later if they decide to start collecting more information.

Choosing Data Base Software. It is almost never necessary for a clinical program to write, or contract to have written, its own microcomputer software for client record keeping. A variety of data base programs can be purchased at local computer stores for $300 to $500.

The first characteristic to look for in choosing a data base program is a system that matches the skill level of the user. This is a tradeoff; typically, the easier a program is to learn and operate, the less flexible it is in performing complex data base functions. A data base program designed for a novice will not have the power and flexibility of one designed for professional programmers; it will be limited and include a number of compromises to keep the process simple. In the simpler systems, users interact with the program via a series of menus. While a menu-driven program is easier to learn and use than a command-driven program, it may take longer to operate, as each menu must be loaded from the disk each time.

It may be difficult for a first-time user to choose a data base program. Often it is not until one uses a program that one becomes aware of critical features that are missing. Computer store salespeople are not always the best sources of information. Dozens of data base programs are available for widely used microcomputers, and unless a supervisor happens to be interested in programs with which the store personnel are very familiar, they are not likely to be able to answer questions. However, they should be willing to let the supervisors look at the documentation, which may answer some questions. Supervisors should choose data base programs that are easy to use. Most people don't want to know how the program works. They just want to be able to put in data and get out reprocessed information.

File managers, computerized versions of the metal file cabinet, are generally easier to use than their more powerful cousins, relational data base programs. All file managers allow the user to set up a client file, enter information, sort and search these records to some degree, and print them.

A special kind of file manager exists (the dedicated file manager) in which the file has already been set up by a commercial firm. In other words, the designer has already decided which pieces of speech, language, and hearing information will be collected. Some dedicated file managers do not allow for customizing client information without reprogramming, a difficult process. These programs can save supervisors the trouble of determining what information to collect, since that is already done by the program author. Of course, problems arise if supervisors want to collect information the author did not, such as social security numbers, test scores, referral sources, tympanogram results, and so on. Also, dedicated file managers will not have as powerful data processing functions as do general file managers.

Relational data base programs have the same features as file managers and often a greater ability to manipulate the data. However, the major advantage of relational software is its ability to compare, manipulate and merge data from separate files. For example, a school speech-language pathologist may have one file of students receiving speech services. The occupational therapist may have a separate file for students receiving O.T. services, and the physical therapist a third file for P.T. records. With a relational data base program, the supervisors can ask questions like, "Which students between the ages of 6 and 18 are receiving speech-language, O.T., *and* P.T. services?" A relational data base can process that information by looking through all three files in one operation; a file manager cannot perform such a complex task.

It is often necessary or advantageous to include information drawn from a client records data base in an administrative report, grant proposal, or research paper. In 1982, several programs were designed so that data from a specific data base program could be easily transferred to a file in a word processing program. By 1984 *integrated software* was developed, so that users could operate two or more applications within the same program. Usually this means that one software package contains a data base program, word processor, spreadsheet, and graphics. The information from the spreadsheet or data base can be easily transferred to a word processing file. Another advantage to integrated packages is that they have a unified command structure, so that if users learn the commands for one module they can also operate the others.

Dozens of data base programs are available for the more widely used microcomputer systems, and more are introduced every year. They vary in cost from $20 to $700. In general, the differences among these programs can be described in terms of (a) capacity, (b) data entry, (c) data retrieval, and (d) report generation.

Only a limited number of words can be typed on a piece of paper, only a finite number of pages can go in a manila record folder, and only a limited number of record folders can fit into a single metal file cabinet. These limits of capacity also hold true for computer record keeping software. To determine what capacity is needed, the clinic should first set up the client record file on paper.

☐ *Number of characters per field:* Many programs limit the length of any particular field. For example, a program that limits field length to 12 characters will not accommodate most names or many addresses. One strategy for reducing the number of characters needed is to use a code system. Instead of requiring a long field for the type of disorder, a two-digit code could be used.

☐ *Number of characters per record:* The record is all the information on a particular individual. Most programs limit the total number of characters in each record. Some programs have record length limits in the 1000-character range. Programs that severely limit the number of characters per record may cause problems. For example, a program may indicate that a record can have up to 70 fields, but only 280 characters. That means the average length of each field could be 4 characters!

☐ *Number of fields per record:* This indicates the total number of specific pieces of information (fields) you can have for each individual. A program with a limit of 10 fields per record would barely get past the name, address, telephone, and date of birth. The file design made on paper will indicate how many fields are required.

☐ *Number of records per file:* Just as a limited number of manila folders can be placed in a metal file cabinet, so the number of records is limited in a computer file. Since clinics often keep both active and inactive records in the computer file, an estimate should be made of the number of clients for whom services will be provided during the next 5 years.

For data entry itself, investigate the ease of (a) setting up a file, (b) changing a file, (c) entering data into a record, and (d) changing information in a record.

☐ *Setting up a file:* Once the file structure has been developed on paper, it is entered in the data base program. Most programs do this interactively. The program asks the user to type in the name of the first field, which could be *Name.* It may then ask how long this field should be. To enter most individuals' last and first names requires 20 to 30 characters. When all the fields are entered, the file is set and data can be entered.

☐ *Changing a file:* When supervisors are first setting up client or supervisee files, they may not think of all the information they will wish to include. Supervisors may decide a year later that it would be valuable to begin including tympanometry results for the clients, or the names, ages, and disorder types of all the clients the supervisee has had. A few programs do not allow the user to change or add new fields after the file has been entered, but many allow the user to change, delete, and add new fields at any time.

☐ *Entering data:* Most programs allow easy entry of record data. Programs that permit customization of the data entry screen can be especially useful when many people are responsible for entering data. For example, without this feature a program in the data entry mode may just say

Name_____

A program for which the user has designed the data entry screen could say

> Type in the name: Last name, first name (*example:* SMITH, David)

This feature can also be useful when codes are used to enter information:

Intelligibility level (enter the number) _____
1 = normal
2 = mild
3 = moderate
4 = severe

The ability to reorganize and process information is the heart of a data base program. This is what separates it from paper record-keeping systems. Three main process functions of data base software are sorting, searching, and frequency of occurrence.

☐ *Sorting:* reorganizes all of the records in a file either alphabetically or numerically. While the most common way to keep records organized is alphabetically by last name, it might prove useful at times to have the file ordered by date of evaluation, date of birth, primary disorder, or some other criterion. This is known as a *single-level sort.* It sorts all of the records based on the information in one field. Many programs can also perform a *multilevel sort:* for example, an alphabetized list of all the clients in each disorder category (see Table 10–3). The pro-

TABLE 10–3
Multilevel sort by disorder and last name

Speech and Hearing Center
Multilevel sort: (1) by disorder and (2) by last name

September 3
Page 1 of 6

Disorder	Name	Date of Birth	File No.
Aphasia	Carr, Dennis[1]	09/12/39	5.0295
	Duffey, Mary	02/04/27	5.0167
	Gordon, David	11/22/32	5.0746
	Jenkins, Stuart	09/03/23	5.0285
Articulation	Barry, Richard	03/12/63	6.1823
	Martin, Jack	11/02/57	6.2295
	Pierce, Robert	03/09/80	6.1090
	Sullivan, Walter	12/24/81	6.2551
	Thompson, Shelly	09/22/82	6.8461
Cleft Palate	Cooper, Julian	02/22/79	1.0827
	Denney, Charles	04/08/80	1.0602
	Harden, Linda	11/14/74	1.8482
Developmental Language	Allen, Michael	06/14/81	3.0112
	Cannon, Jill	11/03/82	3.0330
	Ferguson, Kent	03/09/79	3.0202
	Stone, Raymond	10/30/81	3.0939

[1]All names used in these examples are fictitious.

gram first sorts all of the records by disorder and then, within each disorder category, sorts the names alphabetically. Some programs allow multilevel sorts using several fields at once.

☐ Unlike sorting, which affects all of the records in a file, *searching* finds only those records that meet one or more conditions. *Single searches* are used to find records based on information in one field. For example, the program could be told to find the record of *Smith, David* and that this information will be located in the *name* field. If it is not possible to determine the first name, most programs will allow a partial search of a field: for example, to find everyone whose last name is Smith. The search capability has many applications other than finding an individual's record. Supervisors can find the records of all clients who were given a particular language test, or all clinicians who need voice hours or who have completed a practicum at General Hospital.

One of the most exciting capabilities of data base software is the *multilevel search*. This capability can be used to find the records of individuals who meet a series of criteria (see Table 10-4). For example, the program could find all the males between the ages of 6 and 18 who are dysfluent, have normal hearing, and live within the city limits.

☐ The *frequency of occurrence* function will answer questions beginning "How many...." For example, it could print out a list of all the primary disorders in the client file and indicate how many people have each disorder. This function allows clinical programs to produce percentages for each disorder category, determine the number of clients in each age category who received a particular type of assessment, or find out how many clients were seen by a particular supervisor or student during a specified period and what disorders the clients presented.

While processing the data is at the heart of data base software, the program's ability to print out the information in a useful form is crucial too. Flexibility in report format varies greatly from one program to another. A good program should allow the user to (a) define left, right, top, and bottom margins, (b) print headers and footers (i.e., headings at top or bottom of form; titles, footnotes), (c) put the date on the page,

TABLE 10-4
Multilevel search

Speech and Hearing Center

Multilevel search: Males between the ages of 6 and 21 with an articulation deficit and normal hearing in both ears who have been evaluated within the past 3 years.

Printed out in order of chronological age:

Date of Birth	Name
03/12/68	Barry, Richard
09/03/68	Glover, Jerry
12/02/70	Diamond, Arthur
06/10/73	Sayre, Chris
01/22/74	Brown, George
11/19/77	Wright, William
06/30/79	Meyer, Peter
06/02/81	Simpson, Harlan

and (d) control page numbering. It should also allow the user to save a report format so that it need not be recreated each time a report is required.

Microcomputer-based record keeping systems allow supervisors to generate data needed by others and for their own service projections. The major limitation of microcomputer-based files is the file and record capacity limits imposed by the floppy disk, but new data base programs are being developed that are more powerful and easy to use.

It would be naive to think that a project like maintaining client records on the microcomputer does not present problems.

Problems. The first problem supervisors should expect is in developing the file. The more people involved in choosing what information should be collected, the more difficult the process will be. Some of the client information can be difficult to translate into small bits. Next, since there is a lag between the time when personnel enter information about clients and the time when enough data are in the file to process the information, some personnel may not appreciate at the beginning why they must fill out yet one more form. Finally, as often as the instructions for entering the client data are given, at least one person will not follow them and will try to "wing it." This person will get stuck in some far-flung area of the data base program and not know how to get out.

In addition to the record-keeping applications of microcomputers, telecommunication is creating many new tools for supervisors.

TELECOMMUNICATIONS

Telecommunications is electronic communication involving machines (or people and machines) that use existing telephone, radio, and television systems. Voice, texts, photographs and other images, and handwriting are among the signals that can be sent and received via telecommunication.

The modem connects the microcomputer to any telephone line, with three basic applications for supervisors: (a) file transfers, (b) bulletin boards, and (c) searchable data bases.

File Transfers

In the Professional role, officers of CUSPSPA will find the electronic mail function helpful in keeping in touch with each other and with CUSPSPA members. This not only reduces the paperwork avalanche but also allows instant message transmission. Also, proceedings from conferences and workshops can be put together easily by having participants send their manuscripts to a source that prints the document for publication.

In the Research domain, supervisors can use file transferring to facilitate collaborative research projects. Publications such as *The Clinical Supervisor* or *SUPERvision* may one day be edited by a telecommunication process.

Supervisors operating in the Educator role can monitor supervisees in field sites far from the primary worksite by having them send lesson plans, reports, videotapes, writing samples, and any questions they have. The supervisors can then send back comments and answers to questions. This use of telecommunication opens new options for Clinical Fellowship Year (CFY) positions and student practicum experiences in rural areas. New information about supervision can be disseminated quickly to those supervisors who teach supervision courses, so that the latest information is always available.

For supervisors in the Administrator role, file transferring may be used to send reports to insurance companies and other agencies. Documents such as diagnostic and therapy reports can be quickly transferred from one computer to another over the telephone line, eliminating the photocopying and mailing of multiple copies. Administrators also find the electronic memo capability an efficient way to keep in touch with personnel within house or in satellite facilities.

Supervisors functioning in the Clinician role can transfer reports of clients across town or across the country to other clinicians so that services for clients who relocate are not delayed because necessary paperwork has not been received.

Bulletin Boards

Electronic bulletin boards are the computer equivalent to the posting spaces found in most worksites, especially university settings. Some are specialized; SpecialNet is a network for Special Education information. However, the information it carries is of varying degrees of value. Indeed, much of the same critical information about legislation, employment opportunities, and conference schedules appears in such readily available journals as *Asha* and *Teaching Exceptional Children*.

Data Bases

Data bases are searchable collections of related information. The ones most commonly used in Communication Disorders are Educational Resources Information Center (ERIC), Bibliographic Research Service (BRS), and Medline. It is the search capability that makes these data bases so much more valuable than bulletin boards. They can quickly provide listings of information on very specific topics, such as "treatment programs for stuttering used with adolescents."

Just as it was necessary in the past to work with a computer programmer to use a main frame computer, many universities still require a librarian to query a data base because training is needed to produce a quality query at the minimum cost. However, data bases are becoming easier to use, and it is likely that supervisors and other Communication Disorders personnel will soon be able to access and use these data bases on their own.

CUSPSPA, through the Supervision Network (SUPERnet), has established a data base of supervision presentations made at ASHA conventions since 1985.

OTHER APPLICATIONS

Other applications are being developed every day for modems, data bases, spreadsheets, and diagnostic and therapeutic strategies and materials. These include library card catalogs, research uses, networks, graphics, education/training programs, artificial intelligence, and prosthetics.

Computerized Library Card Catalogs

A computerized library card catalog allows users to search for references in a university or city library from the microcomputers in worksites or homes. Users can search information by topic (e.g., all the books about supervision) or by author and can learn the location and availability of specific books. This function expands opportunities for research from worksites that are not located near major library facilities.

Research and Creative Activity

Beyond the daily use of microcomputer-based client records in speech-language and hearing worksites, the research applications are enormous and exciting. Once hospitals, schools, and clinics around the country begin to maintain client information on microcomputers with hard disk drives, a large data base of individuals with communication disorders comes into being. This large storehouse of information opens new avenues of research. It also increases the potential for collaborative projects, which can have a profound effect on the quality and quantity of Communication Disorders research in general and supervision research in particular.

Much supervision research involves conferences, especially the verbal and nonverbal communication used in conferences. An area that has received minimal attention thus far is the paralinguistic elements (e.g., silence/pauses, inflections, and intonations) of supervisors' oral communication. Advances made in electronics allow researchers to use equipment such as sound spectrographs, the Visi-Pitch (Kay Electronics Corporation), specially constructed instrumentation (Horii, 1983), and software such as the *Computer-Aided Fluency Establishment Trainer (CAFET)* (Goebel, 1986) to examine prosodic features, pause-utterance length and frequency, and breathing patterns. This equipment makes possible a more scientific approach to defining psychologically perceived phenomena such as "warmth" and "sincerity."

Another form of conference is the interview. The *Molyneaux-Lane Interview Analysis System* (Molyneaux & Lane, 1982), discussed in chapter 4, has the capability for computer analysis of data, which makes it valuable for research.

The portability of microcomputers allows them to be taken almost anywhere a speech-language pathologist or audiologist might go. Speech-language pathologists who work on dysmorphology and genetics teams can often get information about unusual syndromes almost instantly by accessing a medical syndrome data base. Not only does this provide immediate information on which to base professional decisions, but the speech-language pathologist can enter data into the bank, thereby expanding the information it contains about unique medical conditions.

With a basic understanding of what microcomputers do and how they do it, plus a good knowledge of personal, program, and/or institutional needs, supervisors can set up data base systems that will do just about anything with the information that is available.

For researchers interested in research using statistics, microcomputer software programs provide the convenience of doing computations at desktop rather than using large computing center facilities.

A common misconception about the use of microcomputers is that users must be proficient in programming. Authoring software such as *SuperPILOT* (Apple Computer, Inc., 1982) helps users to create, without programming, different kinds of programs with graphics, sound, and color. The computer assisted instruction (CAI) program *Microcomputer Assisted Study Partner in Anatomy and Physiology of the Speech and Hearing Mechanism* (Rushakoff, Jackson, Farmer, & Farmer, 1984) was produced with *SuperPILOT*.

Word processing, too, with its capabilities for easy editing, helps supervisors generate works for publication. Multiple authors can edit jointly-produced manuscripts via modem; chapters of a book with multiple contributors can be combined and edited at one central location.

Networking

Although networks have been mentioned before, the concept needs reiterating because it offers so many possibilities for facilitating communication. It has become increasingly important for Communication Disorders training programs, as well as service delivery programs, to keep in touch with alumni or former patients for financial, recruitment, and volunteer support. Mailing lists of alumni can be maintained and easily updated on the computer, allowing for frequent and efficacious contact with former consumers of service. Newsletters, job announcements, and endowment or scholarship requests can be sent easily and cheaply by electronic mail.

With the search and sort capabilities of data base programs, categories of people who should receive certain information can be easily separated, eliminating the need to send specific information to everyone. Mailing lists can be sorted by geographic area (local, state, regional), by worksite type (university, community center, hospital, nursing home, school, preschool, private practice), by discipline (speech-language pathologists, audiologists), by title (therapists, diagnosticians, supervisors, administrators), by year (all 1979 graduates), and in many other ways.

An additional benefit in some data base software is the capability of "blocking out" certain fields of information so that they are not readily accessible to most users. If necessary, personal data (grade point average, scores from the *Na-*

tional *Examination in Speech-Language Pathology and Audiology* (*NESPA*) and *Graduate Record Examination* (*GRE*), annual income, and so on) can be recorded without risk to their confidentiality.

Graphics

A number of programs are available to turn data or images into impressive graphics. These programs produce high-quality results quickly and easily. Although microcomputer graphics in the form of pie charts and bar and line graphs have been used for many years, image scanning is a relatively new application. Photographs, charts, or graphics can be scanned electronically and the images placed on disk, then either printed separately or merged with a text file and printed as part of a narrative document. Pictures, graphs and charts, or schematic diagrams can be beneficial to the supervisor in all five roles.

Education/Training

Computer Assisted Instruction (CAI). More and more CAI programs are emerging in the field of Communication Disorders. Supervisors in the Educator role, in any setting, can use CAIs to help supervisees learn new information or to review (e.g., before taking the *NESPA*). The *Microcomputer Assisted Study Partner in Anatomy and Physiology of the Speech and Hearing Mechanism* (Rushakoff et al., 1984) is a CAI designed specifically for Communication Disorders personnel.

While most of the tools described in this chapter are already being used in some form by supervisors, several new applications of technology to supervision are just on the horizon. One is interactive video disks, which promise to open potent new forms of clinical and supervision training.

Video Disks. A user can interact with a video disk system on three levels (Currier, 1983; Daynes, 1982; Zollman & Fuller, 1982). A Level One video disk program requires the user to watch the lesson passively. At most, the user may have limited control over the video disk and the lesson can direct the learner to a small degree. A Level Two lesson can branch to particular frames depending on the user's response. Although branching allows for more sophisticated programming, Level Two lessons are still rather limiting. Level Three programs (originally termed "intelligent video disks") are the most interactive; the user controls the video disk player through a microcomputer. An early application of this technology won a Scientific Exhibit award at the 1985 ASHA convention. Kopra, Dunlop, Kopra, and Abrahamson (1985) demonstrated how use of an interactive, computer-assisted video disk system could facilitate speechreading. Other possible uses of Level Three programs in Communication Disorders supervision follow.

Students will report that, despite preparing to administer a particular diagnostic test or treatment strategy, they find the initial clinical experience with it difficult. An interactive video disk can help. Several different types of tests or therapeutic strategies could be administered to individuals with various disorders, with the camera recording from the perspective of the clinician. Students could use the disk to practice administering and transcribing an articulation test to a hearing-impaired child, an adult stroke victim, or a teenager with cerebral palsy. The video disk would be designed to respond and remediate the student's errors. The student could continue practicing until competent. In a similar way, Level Three video disks may someday be used to help supervisors develop the skills and dispositions of the four STYLES of supervision discussed in chapter 4. Level Three video disks bring the features of CAI and high-quality video together in a combined system whose promise is greater than the sum of the parts.

Artificial Intelligence. Artificial intelligence (AI) has been defined as "the study of ideas which enable computers to do the things that make people seem intelligent" (Winston, 1979, p. 3). As AI techniques expand the capability of computers into the realm of symbolic processing rather than just numeric processing, computers will be able to solve problems previously beyond their power. One capability germane to supervision would be natural language analysis, the power to decode meaning from pragmatic and contextual elements of communication. Not only would natural language analysis alter research into supervision conference communication, it would also affect the clinical analysis of communication and augmentative communication (nonvocal communication using communication boards, voice synthesizers, etc.).

Prosthetics. Prostheses provide handicapped individuals with compensations for control of the environment (e.g., robotics), sense perception (e.g., bio-ear, artificial vision), and communication (e.g., voice synthesizers). The design and use of prosthetic devices has been, and will continue to be, facilitated by microprocessor technology. The microprocessor enhances independence by adding the possibility of programmed responses to stimuli; the prosthetic device reacts as well as acts (Behrmann, 1984).

Continuing Education. The opportunities are increasing annually to take academic courses via telecommunication systems. Students can attend one university but take courses at others at the same time. Thus, for instance, colleges and universities that do not offer courses in Communication Disorders supervision can have their students receive education in the subject through telecommunications coursework. However, before such courses can be offered, technologically literate supervisors must develop them and get them incorporated into the national telecommunications coursework system.

It behooves present-day Communication Disorders supervisors to expand their knowledge of supervision to include advanced technology. University and continuing education programs should address this area of knowledge when training Communication Disorders supervisors. Supervisors must be able to instruct clinicians and clients in the use of augmentative devices and evaluate supervisees' use of electronic equipment.

Although electronic technology offers supervisors new, exciting opportunities in all five roles, caution must be exercised when implementing the technology.

CONCERNS

High Tech/High Touch

Supervisors must place microcomputers in a proper perspective as they become more common in all supervision settings. Microcomputer technology can add tremendously to the scientific dimensions of supervision. However, Communication Disorders is a person-oriented profession, and the focus of professional efforts must always be on the human connection through communication (the art). Microcomputer technology (part of the science) can facilitate human communication but never replace it. Communicating through physical contact will always be necessary.

Practical Use

Certain tasks may actually take longer on the microcomputer than with paper and pencil. Examples are keeping attendance records, scheduling clients, and recording that lesson plans were turned in. Supervisors must use microcomputers to save time and money, not as their only tool.

Confidentiality and Security of Records

Supervisors must guard against losing client or supervisee records and breaking the confidentiality of the information. For several reasons it is not recommended that microcomputer-based client or supervisee record systems completely replace standard archival records. First, although it does not happen often, it is possible to lose information stored on a disk. Paper records are a bit more resistent to loss. Most microcomputer users are aware of two ways to protect against loss of disk records: (a) keeping a back-up disk of the data, or (b) printing out disk records periodically. Unfortunately, it usually requires the loss of at least one major document to make users follow these safeguards consistently.

Supervisors also need to be concerned about confidentiality of client and staff records. One easy way to maintain confidentiality is to restrict access to the data disks, for example by locking them in a secure area. Even if the disks must be left out during the day, many data base programs require the use of a password to access the data on the disk. If necessary, the password can easily be changed. The password feature should not give supervisors a false sense of security about access to data, however. Many inexpensive programs are available that will scan any data disk to show the user all the information on it. For example, if a clinical educator forgets the password used for an instructional file, the data base program will not allow access to the file without it. However, by using a word processor to load the password file, the supervisor can see the forgotten password and access the data.

Expense

Although microcomputer systems are not inexpensive, the cost of a basic system (keyboard, disk drive, monitor, printer) is affordable to many individuals and institutions in the Communication Disorders profession, especially when viewed as a long-term, cost and time efficient investment. Supervisors need to know what functions their setting needs from a microcomputer system; they can then comparison shop to find the best price for equipment that meets those needs.

Preparation

The last concern about the advent of microcomputer technology to the field of supervision is how to prepare supervisors to be literate users of electronic technology. Preparation includes addressing cyberphobia, as well as providing knowledge, training, and experience for those who have no computer fears.

The first stage is awareness: awareness of microcomputer uses and misuses, advantages and disadvantages, and personal knowledge, skills, and feelings about microcomputers in Communication Disorders. The next step is to identify the personal, professional, program, and institutional needs to be met with microcomputers. The third step is to acquire knowledge of the market—what hardware and software is available—and then to compare what is available with what is needed. The fourth step is to develop the skills necessary to use the equipment. The last step is to locate, and perhaps join, a computer users' group or club. The group support is often beneficial, especially to beginning computer users. The national organization Computer Users in Speech and Hearing (CUSH), with its publications, is a good source of information for Communication Disorders personnel.

SUMMARY

A variety of microcomputer applications is possible in supervision, and most of them can be accomplished with three basic programs: (a) word processing, (b) data base, and (c) spreadsheet. Present-day supervisors need to know about and use electronic technology, but it is even more important that Communication Disorders training programs include such information in supervision curricula. It is critical to the profession in general and to supervisors specifically that Communication Disorders personnel become informed consumers of microcomputer technology.

APPLICATIONS

Discussion Topics

1. Discuss how the confidentiality of clients could be protected if their records were computerized.
2. Discuss who should be responsible for training students to use word processing.
3. Discuss five things you wish microcomputers could do.
4. Discuss the advantages and disadvantages of programs such as spelling checkers in the development of clinical literacy.
5. Discuss the advantages and disadvantages of using telecommunication systems for supervision in rural areas.

Laboratory Experiences

1. Prepare a disorders categorization for operations in a specific worksite.
2. Prepare an outline for implementing a microcomputer-based client records system. Include such steps as creating the file and training supervisors and other personnel.
3. Find out the names of at least two spelling checker programs that will work with the microcomputer system and word processor you use most often.
4. Develop a report-writing CAI to train various areas of clinical report writing (e.g., syntax, semantics, punctuation).
5. Do a language analysis of a supervision conference using one of the programs discussed in this chapter.

Research Projects

1. Design a study to answer the question: Does using a word processor produce higher-quality clinic reports than using a typewriter?
2. Design a study to compare how long it takes to answer a particular question about your clients from paper and computerized records.
3. Use a data base to generate data for a descriptive study of the Communication Disorders supervisors in your state or region.
4. Use the SUPERnet data base of syllabuses for supervision courses taught across the country to compare similarities and differences.
5. Develop a telecommunication network for supervisors in your state (region).

REFERENCES

Apple Computer, Inc. (1982). *SuperPILOT.* Microcomputer software. Cupertino, CA: Apple Computer, Inc.

Behrmann, M. (1984). *Handbook of microcomputers in special education.* San Diego: College-Hill Press.

Bennet, C., & Alter, K. (1985). *Word Class Inventory.* San Diego: College-Hill Press.

Conover, H. (1974). *Conover Analysis System.* Unpublished manuscript, Ohio State University, Columbus.

Currier, R. (1983). Interactive videodisc learning systems. *High Technology, 10* (November), 51–59.

Daynes, R. (1982). The videodisc interfacing primer. *Byte, 7*(6), 48–59.

Elliott, L., Vegely, A., & Falvey, N. (1971). Description of a computer-oriented record-keeping system. *Asha, 13,* 435–443.

Farmer, S. (1985, November). *Supervision in communicative disorders: Metalinguistic analysis of assumptions and predictions. Phase I.* Paper presented at the annual convention of the American Speech-Language-Hearing Association, Washington, DC.

Fitch, J. (1986). *Clinical applications of microcomputers in communication disorders.* Orlando, FL: Academic Press.

Goebel, M. (1986). *A Computer-Aided Fluency Establishment Trainer (CAFET).* Falls Church, VA: Annandale Fluency Clinic.

Harden, R. J., Harden, R. W., & Norris, M. (1977). Computer program for the analysis of clinical enrollment. *Asha, 19,* 472–474.

Holloway, J. (1984). *CONAN: A computerized version of the Conover Analysis System.* Unpublished computer program and manuscript, Zanesville, OH.

Hood, S., & Miller, L. (1984). Administrative applications in microcomputers. In A. Schwartz (Ed.), *Handbook of microcomputer applications in communication disorders* (pp. 219–245). San Diego: College-Hill Press.

Horii, Y. (1983). An automatic analysis method of utterance and pause lengths and frequencies. *Behavioral Research Methods Instruction, 15,* 449–452.

Jackson, C. (1983, November). *Use of microcomputers for school hearing screening and evaluation records.* Paper presented at the annual convention of the American Speech-Language-Hearing Association, Cincinnati, OH.

Kamara, C., & Kamara, A. (1976). Computer billing, service analysis, and financial reporting in a hearing and speech agency. *Asha, 18,* 229–231.

Katz, R. (1984). *Clinical Data Manager.* San Diego: College-Hill Press.

Kopra, L., Dunlop, R., Kopra, M., & Abrahamson, J. (1985). *Laser videodisc interactive system for computer-assisted instruction in speechreading.* Scientific exhibit presented at the annual convention of the American Speech-Language-Hearing Association, Washington, DC.

Lashbrook, W., & Lashbrook, V. (1975). *Proana 5: A computer analysis of small group discussion.* Minneapolis: Burgess.

Lissner, R. (1983). *Appleworks.* Microcomputer software. Cupertino, CA: Apple Computer, Inc.

Mahaffey, R. (1973). A computerized procedure of keeping student records for ASHA-CCC requirements. *Asha, 15,* 590.

Miller, J., & Chapman, R. (1982). *Systematic Analysis of Language Transcripts (SALT)*. Unpublished manuscript, University of Wisconsin—Madison, the Language Analysis Laboratory, Waisman Center of Mental Retardation and Human Development.

Molyneaux, D., & Lane, V. (1982). *Effective interviewing: Techniques and Analysis*. Boston: Allyn & Bacon.

Mordecai, D., Palin, M., & Palmer, C. (1982). *Lingquest 1: Language Sample Analysis*. Columbus, OH: Charles E. Merrill.

Mueller, P., & Peters, T. (1976). A clinical record-keeping system. *Asha, 18,* 352–353.

Oratio, A. (1979). *Pattern Recognition*. Baltimore: University Park Press.

Peterson, H. (1977). More about computer assisted clinical record keeping. *Asha, 19,* 617–618.

Rushakoff, G., Jackson, C., Farmer, S., & Farmer, J. (1984). *Microcomputer Assisted Study Partner in Anatomy and Physiology of the Speech and Hearing Mechanism*. San Diego: College-Hill Press.

Rushakoff, G., & Lombardino, L. (1984). Microcomputer applications. *Asha, 26,* 27–31.

Rushakoff, G., Vinson, B., Penner, K., & Messal, S. (1979, November). *Clinical decision making through electronic information processing*. Paper presented at the annual convention of the American Speech-Language-Hearing Association, Atlanta.

Schwartz, A., & Rushakoff, G. (1985). *The Clock Hours Program*. Computer software. Las Cruces: New Mexico State University.

Silbar, J., & Konarska, K. (1984, November). *Reports with ease: Word processing for fast and easy reports*. Paper presented at the annual convention of the American Speech-Language-Hearing Association, San Francisco.

Weiner, F. (1984). *Computerized Language Sample Analysis (CLSA)*. State College, PA: Parrot Software.

Weller, R. (1971). *Verbal communication in instructional supervision*. New York: Teachers College Press, Columbia University.

Winston, P. (1979). *Artificial intelligence*. Reading, MA: Addison-Wesley.

Zollman, D., & Fuller, R. (1982). The Puzzle of the Tacoma Narrows Bridge Collapse: An interactive videodisc program for physics instruction. *Creative Computing, 2,* 100–109.

11
Assessment in Supervision

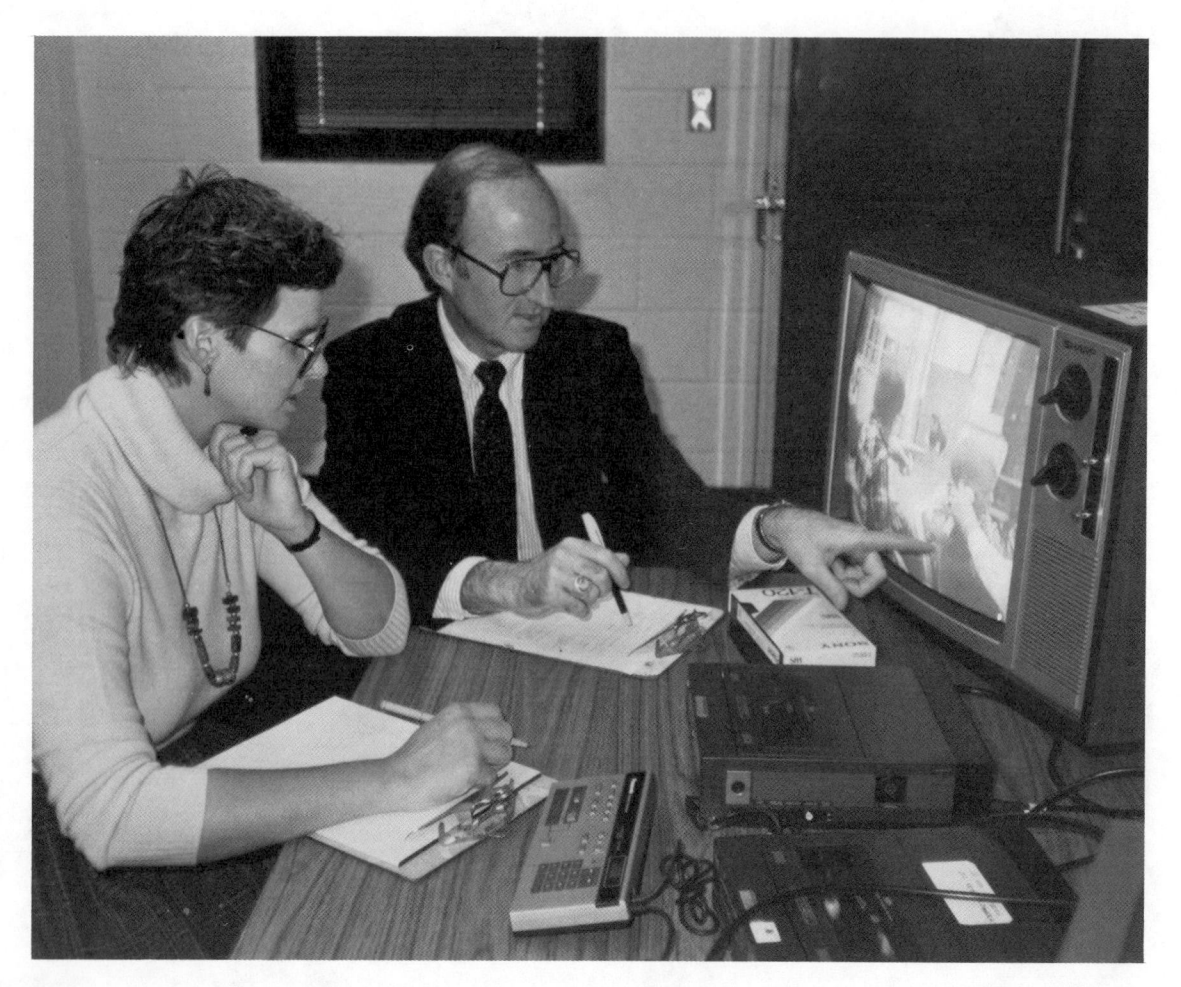

CRITICAL CONCEPTS

- *Assessment in Communication Disorders supervision is a system that includes preparation, planning, and an evaluation-feedback process.*
- *Supervisors need training in assessment.*
- *Personal biases affect the assessment process.*
- *Supervising marginal personnel, minority language-multicultural personnel, communication-impaired personnel, and peers, as well as doing generic supervision, require special consideration.*

OUTLINE

INTRODUCTION

THE ASSESSMENT SYSTEM

Preparation

Planning

The Evaluation-Feedback Process

SPECIAL CONSIDERATIONS

Marginal Personnel

Nontraditional Learners

Evaluating and Grading Peers

Generic Supervision

SUMMARY

APPLICATIONS

INTRODUCTION

Major decisions are made daily about people's lives—whether they should remain in school, enter professional or graduate institutions, be given jobs. Because the decisions are made partially on the basis of assessment statistics, the entire assessment enterprise merits attention. In Communication Disorders, supervisors assess personnel (e.g., student clinicians, staff clinicians, office staff) and programs, both those that train clinicians and those that simply provide services. Personnel and program assessment may have stronger consequences than any of the other tasks supervisors perform. Unfortunately, assessment is also the area for which most supervisors are least prepared. The same assumption seems to be made as is made about supervision in general: Anyone who is a competent clinician can supervise; anyone who is a competent clinician can assess personnel and programs. As the present cadre of supervisors knows, assessment in supervision is complex and requires preparation.

Although the terms *assessment* and *evaluation* are often used synonymously, they are differentiated in this text. *Evaluation,* one kind of assessment, is a combination of testing and grading. *Assessment,* as applied to supervision, is a system that includes (a) preparing to be a competent assessor; (b) planning the assessment (establishing policies and procedures, purpose(s), competencies to assess, goals/objectives, and consequences); and (c) the evaluation-feedback cycle. Unless all three steps are included, the risk of inappropriate personnel and program assessment is high, because the evaluation-feedback cycle can occur by itself. In that case, supervisors may not be assessing the most relevant competencies, goals, and objectives.

This chapter was contributed by Stephen S. Farmer, New Mexico State University.

The evaluation-feedback cycle should be considered a subprocess within a system. This view makes it easier to see the interdependence of the system's components and to understand why supervisors should learn about and use them as a unit.

All five domains of Communication Disorders supervision employ assessment in some form. The Professional domain requires supervisors to assess the attributes of potential candidates for offices of ASHA, CUSPSPA, and state, regional, or local organizations. In addition, active members of groups must evaluate conferences, continuing education programs, and written documents such as the constitution and by-laws of the organization.

In the Research domain, supervisors maintain high assessment standards for personal and colleague research and creative activity and strive for works with strong validity and reliability.

The Educational domain uses the evaluation-feedback cycle continually at two levels: academic and clinical. Supervisors who teach academic classes constantly evaluate academic performance and provide feedback to the students; supervisors also spend much of their clinical education time evaluating the clinical competence of supervisees and giving them feedback. At the preservice level, the development of skills will take top priority and the development of dispositions will be secondary. At the service level, supervisors mainly assess dispositions: are the personnel applying what they learned at the preservice level?

The Administrative domain often carries the onus of conducting evaluation and feedback for hiring, promotion, tenure, salary increments, and merit pay, as well as for the less frequent necessities of personnel or program termination.

The Clinical domain has always included evaluation of client/patient progress, and has recently come to include assigning grades to students enrolled in communication therapy classes in secondary or postsecondary educational settings. Feedback is an integral part of both situations.

Even with heavy use of the evaluation-feedback cycle in all aspects of the supervisor's job, minimal attention has been paid to defining productive assessment. But the study of educational evaluation and feedback procedures in general and in Communication Disorders specifically has identified a number of variables that can affect the process. These factors include (a) the purpose of the assessment; (b) whether the supervisor is trained in observing, evaluating (testing/measuring, grading), or providing feedback; (c) whether the supervisor is trained in developing criterion-referenced goals and objectives, Professional Development Plans, or job descriptions; (d) biases, including the supervisor's preferences about the teaching-learning process as well as more general factors such as grade point average, supervisor-supervisee familiarity, and preconceived notions of what competence is; and (e) the *who, what, when, where,* and *how* of the assessment process. Each of these factors will be discussed below.

THE ASSESSMENT SYSTEM

Preparation

Productive participation in assessment requires education and training in communication (chapter 5), observation (chapter 6), decision making (chapter 7), problem managing (chapter 8), clinical literacy (chapter 9), and technology (chapter 10). It also requires work in planning, establishing policies and procedures, establishing competencies, setting goals and objectives, writing a Professional Development Plan and job descriptions, and evaluating (testing/measuring and grading).

Observation Competence. Observation forms a major part of the evaluation and grading system. After the purpose of evaluation has been established, various modes of observation and data recording will need to be implemented to achieve the purpose. Therefore, supervisors must have the skills and dispositions of gathering data in place. It is assumed that most supervisors do not have the innate ability to be critical observers in all modes nor accurate data recorders and therefore will benefit from training to hone these abilities.

Communication Competence. Recording and interpreting data from observations are two important functions in the evaluation-grading-feedback process. Both depend on using a symbol system, language, to develop a message to impart to the person who has been observed. The feedback process is based entirely on communication. Therefore, the success of the feedback hinges on the communication competence of the personnel involved.

Decision Making. Decisions are made continuously during all phases of assessment. Some decisions will be immediate, others will be made over a span of time; some decisions will be simple and clear-cut, others will be more complex and will require some problem managing.

Problem Managing. The assessment process often leads to problems and conflicts; both conditions require vertical and lateral thinking strategies (to manage problems either logically or creatively), as dictated by the conditions of the situation. A competent supervisor needs to (a) know when to use vertical strategies and when to use lateral ones, and (b) have a workable repertoire of strategies of both kinds for productive management of problems and conflicts.

Clinical Literacy. Clinical reading and writing are dimensions of communication competence that need to be emphasized in assessment training. Supervisors conducting assessments must often read (e.g., lesson plans and reports) and write (e.g., to critique the lesson plans or reports or mark an observation recording form). The reliability of the data they gather depends upon the accuracy of their manipulation of the symbols: clinical literacy.

Technology. Supervision is beginning to explore the possibilities of using electronic technology in the assessment process. Microcomputer-based clinical assessment, spreadsheets, data bases, and the multitude of other software discussed in chapter 10 are important advances. Videotape and videodisc recorders and acoustic analysis equipment require technological competence for the supervisor.

Planning

All worksites, including college and university clinical and supervision training programs, should have policies and procedures for assessment. These assessment procedures should be developed only after well-developed job descriptions, Professional Development Plans, and goals and objectives are in place (Kamara, 1987). Policies and procedures are guidelines that all personnel can use to assure that they are developing high-quality competencies and using them in the delivery of services. Since programs must be assessed too, supervisors should develop guidelines for evaluating and providing feedback about them as separate from personnel.

Policies and Procedures. It is important for each Communication Disorders program to have policies and procedures that define its specific assessment process. Suggested policy and procedure propositions are presented in Table 11–1.

The next step in the planning phase of assessment is to identify the purpose(s) for engaging in the process.

Purpose. In general, assessment is used by someone (supervisor, supervisee, or other) to evaluate a person's competence (skills and dispositions) in some professional area (clinical or interpersonal) or to examine a program, for some outcome (a grade, a pay raise, a promotion, continuing or discontinuing a program, and

TABLE 11-1
Policies and procedures propositions

Communication Disorders programs have a responsibility:
1. To evaluate (grade), and provide feedback to all preservice and service personnel about their professional performance.
2. To develop statements of consequence that protect an individual's right to due process.
3. To prepare and maintain practitioners who are careful not to hurt patients/clients.
4. To preserve educational and professional integrity.
5. To uphold each person's right to fair and impartial treatment.
6. To uphold each person's reputation.
7. For the services provided by all personnel within the worksite.
8. To acknowledge each person's feelings of failure and rejection.
9. To acknowledge each person's perceptions of time lost in a nonproductive work/learning endeavor.
10. To acknowledge negative feelings, toward the program or individuals, associated with nonproductive work/learning endeavors.
11. To acknowledge any feelings of failure supervisors have as a result of supervising individuals involved in nonproductive work/learning endeavors.
12. To evaluate and provide feedback about programs, as well as personnel.

Guidelines for meeting those responsibilities:
1. Develop clearly stated job descriptions or work expectations.
2. Develop clearly documented and comprehensive procedures for evaluating (grading) and providing feedback.
3. Plan for periodic review of the procedures for appropriateness and uniformity of application.
4. Employ objectivity.
5. Base decisions primarily on documented observed occurrences or behaviors.
6. Be prepared for and be skillful in handling emotional reactions to clinical and interpersonal problems and conflicts.
7. Answer all personnel questions in a direct manner.
8. Develop realistic consequences for the evaluation-grading-feedback process; focus on what can be done next.
9. Help personnel who are asked to leave because of negative evaluation to leave with positive feelings and attitudes about the program and the profession.
10. Recognize that establishing and maintaining high levels of competence through an active, productive assessment process will have a positive effect on personnel and programs by demonstrating the integrity of the program and the high standards of the profession.

so forth). However, a specific purpose for assessment must always be defined because the purpose clarifies who will be involved in the process and how, when, and where it will be done. At least 13 specific purposes exist for assessment:

1. To facilitate a supervisee's or supervisor's self-confrontation.
2. To help a supervisee or supervisor learn self-evaluation.
3. To help a supervisee or supervisor learn to supply and receive constructive criticism.

4. To help a supervisee or supervisor learn to establish appropriate goals and objectives for self and client.
5. To help a supervisee or supervisor to develop criterion-referenced competencies.
6. To help a supervisee or supervisor to relate a grade objectively to a level of competence.
7. To convey or receive information that will culminate in a grade, a job, a raise, or a change of status.
8. To document success or progress, or lack thereof.
9. To develop or change the supervisee-supervisor relationship.
10. To nurture a supervisee's clinical development.
11. To nurture a supervisor's supervision development.
12. To nurture a supervisee and supervisor's interpersonal skills development.
13. To restructure, strengthen, or eliminate a clinical program.

Each of these 13 purposes requires a somewhat different approach. For example, Purpose 1 dictates that videotape recording be used, whereas Purposes 6 and 8 may not.

Each purpose must be guided by a set of competencies or standards and then written into a goal or objective(s), a Professional Development Plan (PDP), or a job description that states clearly who does what to whom, how is it done and for how long, how you will measure success, and the consequences of the outcome. Once the appropriate goals/objectives, PDP, or job description have been developed, evaluation, grading, and feedback should be done using a type (STYLE + form) of supervision congruent with the one that has been used during conferences based on the supervisee's readiness state (refer to Table 3-3, p. 72-73, for information on supervision types and readiness states in differential supervision). Even with this supervision type guideline, it is no simple feat to become competent in evaluation and feedback; extensive training is required.

Establishing Competencies. Statements defining professional competence are used as yardsticks to measure clinical and interpersonal proficiency. Competencies can be stated for clinicians and for supervisors. The statements for clinicians may be standardized, like the *Wisconsin Procedure for Assessing Clinical Competence (W-PACC)* (Shriberg, Filley, Hayes, Kwiatkowski, Schatz, Simmons, & Smith, 1975), or may be criterion-based statements developed by educational and professional institutions. Competence for clinicians is measured at three levels: (a) academic knowledge, (b) clinical skills and dispositions, and (c) interpersonal skills and dispositions. There are eight types of clinician competence, based on combinations of the professional knowledge, clinical, and interpersonal variables. The types of clinician competence are shown in part A of Table 11-2.

Totally competent clinicians are classified as "Ideal." Those who have the necessary professional knowledge and clinical competence but do not have the interpersonal skills and dispositions are referred to as "Cold" clinicians. "Warm" clinicians are professionally knowledgeable and interpersonally competent but not clinically competent. The knowledgeable but unskilled "Scientific" clinicians know the theories and concepts, but they do not use them well or in appropriate contexts. Clinicians without the professional knowledge but who have some clinical and/or interpersonal skills and dispositions are referred to as "Natural," "Nice but ineffective," or "Technical" clinicians, depending on their area(s) of competence. The "Incompetent" speech-language pathologist or audiologist has neither adequate professional knowledge nor adequate clinical or interpersonal skills and dispositions.

Supervisor competency statements have been developed by the ASHA Committee on Supervision (ASHA, 1985) and appear in appendix A. Supervisor competence profiles similar to the clinicians' are shown in part B of Table 11-2. The difference between clinical competence and supervision competence is that interpersonal com-

TABLE 11-2
Types of competence

Part A: Clinician Competence

Type	Knowledge	Clinical[1] Competence	Interpersonal[2] Competence
"Ideal" clinician	+	+	+
"Cold" clinician	+	+	−
"Warm" clinician	+	−	+
"Scientific" clinician	+	−	−
"Natural" clinician	−	+	+
"Nice but ineffective" clinician	−	−	+
"Technical" clinician	−	+	−
"Incompetent" clinician	−	−	−

Part B: Supervisor Competence

Type	Knowledge	Supervision Competence[3]
"Ideal" supervisor	+	+
"Scientific" supervisor	+	−
"Natural" supervisor	−	+
"Incompetent" supervisor	−	−

+ = Competent
− = Not competent

[1] Clinical competence = skills and dispositions of diagnosing and treating problems of speech, language, and hearing.
[2] Interpersonal competence = skills and dispositions of interpersonal communication.
[3] Supervision competence = skills and dispositions of communication, observation, decision making, problem managing, clinical literacy, technology, and assessment.

munication is an integral part of supervisors' skills and dispositions. This allows for four, rather than eight, types of supervisor competence.

Initial planning for what to include in goals and objectives is the first step of the process of evaluation and grading. It may be accomplished by following the three-part sequence presented in Table 11-3.

Part 1 of the sequence involves identifying the present levels of professional competencies for all personnel. College and university training programs will have clinical competencies for speech-language pathology and audiology trainees, and supervisor competencies for supervisor trainees. For the sake of brevity, the process will be described only for use with clinical supervisees. Supervisor trainees, however, would go through the same process.

It is possible to use the 13 tasks and 81 competencies for supervisors (see appendix A) as goals and objectives for clinicians. Minor rewording makes a compatible set of competencies for both supervisors and supervisees. Each institution can also develop its own competencies or use existing ones such as the W-PACC.

The categories in Part 1 of Table 11-3 include competence levels from novice (column A) to expert (column D). Each competency item is to be marked in the appropriate column. For Part 2, a maximum of 12 items (a minimum of 3) from columns A, B, and C in Part 1 are selected. Depending on the type of supervision being used (type = STYLE + form), the supervisor and supervisee may work together at this stage or the supervisor may assume responsibility for Part 2. (Refer to Table 3-3 for a description of types of supervision.) For example, if supervision type 1, 2, 3, or 4 is used, then the supervisor will rank in importance each of the items selected from Part 1 and place them in column

E; if supervision type 5, 6, 7, or 8 is used, then the supervisor ranks the items in column E, the supervisee ranks them in column F, and then the supervisor and supervisee negotiate a mutual list for column G. These items are the competencies from which the goals and objectives are developed. After the goals (a maximum of 12, a minimum of 3) have been developed and implemented, Part 3 is used to evaluate the status of each competency. If supervision type 1, 2, 3, or 4 is used, then the supervisor evaluates the targeted competencies using some value system (e.g., numerical, alphabetical). If supervision type 5, 6, 7, or 8 is used, then the supervisor evaluates the competencies and places the value in column H, the supervisee also evaluates and places the values in column I. The supervisor and supervisee then negotiate mutual values for column J. Based on the values, recommendations are made in column K.

Another way to target competencies to be developed is to use the self-assessment inventories discussed in chapters 2 and 5.

Goals and Objectives. Goals and objectives can be used at all levels of the profession, from preservice to service. If goals and objectives are developed adequately, they provide a natural map for what to observe in order to evaluate. The key word is *adequately;* goals and objectives are sometimes developed based on categorical percentages from an interaction analysis with no regard for context. For supervisors to state, for example, that they will decrease their use of questions during conferences is not a totally appropriate goal; some conferences, to be pro-

TABLE 11-3
Sequence of identifying target competencies for professional development

PART 1 (Identifying levels of competence)

A	B	C	D
I am not familiar with the item	I have heard of the item but I don't understand it completely	I know about the item but am not competent at application	I understand the item and can apply it in clinical situations appropriately

Items[1]

TABLE 11-3
continued

PART 2 (Ranking and targeting specific competencies)

	E Supervisor's ranking of importance	F Supervisee's ranking of importance	G Mutually negotiated ranking of the number to be targeted for development during evaluation period
Items[2]			
	_____	_____	_____
	_____	_____	_____
	_____	_____	_____
	_____	_____	_____
	_____	_____	_____
	_____	_____	_____

PART 3 (Evaluating the target competencies)

	H Supervisor's evaluation of competence development	I Supervisee's evaluation of competence development	J Mutual agreement	K Recommendations
Items[3]				
	_____	_____	_____	_____
	_____	_____	_____	_____
	_____	_____	_____	_____
	_____	_____	_____	_____
	_____	_____	_____	_____
	_____	_____	_____	_____

[1] Twelve items to be developed by each organization. Personnel rate own competence for each item by placing an X in the appropriate column across from each item.
[2] Select 6 items from columns A, B, C in Part 1. Supervisor ranks importance; supervisee ranks importance. Negotiate the number of items to be targeted for development.
[3] List the items from column G (for supervision types 5, 6, 7, 8) or E (for supervision types 1, 2, 3, 4).

ductive, require numerous questions. A more beneficial goal would include a statement about contextual appropriateness. Omitting context may be a reason why supervisors do not make significant behavior changes that have been targeted from interaction analysis systems. Context is crucial to goals and objectives in any aspect of Communication Disorders. Goals and objectives depend on the written language used to define time, direction, criteria, and measures of success. Although most speech-language pathologists and audiologists develop the skill to follow the formula for writing goals and objectives, they do not all develop the disposition to employ that skill in supervision. The result is that inadequate evaluations are done because it is unclear what is expected of the supervisee.

The supervisor should develop personal goals

and objectives in all domains: Professional, Research, Educational, Administrative, and Clinical. Developing goals and objectives is part of supervision competence and should be addressed in a Communication Disorders supervision training program. (See chapters 5 and 9 for additional discussions of goals and objectives.)

Matrix Management. When goals and objectives are written, it is generally not productive simply to write down intentions to increase or decrease specific behaviors; the goals and objectives should be relevant to the diversity of situations that confront Communication Disorders personnel from day to day. Chapter 3 described four STYLES of supervision predicated on strand continua that can be transformed into a matrix configuration. Goals and behavioral objectives can be conceived in the same way. Suppose a supervisor sets a goal to improve communication during conferences. An objective of increasing the use of supervisee ideas during conferences is insufficient, because at times a supervisee is either unable or unwilling to share ideas and a conference develops from the supervisor's agenda to meet the needs of a client, supervisee, supervisor, or program. Competence in conference communication hinges on the ability to use the most productive type of communication for each situation. Therefore, goals and objectives should be so stated as to reflect that flexibility; evaluation and feedback should then be congruent with the goals and objectives.

The top portion of Figure 11-1 shows the continuum for improving productive communication, ranging from high use of supervisor ideas (SI) to high use of supervisee ideas (si), and how that continuum is transformed into a two-by-two matrix.

This configuration allows for four kinds of communication. The upper left quadrant reflects high use of supervisor ideas and low use of supervisee ideas (HSI/Lsi); the lower left quadrant reflects low use of both supervisor and supervisee ideas (LSI/Lsi); the lower right quadrant reflects low use of supervisor ideas and high use of supervisee ideas (LSI/Hsi); and the upper right quadrant reflects high use of both supervisor and supervisee ideas (HSI/Hsi). The bottom portion of Figure 11-1 shows how the supervisor can best meet the needs of supervisees in fulfilling the objective by using the most appropriate type of supervision for each supervisee's readiness state; the quadrants of the two figures correlate. If Supervisee A is at Readiness State 1 (unable and unwilling or insecure), the most productive use of ideas will result from Type 1 (STYLE I/dyad) or Type 2 (STYLE I/group) supervision. This means that many of the supervisor's ideas and few of Supervisee A's ideas will be used. On the other hand, if Supervisee B is at Readiness State 3 (able but unwilling or insecure), the most productive use of ideas will emerge from Type 5 or Type 6 supervision, in which many of Supervisee B's ideas are used and fewer supervisor ideas will be necessary.

A second rule for professional growth is to develop competencies in pairs, so that each competency is related to something else and is not an isolate. A matrix can be developed for any combination of two competencies to provide some idea of what a person does well and what needs to be developed. Coordinating two competencies helps supervisors develop dispositions, because of the difficulty of using competencies developed out of context or without relation to each other. An example of paired objectives within a matrix is shown in Figure 11-2.

In this example, a supervisor sets the objectives of using supervisee ideas and asking questions in ways that are congruent with the context of conferences (pairing the type of supervision with the supervisee's Readiness State). It is not productive to attempt never to ask questions or always to use a clinician's ideas. The two strategies should be used in the total supervision context, differently for each supervisee. Quadrant 1 (Q1) represents frequent questioning and low use of supervisee ideas, a combination appropriate for supervision types

FIGURE 11-1
Matrix Management

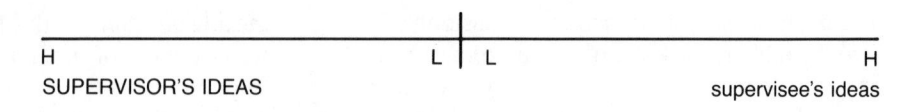

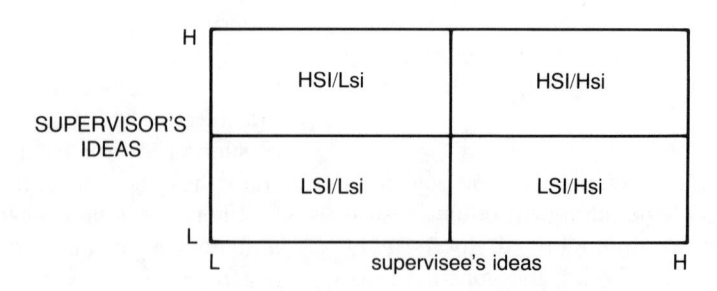

```
              H              L | L              H
        SUPERVISOR'S IDEAS       supervisee's ideas
```

SUPERVISOR'S IDEAS H	HSI/Lsi	HSI/Hsi
L	LSI/Lsi	LSI/Hsi
	L supervisee's ideas H	

HSI = Frequent use of supervisor's ideas
LSI = Infrequent use of supervisor's ideas
Hsi = Frequent use of supervisee's ideas
Lsi = Infrequent use of supervisee's ideas

STYLE I	STYLE IV
Type 1 (Dyad)	Type 8 (Group)
Type 2 (Group)	Type 7 (Dyad)
RS1 and RS2	RS4
STYLE II	**STYLE III**
Type 3 (Dyad)	Type 6 (Group)
Type 4 (Group)	Type 5 (Dyad)
RS2	RS3

RS = Readiness State
RS1 = Unable and unwilling or insecure
RS2 = Unable but willing or confident
RS3 = Able but unwilling or insecure
RS4 = Able and willing or confident

1 (STYLE I/dyad) and 2 (STYLE I/group) and for RS1 (unable and unwilling or insecure) and RS2 (unable but willing or secure). Quadrant 2 (Q2) allows for low questioning and low use of supervisee ideas, a pattern congruent with supervision types 3 (STYLE II/dyad) and 4 (STYLE II/group) and with RS2. Quadrant 3 (Q3) shows high use of supervisee ideas and low use of questions, appropriate for supervision types 5 (STYLE III/dyad) and 6 (STYLE III/group) and for RS3 (able but unwilling or insecure). Quadrant 4 (Q4) represents high use of questions and high use of supervisee ideas, a pattern consistent with supervision types

7 (STYLE IV/dyad) and 8 (STYLE IV/group) and with RS4 (able and willing).

The point here is that goals and objectives should not be developed in a vacuum. They must be related to companion areas of professional competence. In this example, a supervisor could tally, in the appropriate quadrants, the data from a supervision conference. If the resulting picture shows the appropriate type of supervision for the supervisee's Readiness State, then the goal has been accomplished and the supervisor should evaluate his or her work accordingly. For instance, if a supervisor has decided to use type

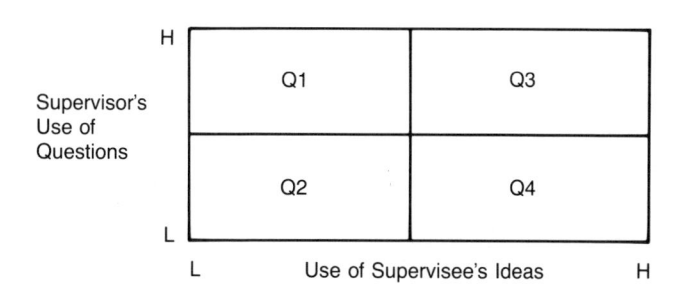

FIGURE 11-2
Pairing supervisor goals and objectives through Matrix Management

```
                H  ┌─────────────┬─────────────┐
                   │             │             │
                   │     Q1      │     Q3      │
Supervisor's       │             │             │
Use of             ├─────────────┼─────────────┤
Questions          │             │             │
                   │     Q2      │     Q4      │
                   │             │             │
                L  └─────────────┴─────────────┘
                   L    Use of Supervisee's Ideas    H
```

Q1 = Supervisor asks questions frequently, uses supervisee's ideas infrequently
Q2 = Supervisor asks questions infrequently, uses supervisee's ideas infrequently
Q3 = Supervisor asks questions infrequently, uses supervisee's ideas frequently
Q4 = Supervisor asks questions frequently, uses supervisee's ideas frequently

1 supervision (STYLE I/dyad) and the supervisee manifests a RS1 (unable and unwilling or insecure), then it will be congruent for the supervisor to ask many questions and use few of the supervisee's ideas. On the other hand, if type 5 (STYLE III/dyad) is being used with a supervisee whose readiness state is 3 (able but unwilling or insecure), it will be congruent for the supervisor to use many of the supervisee's ideas and to ask few questions. Again, if goals and objectives are to help supervisors change behavior on which their evaluation is based, the goals and objectives must reflect the context.

A third kind of Matrix Management can be used with individual supervisors and supervisees or with organizations. A graticule (Bess, 1987) is a way of prioritizing goals and objectives (see Figure 11-3).

The system, modified for Communication Disorders supervision, includes these steps:

1. Identify all personal or organizational objectives.
2. Rate the importance of each objective from 0 (least important) to 9 (most important).
3. Estimate the individual's present performance level for each objective using a 0-9 point scale (0 = no skill and no disposition; 9 = good skill, poor disposition).
4. Analyze the matrix and prioritize objectives.
5. Implement the plan to accomplish goals and objectives.

a. Assess objectives periodically.
b. Identify problems.
c. Analyze problems.
d. Manage problems; develop possible outcomes.
e. Implement new outcomes.
f. The audit cycle continues.

Using the graticule presented in Figure 11-3, plot in the upper left quadrant objectives that are valued highly but not performed well or used consistently. Plot in the lower left quadrant those that are less valuable, not well developed, and not used often. Plot in the lower right quadrant objectives of low relative value for which the individual has the skill but not the disposition. Plot in the upper right quadrant objectives that are

```
High  9 ┌─┬─┬─┬─┬─┬─┬─┬─┬─┐
      8 ├─┼─┼─┼─┼─┼─┼─┼─┼─┤
      7 ├─┼─┼─┼─┼─┼─┼─┼─┼─┤
V     6 ├─┼─┼─┼─┼─┼─┼─┼─┼─┤
A     5 ├─┼─┼─┼─┼─┼─┼─┼─┼─┤
L     4 ├─┼─┼─┼─┼─┼─┼─┼─┼─┤
U     3 ├─┼─┼─┼─┼─┼─┼─┼─┼─┤
E     2 ├─┼─┼─┼─┼─┼─┼─┼─┼─┤
      1 ├─┼─┼─┼─┼─┼─┼─┼─┼─┤
Low   0 └─┴─┴─┴─┴─┴─┴─┴─┴─┘
        0 1 2 3 4 5 6 7 8 9
        Poor    PERFORMANCE    Good
```

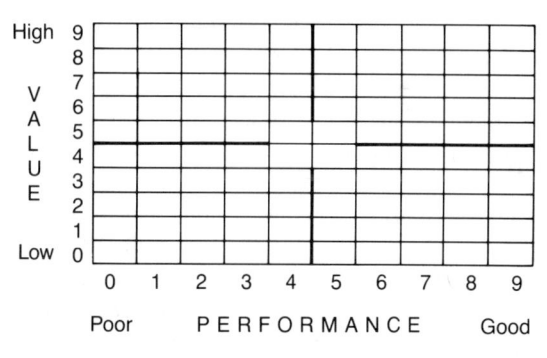

FIGURE 11-3
Goals and objectives priority graticule

considered very important and for which the individual has the skill but not the disposition.

Prioritizing goals and objectives, then, becomes a matter of deciding whether the person (e.g., a beginning employee or student) needs to develop skill for valuable objectives (the upper left quadrant) or whether the person (e.g., an advanced graduate student or experienced employee) needs to polish and integrate those objectives that separate the most competent professionals from the less competent ones. This view of goals and objectives emphasizes that acquisition of professional competence is a lifelong process and that no matter how good an individual is at a job, or how good a service delivery agency is, opportunities exist for improvement based on new knowledge and the transactional nature of the Communication Disorders profession.

The graticule shown in Figure 11-3 coordinates with the types of supervision and with supervisee Readiness States. For example, if a student or employee has a preponderance of objectives in the upper left quadrant and is operating at either RS1 or RS2, then supervision types 1 or 2 will be appropriate. If, on the other hand, a student or employee shows many objectives in the upper right quadrant and is at RS4, then supervision types 7 and 8 are appropriate. Once again, goals and objectives should be developed and used in context and coordinated with each other.

Professional Development Plans. A Professional Development Plan (PDP) is a set of goals and objectives negotiated between an employee and an administrator. The plan may be based on the employee's existing job description or used to develop or modify the job description.

Job Descriptions. Job descriptions have a similar purpose to goals and objectives and PDPs: to define what is expected of personnel. Goals and objectives and PDPs are often precursors to upgrading or promotion. Job descriptions should be flexible, rewritten as the nature of jobs changes or as the persons filling the positions add new competencies to their professional profiles. Job descriptions can be negotiated regularly as specific goals and objectives are accomplished. As with goals and objectives and PDPs, if job descriptions are not comprehensive and clearly stated, appropriate and accurate evaluation and grading of personnel is impossible. Many Communication Disorders supervisors benefit from instruction, through a clinical literacy module, in how to write good job descriptions. (Guidelines for developing job descriptions are presented in chapter 2).

Consequences. The policies and procedures component of the assessment system must clearly state what will happen if goals and objectives or professional competencies are not attained or if Professional Development Plans or job descriptions are not fulfilled. Three requirements for the use of consequences are important: (a) both positive and negative consequences should be stated clearly in advance, (b) personnel should be told about consequences of their work through some type of formal communication system, and (c) stated consequences should be upheld. These conditions can be met through an assessment process.

The Evaluation-Feedback Process

A central part of the assessment system is the evaluation-feedback process. Although the two components should be considered as a unit rather than as separate entities, they are discussed separately.

Evaluation. Two types of evaluation are used in supervision: formal and naturalistic. *Formal* evaluation is a combination of testing (or measuring) and grading. Testing and measuring are done in Communication Disorders mainly at the preservice level; all preparation programs in some way test academic knowledge and measure clinical and interpersonal skills and dispositions. At the Clinical Fellow and service levels, the National Examination in Speech-Language Pathology and Audiology (NESPA) is required for personnel who want to attain the Certificate of Clinical Competence. Evaluation requires the ability to observe a situation and to judge it based on established testing criteria, goals and objectives, or a job description so as to record the presence or absence, frequency, and quality of the targeted skills and dispositions. High levels of intra- and interobserver reliability are an essential part of evaluation competence. After a situation is observed or a person tested or measured in some way, the results must be recorded in writing or on audiotape for documentation and for providing feedback to the person who was observed, tested, and perhaps graded.

Grading means quantifying or classifying documented observation data by assigning a number, a letter, or an indication of satisfactory or unsatisfactory performance according to established criteria. Grades, then, are evaluative symbols related to criteria for specific knowledge or behavior. Learning to classify behavior by *degree* of success relative to criteria can be difficult without the guided experiences provided in supervision training programs; the priority graticule can help in this part of the process.

Matrix Management can also be used in grading, starting from inventories of clinical competencies. For example, the competencies on the selected inventory can be rated on a point system based on the amount of supervision required over time to attain each one. The supervisee's ultimate goal is to attain ratings equivalent to "minimum supervision required to perform the task competently" for a majority of the tasks.

The system is based on two premises: (a) each supervisee competency develops with some amount of supervisor assistance (total supervision, maximum supervision, moderate supervision, minimum supervision); (b) different supervisee competencies will require differing amounts of help from a supervisor. Figure 11-4 presents three ways that Matrix Management can be used in evaluation.

As an example, if supervisors work with five clinical competencies (lettered V, W, X, Y, and Z) in Section A, *each competency* is ranked for the amount of supervision required to assist the supervisee in attaining it. The letters of competencies rated 1 are entered into the upper left quadrant, those rated 2 into the lower left quadrant, and so forth. The result is an overall picture of the amount (total in Q1, maximum in Q2, moderate in Q3, or minimum in Q4) of supervision that was provided to an individual supervisee during an evaluation period. Competencies that were not attained (rated *0*), those that were not applicable (rated N), or those for which the supervisor did not have enough information to rate (rated I) will be minimal but can be accounted for. Overall proficiency is measured in an average (mean score) of all item ratings. Alphabetic grades (A, B, C) can be assigned differentially by clinician Readiness States through some system developed by individual institutions to meet their needs. After each competency has been rated and tallied, the information can be analyzed and discussed by the supervisor and the supervisee.

The second way to use the matrix (Figure 11-4), Section B) is for supervisors to monitor their ratings of competencies for all their supervisees. For example, if five supervisees were evaluated and competency Y was rated 1 for one of the supervisees, 2 for one of the supervisees, 3 for one of the supervisees, and 4 for the remaining two supervisees, then the letter Y would be entered once into quadrants 1, 2, and 3, and twice into quadrant 4. This type of analysis shows the supervisor which competencies are being attained through minimum (Q4), moderate (Q3), maximum (Q2), or total (Q1) supervision, as well as which items are not being developed successfully (those with *0* ratings), which items are not being attended to (N), and which items require more information (I). This helps supervisors identify specific competencies that clinicians need more (or less) help attain-

FIGURE 11-4
Matrix Management for evaluation

SECTION A: Item Analysis for Individual Supervisees

Q1 Rating 1 (Write the letter of each competency rated 1)	Rating 4 Q4
Q2 Rating 2	Rating 3 Q3

0 = _____   N = _____   I = _____

Mean rating _____ (Multiply the number of items in each quadrant by the rating value of the quadrant; divide by the total number of competency items.)

RATINGS:

1 = Total supervision
2 = Maximum supervision
3 = Moderate supervision
4 = Minimum supervision
0 = Failed to attain
N = Not applicable
I = Insufficient information

SECTION B: Analysis of Competencies per Rating for All Supervisees

Q1 Rating 1	Q4 Rating 4
Q2 Rating 2	Q3 Rating 3

Percents of Ratings

Competency   1   2   3   4   0   N   I
V
W
X
Y
Z

# of supervisees: _____
# of items marked: _____
% of 1 ratings: _____
% of 2 ratings: _____
% of 3 ratings: _____
% of 4 ratings: _____
% of 0 ratings: _____
% of N ratings: _____
% of I ratings: _____

SECTION C: Longitudinal Monitoring of Ratings and Competencies

Q1 Rating 1	Q4 Rating 4
Q2 Rating 2	Q3 Rating 3

Ratings   Competencies
Period 1   A   B   C   D   E
0 (Red)   %
1   %
2   %
3   %
4   %
N   %
I   %

Period 2
0 (Blue) %
1   %
2   %
3   %
4   %
N   %
I   %

ing, which in turn helps the supervisor develop better ways of facilitating supervisees' acquisition of the difficult competencies. Section B analysis also presents a pattern of supervisor time expenditure (e.g., a majority of competencies rated 1 requires more supervision time than a majority of competencies rated 4).

The third way a supervisor can use the evaluation matrix is to monitor personal evaluation patterns over time. Section C of Table 11-4 allows for a comparison of competencies and their ratings for two evaluation periods. The competency letters are entered into the matrix as they are for Sections A and B, but they are color coded by evaluation period (e.g., red for Period 1, blue for Period 2). Analysis will help identify idiosyncratic supervision patterns, which may reflect overall supervision biases, or biases related to supervisee Readiness States or supervision STYLES.

Supervisees can use the same procedures. The tally procedure shows the amount (minimum, moderate, maximum, total) of supervision that the supervisee required during an evaluation period to attain a certain level of overall competence. The item count for 0 ratings shows which competencies need to be targeted for future development. The supervisee can track specific items longitudinally by monitoring the progression of the item number through the four quadrants. The ultimate goal for supervisees is to have a majority of the competencies tallied or enumerated in quadrant 4.

Supervisors can always classify supervisees into the four quadrants in terms of their Readiness States, which in turn should direct what types of supervision are used. If Supervisee A, at the end of a graduate program in audiology, is at Readiness State 4 (able and willing), then supervision types 7 (STYLE IV/dyad) or 8 (STYLE IV/group) are most appropriate for the supervisor to use. However, during Supervisee A's first professional position in a rehabilitation center as a staff audiologist, the new constituents, concepts, and context will require new competencies. Therefore, A's readiness state may be 2 (unable but willing), which requires a different type of supervision. Matrix Management allows the supervisor to identify the readiness state, match an appropriate type of supervision, set goals and objectives, and monitor the supervisee's and supervisor's activities throughout supervision.

Naturalistic evaluation, as described by Sergiovanni and Starratt (1979), has a different purpose. Rather than to determine or judge—the purpose of standardized evaluation procedures—naturalistic evaluation is used to discover or understand. Sometimes supervisors become too serious about the scientific and objective documentation of events, too serious about predetermined objectives or specified blueprints of personnel effort. The evaluation-feedback cycle should strike a balance between discovering/understanding and judging. Supervisors use three types of naturalistic evaluation: connoisseurship, artifacts analysis, and portfolio development.

Connoisseurship is the qualitative ability of a supervisor to appreciate, infer, describe, and disclose things about supervision constituents, concepts, and contexts. Connoisseurship is the scientific and artistic expertise some supervisors use to understand a situation and know how to manage it productively. Connoisseurship has as its foundation the knowledge and competencies discussed in parts I, II, and III of this textbook.

Artifacts analysis is the random, unplanned examination of materials, records, photographs, audio- and videocassettes, and other artifacts used by personnel in their personal and professional endeavors. Its purpose is to show how they approach their jobs and to help a supervisor understand their needs as personnel.

Portfolio development is similar to artifacts analysis but is planned. The person being evaluated assembles a collection of materials, records, reports, publications, cassettes, and other artifacts, intended to present an overview of his or her achievements.

Feedback. Like the evaluation components of assessment, feedback should be guided by a purpose or intended outcome. The purpose will help determine the most appropriate channel, method, type, timing, location, personnel, and follow-up procedures to use. Feedback should follow the unilateral-bilateral communication patterns associated with the four STYLES of supervision: STYLE I = high unilateral/low bilateral; STYLE II = low unilateral/low bilateral; STYLE III = low unilateral/high bilateral; STYLE IV = high unilateral/high bilateral.

The *who, what, when, where,* and *how* variables of evaluation and feedback have different degrees of importance in the five roles of Communication Disorders supervision. It is a scientific/artistic challenge for supervisors to select the components that will combine to produce the most productive assessment system. Productive evaluation and feedback depend on these five variables. Supervisors need competence to combine all dimensions of the Communication Disorders supervision assessment process successfully. The interaction of each element with another increases the power of the process exponentially.

TABLE 11-4
Patterns of evaluation

Supervisor Role	Supervisee Role
A. Staff (clinical) supervisor	1. Staff (clinical) supervisor
B. Supervisor trainee	2. Supervisor trainee
C. Student supervisee (preservice)	3. Student supervisee (preservice)
D. Staff clinician	4. Staff clinician
E. Other	5. Other

Level	Pattern	Example
I (Supervisor-Supervisee Evaluation)	A-3	A supervisor in a university affiliated speech-language-hearing training program evaluates students.
	A-4	A supervisor in a worksite (e.g., school, hospital) evaluates a staff member.
	A-1	An employer/administrator evaluates the staff supervisor in a worksite.
	B/A-3	A supervisor trainee coevaluates a student clinician with a staff supervisor.
	A-2	A supervisor instructor in a supervisor training program evaluates a supervisor trainee.
II (Self-Evaluation)	1.	A staff supervisor self-evaluates.
	2.	A supervisor trainee self-evaluates.
	3.	A student supervisee self-evaluates.
	4.	A staff clinician self-evaluates.
	5.	Other personnel (e.g., family member, aide) self-evaluate.
III (Peer Evaluation)	A-1	Staff supervisors conduct peer evaluations.
	B-2	Supervisor trainees conduct peer evaluations.
	C-3	Student supervisees conduct peer evaluations.
	D-4	Staff clinicians conduct peer evaluations.
IV (Generic Supervision Evaluation)	A-5	A Communication Disorders supervisor, as a generic supervisor, evaluates personnel from other disciplines.
	B/A-5	A Communication Disorders supervisor, with

ASSESSMENT IN SUPERVISION

Who. Evaluation is done in many different patterns based on which of five types of participants are involved—staff supervisor, supervisor-trainee, student supervisee, staff clinician, other (other disciplines, paraprofessionals, aides)—and in which role, supervisor or supervisee. Table 11-4 shows the patterns of evaluation.

The five participant types can be combined into five levels of evaluation patterns based on frequency of use. Level 1 is made up of supervisor-supervisee patterns. They include the staff supervisor (A) evaluating (and perhaps grading) student supervisees (3) or staff clinicians (4). These patterns are represented as A-3 and A-4. The A-3 pattern occurs in college and university speech-language-hearing training programs, both on campus and at field sites. Supervisors evaluate or grade supervisees to help them develop preservice professional competence. The A-4 pattern involves a staff supervisor in a worksite evaluating a staff member. A second kind of Level I pattern is the employer/supervisor (A) evaluating the Communication Disorders supervision staff, who are now super-

TABLE 11-4
continued

Level	Pattern	Example
	E-1	a Communication Disorders supervisor-trainee (as generic cosupervisors), coevaluate personnel from other disciplines.
	E-2	A supervisor from another discipline, as a generic supervisor (e.g., physiatrist, director of special education) evaluates Communication Disorders personnel (and perhaps other personnel).
	E-3	
	E-4	
	E-5	
	A-E-1-5	Wholistic Supervision (all members of a clinical team, including the clients who are capable, evaluate each other).
V (Supervisee-Supervisor Evaluation)	3-A	A student supervisee in a university affiliated speech-language-hearing training program evaluates staff (clinical) supervisors.
	3-B	A student supervisee in a university affiliated speech-language-hearing training program evaluates a supervisor trainee who is cosupervising with a staff supervisor.
	1-A	A staff supervisor evaluates an administrator-supervisor.
	1-B	A staff supervisor evaluates an administrator-supervisor trainee.
	2-A	A supervisor trainee evaluates a supervisor instructor in a supervision training program.
	5-A	Other personnel (e.g., family member, aide) evaluate a staff supervisor.
	5-B	Other personnel evaluate a staff supervisor trainee.

visees (1) for purposes of continued employment, tenure, advancement, pay increases, merit pay, and so forth. This is an A-1 pattern. A major part of this type of evaluation is documenting patterns of supervision: how much time is being devoted to each of the various duties of the supervisor. Laccinole and Schill (1982) stated that good time management is one characteristic of efficient, high-quality supervision and presented a supervision time audit system. A supervision hours summary form, such as the one shown in Table 11-5, can be used to record work time in the five supervision roles.

These data can be compared with goals and objectives, Professional Development Plans, or job descriptions, or used to identify personal patterns of supervision. They can also be used by administrators to justify requests for additional supervision staff.

In one modification of this supervisor-supervisee evaluation pattern, a supervisor trainee (B) cosupervises a student supervisee (3) with a staff supervisor (A). This triangular pattern is represented as B/A-3. The purpose is to provide an evaluation/grading experience for the supervisor trainee.

The last example of a supervisor-supervisee pattern has the supervisor instructor in a Communication Disorders supervision training program (A) evaluating the supervision competence of a supervisor trainee (2) (who then becomes the supervisee). This pattern is represented as A-2. The supervisor-supervisee format requires some personnel to operate in multiple roles, sometimes as supervisors, at other times as supervisees. The multiple role-taking requires these personnel to produce and receive evaluation/grading information equally well, a competency that takes preparation.

In Level II patterns, supervisees evaluate or grade their own competence. The purpose is to facilitate the development of self-supervision in all levels of personnel; participants must define appropriate goals and objectives, work to accomplish them, and then evaluate their success. They then begin the cycle again by evaluating their broad areas of competence.

Self-evaluation leads eventually to self-management, or self-supervision, a process in which learners who are changing their own behavior decide on the direction, extent, or method of change.

Level III patterns represent peer evaluation, which is done on two sublevels. Preservice student supervisees (C) evaluate each other's (3) clinical and interpersonal competence (a C-3 pattern) in order to facilitate the development of objectivity in evaluation/grading, because these supervisees will be the next generation of staff supervisors (A). Another form of peer evaluation is the staff supervisor-staff supervisor (A-1) pattern. It emphasizes supervisors' continued development in all the Communication Disorders supervision roles. In other forms of peer evaluation, supervisor trainees (B-2) and staff clinicians (D-4) evaluate each other.

Level I, II, and III patterns occur in categorical supervision. Level IV patterns typify generic supervision. In these patterns, a staff Communication Disorders supervisor (A) may evaluate some other professional, as in the Multi-, Inter-, or Transdisciplinary team formats, or evaluate paraprofessionals or aides (5). This process is represented as A-5. If a supervisor trainee (B) is involved, the configuration is B/A-5. Another possibility for generic evaluation is to have a supervisor from another discipline (E) evaluate personnel from Speech-Language Pathology and Audiology, as a physiatrist in a medical setting or a director of special education in the schools might do. This pattern of evaluation is represented as E-1, E-2, E-3, E-4, and/or E-5 (if professionals from other disciplines such as occupational and physical therapy are also evaluated). The last Level IV pattern is used in the wholistic model of supervision, discussed in chapter 3. Wholistic Supervision (Farmer, 1986) involves any number of participants (including

TABLE 11-5
Supervision hours summary

Supervisor_____   Data period_____

Week of:
(Enter amount of time devoted to each activity)

Roles/Tasks		Date											T
1.0 Professional													
1.1	Attend Meetings												
1.2	Officer												
1.3	Committee												
1.4	Presentation												
1.5	Other												
2.0 Researcher													
2.1	Develop Project												
2.2	Execute Project												
2.3	Analyze Data												
2.4	Write												
2.5	Disseminate												
2.6	Other												
3.0 Educator													
3.1 (Classroom)													
3.1.1	Prepare Class												
3.1.2	Teach												
3.1.3	Evaluate												
3.1.4	Other												
	Total												
3.0 Educator													
3.2 (Clinical)													
3.2.1	Observe/Monitor												
3.2.1.1	On Site (Direct)												
3.2.1.1.1	Participant												
3.2.1.1.2	Nonparticipant												
3.2.1.2	On Site (Indirect)												
3.2.1.3	Closed Circuit												
3.2.1.4	Videotape												
3.2.1.5	Audiotape												
3.2.1.6	Lesson Plans												
3.2.1.7	Telecommunication												

TABLE 11-5

continued

3.2.2	Conference	
3.2.2.1	Group	
3.2.2.1.1	Academic	
3.2.2.1.2	Procedural	
3.2.2.1.3	Case Staffing	
3.2.2.1.4	Treatment	
3.2.2.1.5	Prediagnostic	
3.2.2.1.6	Postdiagnostic	
3.2.2.1.7	Family/Client	
3.2.2.1.8	Ancillary Personnel	
3.2.2	Conference	
3.2.2.2	Dyad	
3.2.2.2.1	Academic	
3.2.2.2.2	Procedural	
3.2.2.2.3	Personal	
3.2.2.2.4	Treatment	
3.2.2.2.5	Prediagnostic	
3.2.2.2.6	Postdiagnostic	
3.2.2.2.7	Family/Client	
3.2.2.2.8	Ancillary Personnel	
3.2.2.2.9	Other	
4.0 Administrator		
4.1	Paperwork	
4.2	Staff Meetings	
4.3	Personnel	
4.3.1	Interview	
4.3.2	Employment	
4.3.3	Evaluation	
4.3.4	Termination	
4.4	Public Relations	
4.5	Program Development	
4.6	Other	
5.0 Clinician		
5.1	Diagnosis	
5.2	Treatment	
5.3	Counseling	
5.4	Reports	
5.5	Staffings (EA&R)	
5.6	Case Management	
5.7	Other	
	TOTALS	

clients, parents, and teachers) in the supervision (including evaluation) process. The wholistic pattern is represented as A . . . E–1 . . . 5.

Level V patterns are those in which supervisees evaluate supervisors. Student supervisees (3) should evaluate staff supervisors (A) and supervisor trainees (B) when cosupervision occurs. Staff supervisors (1) should evaluate administrator-supervisors (A) and administrator-supervisor trainees (B) when they are used. Supervisor trainees (2) should evaluate their supervisor instructors (A). Other personnel (5) should evaluate the supervisors with whom they interact (e.g., A or B).

A number of constituents may be included in feedback: the person who has been evaluated and the evaluator(s), such as chief administrator(s), immediate superior(s), peer(s), and others (e.g., clients, families, ancillary personnel associated with Wholistic Supervision). Who is included in the feedback will determine the form (dyadic or group).

The evaluation-feedback cycle is complex because of the potential participants. The process becomes more complex as the variable of *when* evaluation and feedback occur is considered.

When. The question of when evaluation and feedback are done has three elements: frequency, period, and duration. How often evaluation occurs (*frequency*) will depend on the purpose of assessment and will range from daily to annually, with weekly, monthly, midterm, and midyear in between.

The *period* of evaluation refers to whether it occurs at the beginning, middle, or end of a diagnostic or treatment session, a conference, an interview, a class lecture, or a staff meeting. It can also refer to the period within the day, month, or semester. Different information may be obtained at each checkpoint, so supervisors need to use a spread of times for accurate evaluations. The period is usually dictated by the purpose.

Duration of evaluation includes pre-observation conferences and planning, observation time, and reporting time (writing or conference time). How long an evaluation process lasts depends on a number of variables but should be directed by the purpose. If the evaluation involves obtaining data from microfocus, then small increments of time (3–5 minutes) will suffice, but if macrofocus data are needed, then longer periods of observation or more of the brief samples are required. Duration of the feedback should be guided by the purpose of the evaluation.

When feedback is provided includes questions like whether the information should be immediate or delayed, the time of day, the day of the week or month, and what events should precede and follow the feedback. One principle from learning theory is that immediate feedback is more effective than delayed feedback in changing behavior quickly (Hagler & Holdgrafer, 1987). In situations where immediate feedback is desirable, an FM transmitting system or "bug-in-the-ear" device can allow the supervisor to modify a clinician's behavior immediately. However, if the goal is to have a person develop more effective problem managing skills, then delayed feedback may allow the supervisee to try some self-directed problem managing strategies, contributing more to the goal than supervisor-directed feedback might. Buckberry (1980) found that delayed written feedback enhanced self-supervision and helped participants to assign a mutually acceptable grade.

The time of the day, week, or month when feedback is imparted can affect the salience and consequent productivity of the feedback. Psychological and physical states should also be considered when making decisions about timing feedback.

Where. The contexts of assessment include the environment(s) where data are gathered and conferences held. Assessing supervisors includes evaluating professional competence in all five domains. Such a task requires that data be secured from different environments. Assessing clinical supervisees includes evaluating their competence in a variety of clinical and interpersonal skills and dispositions within a number of contexts.

Conferences can be held in different places to maximize the success and productivity of the reporting. A space could be chosen that is considered evaluator-dominant, personnel-dominant, or neutral. Possible sites include primary work areas such as the supervisor's office or supervisee's office (each carries with it a degree of dominance), or a neutral area such as a conference room or lounge. Outside areas like restaurants or faculty clubs may be even better for providing feedback. Environment, coordinated with the psychological and physical states of participants, may determine the success of the assessment. Even negative feedback, such as firing for a staff member or failure of a course for a student, can be given and received productively if the environment, constituents, and timing are mutually supportive.

What. What gets evaluated should be clear from a job description, goals and objectives, or from purpose statements. Supervisors might evaluate supervisees' competencies associated with diagnostic and therapeutic work, counseling, interviewing, conferences, staffings, case management, reporting, and intra- and interprofessional relations. When a supervisor receives an evaluation, it will include the skills and dispositions associated with the supervision roles defined by the job description. (With minor modifications, the 1985 ASHA tasks and competencies for supervisors can be used by supervisees or administrative superiors to evaluate supervisors' competencies; see appendix A.)

Programs are also evaluated, and the Communication Disorders supervisor operating in the Administration domain is often the person responsible for conducting the evaluation. Well-developed program goals and objectives, complete with criteria for evaluating them, facilitate the process. The Program Planning Evaluation (PPE) (Dublinske & Grimes, 1971), Comprehensive Assessment and Service Evaluation (CASE) (ASHA, 1976), and numerous auditing systems can help administrators evaluate programs. One part of many program evaluations is documenting the services delivered. The importance of program evaluation for quality assurance, as well as for documentation for funding sources, cannot be underestimated. The supervisor operating as Administrator must know the available program evaluation tools, their relative advantages and disadvantages, and how to use them effectively and efficiently. For most supervisors, that requires preparation.

What the feedback consists of depends on its purpose. If the purpose is to give information about overall performance, then the feedback will be general; if the purpose is to give information about a specific competency, then the focus will be narrow.

How. Various methods, modes, materials, and instruments exist for evaluating and grading the various aspects of Communication Disorders supervision. The watching/moving, listening/speaking, and reading/writing channels of communication can be the focus of evaluation or the means of providing feedback in the forms of critiques and grades. This means that the verbal and nonverbal dimensions of supervisees' communication (discussed in detail in chapters 5 and 6) that manifest clinical and interpersonal skills and dispositions may be evaluated by the supervisor; the verbal and nonverbal dimensions of supervisors' communication can also be evaluated by supervisees. Supervisors (or supervisees) will use various modes of communication to collect data for the evaluation and then to report the results to the supervisee (or supervisor). Therefore, supervisors (and supervisees) must know the advantages and disadvantages of each mode of observation presented in chapter 6 (e.g., live, audio- and videotape, lesson plans) and use them all competently so that they can choose the best mode(s) for a productive evaluation. Table 11–6 summarizes the relative value of various modes in gathering data for evaluation.

TABLE 11-6
Relative values of observation modes for generating evaluation data

Competence Areas	A	B	C	Modes D	E	F	Total	Mean
I. Interpersonal Communication: Verbal								
A. With client	5	6	5	5 + 1	4	5 + 1	32	5.3
B. With family	4	6	5	4 + 1	4	5 + 1	30	5.0
C. With others	3	6	4	4 + 1	3	5 + 1	27	4.5
II. Interpersonal Communication: Nonverbal								
A. With client	6	6	5	5 + 1	4	2 + 1	30	5.0
B. With family	5	6	5	5 + 1	4	2 + 1	29	4.8
C. With others	4	6	4	4 + 1	3	2 + 1	25	4.2
III. Planning	1	4	2	2	2	3 + 1	15	2.5
IV. Clinical Competence								
A. General	5	6	5	5 + 1	4	2 + 1	29	4.8
B. Diagnostic	5	6	5	5 + 1	4	2 + 1	29	4.8
C. Therapeutic	5	6	5	5 + 1	4	2 + 1	29	4.8
V. Decision Making/ Problem Managing	4	6	4	4 + 1	4	3 + 1	27	4.5
VI. Clinical Reporting								
A. Oral	3	6	5	4 + 1	4	5 + 1	29	4.8
B. Written	1	6 + 1	4 + 1	1	1	1	16	2.7
VII. Case Management	3	6	5	1	1	3 + 1	20	3.3
VIII. Associated Professional Qualities	4	6	5	3 + 1	3	2	24	4.0
Total	58	89	69	69	49	57		
Mean	3.9	5.9	4.6	4.6	3.3	3.8		

Modes:

A = Live (indirect)

B = Live (direct/participant)

C = Live (direct/nonparticipant)

D = Videotape

E = Closed circuit television

F = Audiotape

Ratings:

6 = A sufficient sample of behavior can be observed easily within 5 minutes

5 = A sufficient sample of behavior can be observed with minimum effort

4 = A sufficient sample of behavior can be observed with moderate effort*

3 = A sufficient sample of behavior can be observed with maximum effort

2 = Questionable whether behavior can be observed

1 = Unable to observe behavior

+1 = Extra point for opportunity to review observation data

*Effort = Additional times, additional length of time, more settings, special arrangements

Supervisors also need to know the advantages and disadvantages of feedback procedures (e.g., conferences, written documents including competency rating forms, or audiotape recorded critiques) and be competent in their use. The development of competence in observation and communication must begin early in the preparation of all Communication Disorders personnel.

Major concerns for Communication Disorders personnel evaluation include the validity of the instruments available for evaluating professional competence and their intra- and inter-evaluator

TABLE 11-7
Evaluation instruments

Author	Instrument	Use
Bales (1950)	Interaction Process Analysis (IPA)	Analyzes content of group verbal interaction patterns
Blumberg (1974)	Blumberg Analysis System	Analyzes supervisor-teacher (supervisee) verbal conference interaction
Boone and Prescott (1972)	Boone and Prescott Content and Sequence Analysis System	Analyzes content and sequence of client-clinician verbal interaction
Brasseur and Anderson (1983)	Individual Supervisory Conference Rating Scale (ISCRS), Modified	Rates elements of Direct/Indirect conferences; validated
Conover (1974)	Conover Analysis System	Analyzes content of client-clinician verbal interaction
Culatta and Seltzer (1977)	Culatta and Seltzer Content and Sequence Analysis System	Analyzes content and sequence of supervisor-supervisee verbal conference interaction
Farmer (1980)	Interview Analysis System (IAS)	Analyzes verbal content of interviewer-informant interaction during an interview
Farmer (1981)	Conversation Assessment Technique (CAT)	Analyzes nonverbal and verbal communication (sequence and content) of client-clinician interaction
Farmer (1983)	INREAL Training Evaluation Model —Interpersonal Communication Pacing (ITEM-ICP)	Analyzes supervisor's nonverbal and verbal interpersonal communication pacing (content and sequence) during conferences
Farmer (1987)	Conversation Analysis System (CAS)	Analyzes nonverbal and verbal content and sequence of client-clinician interaction
Flanders (1965)	Flanders Interaction Analysis System	Analyzes verbal content of teacher-student classroom interaction
Klevans and Volz (1974)	Practicum Evaluation Procedure	Rates clinicians' clinical and interpersonal competencies

reliability. Two types of instruments are used for evaluation: interaction analysis (IA) systems and procedures, and clinical competency rating forms.

Interaction analysis systems are used to evaluate clinician-client interaction in clinical situations, clinician-informant interaction during interviews and conferences, interaction among group participants, and supervisor-supervisee interaction during conferences. The most common of these instruments are shown in Table 11-7.

As noted in chapters 5 and 12, most interac-

TABLE 11-7
continued

Author	Instrument	Use
Lashbrook and Lashbrook (1975)	Proana 5	Computer analysis of frequency of verbal interaction patterns during small-group (5) discussion
Lougeay-Mottinger et al. (1984)	UTD Competency-Based Evaluation System	Rates clinicians' clinical and interpersonal competencies
McCrea (1980)	McCrea Adapted Scales	Analyzes verbal content of supervisee-supervisor conference
Oratio (1977)	Oratio's Supervisory Transactional System	Analyzes verbal content and sequence of supervisee-supervisor conference
Oratio (1979)	Pattern Recognition (computer program)	Analyzes verbal content and sequence of supervisee-supervisor conference or client-clinician interaction
Schubert et al. (1973)	The Analysis of Behaviors of Clinicians (ABC) System	Rates clinicians' clinical and interpersonal competencies
Shriberg et al. (1975)	The Wisconsin Procedure for Appraisal of Clinical Competence (W-PACC)	Rates clinicians' clinical and interpersonal competencies
Smith (1982)	Individual Supervisory Conference Rating Scale (ISCRS)	Rates elements of Direct/Indirect conferences; validated
Thorlacius (1980)	Supervisor-Teacher Analogous Categories System (STACS)	Analyzes supervisor-teacher (supervisee) verbal conference interaction
Underwood (1979)	Underwood Category System for Analyzing Supervisor-Clinician Behavior	Analyzes verbal content and sequence of supervisor-supervisee interaction during conferences
Weiss (1983)	INREAL Training Evaluation Model (ITEM)	Analyzes linguistic and nonlinguistic content and sequence of interactant-partner interaction during INREAL training
Weller (1971)	Multidimensional Observational System for the Analysis of Interactions in Clinical Supervision (M.O.S.A.I.C.S.)	Analyzes verbal content and sequence of supervisee-supervisor interaction during conferences; validated

tion analysis instruments do not have strong validity and reliability data to support them. (The *Individual Supervisory Conference Rating Scale* [Brasseur & Anderson, 1983; Smith, 1982], a notable exception, is considered to be a valid and reliable instrument for judging conferences.) An associated problem is that lack of evaluator training to use specific tools results in alarmingly low intra- and inter-evaluator agreement and reliability. Reliability audits conducted on supervisors in a university setting (Sbaschnig & Williams, 1983) and in field sites (Sbaschnig & Williams, 1984) and reported through the Communication Disorders supervision network substantiate the concern many supervisors express about the quality of available instruments and the lack of training in their use. On the positive side of this negative situation is the growing awareness of the problem and the resultant pressure for research that will help rectify the problem.

Clinical competency rating forms present another problem for the supervisor. Although virtually every college and university preparation program uses some type of checklist to evaluate the clinical and interpersonal skills (and maybe dispositions) of its trainees, the instruments suffer from the same problems as the IA tools. One published instrument, the *Wisconsin Procedure for Appraisal of Clinical Competence* (W-PACC) (Shriberg, Filley, Hayes, Kwiatkowski, Schatz, Simmons, & Smith, 1975) is the only instrument that provides empirical data to support its effectiveness. The standardization makes this instrument useful for comparing, screening out, or assigning individuals to different levels. Although many consider it a good tool, it is not easily adapted to the variety of philosophies about what constitutes a competent Communication Disorders professional. It may not include enough of some competencies for some programs, or may emphasize a certain type of competency too much for others. Thus, most Communication Disorders training programs develop their own competence assessment tool to reflect the philosophy of the institution. This allows individuals to set specific objectives, interpret progress directly relative to specific objectives, compile comprehensive records of personnel progress, and check progress regularly without having to administer the entire instrument. It also enables instructors to evaluate the effectiveness of different instructional methods, materials, and strategies. An impressive array of institution-developed tools was presented as a poster session at the 1984 annual convention of the American Speech-Language-Hearing Association. From that national presentation supervisors could compare instruments and identify the features that qualified them as exemplars. None of the forms met all the criteria, but as a group the exemplary forms

1. evaluated both skills and dispositions.
2. were of sufficient length to cover essential components of competence as defined by the individual institutions.
3. were relatively easy and efficient to complete.
4. were formatted logically and attractively and reproduced clearly.
5. combined qualitative and quantitative grading.
6. used descriptors or definitions to clarify terminology.
7. were flexibly designed to be used with a range of personnel levels.
8. provided information that would be useful feedback to assist personnel in professional development.

Criterion-referenced tools can be effective in assessing personnel and providing direction for development if the tools adhere to the eight criteria listed above.

An innovative approach to self-evaluation of academic information has been used by Hunt (1985). The *Multiple Choice Self-Assessment* (McSAT) requires test takers first to select an answer on a multiple choice test and then to indicate how sure they are that the answer is correct (almost guess, probably guess, neutral, fairly certain, almost certain). Test takers gain or lose self-assessment (SA) points (−60 to +50) on each question depending both on the correctness of the answer and on the accuracy of the self-assessment. The number of points available on each question is selected so that a test taker can get the highest SA test score only by being as accurate in the self-assessments as possible. Attempts by the test taker to "beat the system" produce lower SA test scores.

It is suggested that an incentive bonus of 1/3 letter grade (e.g., from a C+ to a B−) be awarded on the test if the self-assessment score is higher than the correctness score, with no penalty for a low SA score. In other words, learners are reinforced for developing accuracy of self-assessment as well as for learning academic material. McSAT has advantages for both teaching and learning. For learners, self-assessment has been shown to

1. improve ability to assess self-knowledge and competence.
2. improve learning of academic information.
3. improve grades if alphabetic or numeric grading is used.

Test results can help instructors to

1. Decide if material has been learned by specific individuals or a group and remedy the situation if it has not. Information about student answers is grouped into four categories: *sure-but-wrong, sure-and-correct, unsure-and-correct,* and *unsure-and-wrong.* It is not uncommon to find a high percentage of *sure-but-wrong* answers on a few questions. Once these questions are identified, the reason for the high false alarm rate should be identified. The most common reasons are learner misinformation (in which case instruction can be provided to correct the misinformation) and misleading test questions (in which case the items should be revised or eliminated).
2. identify guesses.
3. provide an incentive to increase grades.

How evaluations are conducted thus seems to present the greatest problems for Communication Disorders supervisors. Ongoing management of the problems must address the primitiveness of the available instruments as well as the lack of prepared evaluators. These two limitations will reduce the usefulness of feedback.

How feedback is to be provided to personnel is another important consideration that includes (a) the channel (watching/moving, listening/talking, reading/writing), (b) the method (role modeling, face-to-face conference, audio- or videotape reporting, evaluation forms, written narrative), and (c) the type or valence (positive, negative, or neutral).

Geoffrey (1973) reports that when supervisors observe frequently they use the verbal channel most often, but when their observation is less frequent they use some form of written feedback. The choice of channel(s) should be based on the purpose of the feedback. Advantages and disadvantages exist for all channels and methods. Therefore, to create the most productive feedback context, supervisors need to coordinate channels and methods with the purpose of the feedback and with the recipient's learning style.

Research about the effect of valence is not definitive. Edwards (1980) suggests that feedback should include both positive and negative valence. However, the concept of valence is more complex than a simple dichotomy of positive and negative. Farmer (1982) found that the valence of written feedback can be affected by the color of ink used, which can even determine the outcome of the feedback. Some supervisees considered red ink to have negative connotations, regardless of the content of the message; other supervisees reported that colored ink indicated importance. The data supported these statements. If feedback was provided in certain colors of ink (green, orange, purple, peacock blue), the supervisees read and reacted to it immediately; if the feedback appeared in pencil or black ink, it was considered less important and not requiring immediate attention.

Peaper and Mercaitis (1987) found that written feedback was more evaluative than oral feedback and that supervisors asked fewer questions through writing.

An additional perspective on the complexity of valence (positive or negative) in supervision feedback is provided by Stuve (1977). In a study of the effect of supervisors' positive, negative, and neutral oral and written feedback on clinician performance, attitudes, and client performance, Stuve found that client performance improved significantly under all conditions of reinforcement given to supervisee subjects. Remaining results were statistically insignificant but suggested that neutral feedback decreased supervisees' performance as perceived by the supervisors; that supervisees' attitudes toward supervisors were more favorable after positive feedback and less favorable after negative or neutral feedback; and that supervisees' attitudes toward clients were least favorable after negative feedback.

Feedback in self-supervision takes a somewhat different form. Markel (1981) summarized the research on self-management effectiveness and found experimental support for six strategies of self-supervision:

1. *Self-instruction:* learners tell themselves what to do, when, and how to change behavior, gain information, or develop competencies.
2. *Problem managing:* learners work through a systematic sequence of activities including problem definition, identification of barriers to productive management, generating and evaluating alternatives, selecting an outcome or outcomes, trying it (or them), observing and evaluating the consequences, selecting other outcomes, or redefining the problem.
3. *Modeling:* learners receive direct or mediated presentation of appropriate behavior by a peer or role model.
4. *Rehearsal:* learners practice desired behavior, first with assistance and support, then more and more independently.
5. *Self-determination of criteria or objectives:* learners set their own criterion-referenced objectives and then observe themselves and record the degree to which they are meeting their objectives.
6. *Self-contracting:* learners set their own objectives, methods of assessment, timelines, and consequences or reinforcers.

Feedback, too, must be evaluated for its effectiveness relative to the desired outcome or purpose. The evaluation-feedback process should always be an ongoing cycle rather than a series of episodes.

Biases. Communication Disorders researchers have explored a number of biases that affect the evaluation-feedback process. Andersen (1981) found that supervisors who were told that a clinician had a high grade point average (GPA) rated the clinician higher on factors of Responsibility and Conference Behavior than did supervisors who were told that the clinician had less than acceptable supervisor evaluations. Shriberg, Bless, Carlson, Filley, Kwiatkowski, and Smith (1976) reported that grade point average accounted for 25% to 50% of the variance in clinical performance (the higher the GPA, the higher the ratings of clinical performance). Whereas Andersen's study suggests that perceptions of competence may be biased by prior knowledge of academic ability, the Shriberg et al. study suggests that GPA is a robust correlate and predictor of clinical competence.

In a vein similar to Andersen's, Blodgett, Schmitt, and Scudder (1987) found through their research that identical clinician behavior may be judged appropriate or inappropriate depending on the supervisor's point of view and degree of acquaintance with the supervisee.

Andersen's study (1980) also suggested that supervisors trained in supervision rated conferences differently from those who had not received training. Similarly, the results of a study by Mercaitis and Peaper (1984) showed a trend for supervisors' rating of clinician competence to increase with additional supervision experience.

Thompson (1988) discussed actor-observer

bias, positivity bias, the halo effect, and the Rosenthal effect in relation to observation modes for trained supervisors. She found that bias patterns of supervisors trained in critical observation were different from those of untrained supervisors.

The effect of personal biases, causal attributions, and reactivity on observation competence is discussed in chapter 6. The same premises hold for the effect of personal bias on evaluation. The professional tasks a supervisor likes to do tend to receive more attention than the ones the supervisor does not like to do. If supervisors make lists of likes and dislikes to help them work on this problem, they must take care not to overemphasize the tasks they dislike to compensate for past neglect. The awareness of personal biases (positive and negative) should lead to a better balance.

It seems clear that personal and situational biases can affect observation, evaluation, and feedback. It is unclear just what effects the biases can have, and studies of the topic recommend further investigation. The developing awareness of bias as a variable in evaluation and feedback has been a major step. A second step has been to identify biases that exist. The third step will be to determine how the biases affect the evaluation-feedback process; the final step will be to explore ways of controlling the effect of biases.

Although not exactly a bias, the number of supervisees a supervisor is responsible for at a time has been found to affect the evaluation of their clinical competence (Ghitter, 1987).

Effects of the Evaluation-Feedback Cycle. The evaluation-feedback process in Communication Disorders has advantages and disadvantages for both the supervisee and the supervisor. Some advantages of feedback in the forms of evaluative comments, letter grades, numerical ratings, and rankings do exist. In general, such evaluation

1. motivates people to learn.
2. reinforces learning.
3. motivates and reinforces the mastery of basic information and skills that will lead to acquisition of specific professional concepts and abilities.
4. motivates self-competition.
5. necessitates clear statements of purpose, goals, objectives, and evaluation/grading criteria to identify strengths and weaknesses; these statements help supervisees to improve performance.

Disadvantages of evaluation also exist. In general, evaluation

1. limits creativity and individuality of expression; the process may discourage rather than encourage learning that is personally relevant to the supervisee or the supervisor.
2. motivates unproductive competition among group members, which can lead to excessive pressure and decreased enjoyment of learning.
3. motivates people to memorize for short-term but not for long-term retention.
4. encourages "regurgitation of facts" rather than synthesized, integrated, applied learning.

Alphabetic and numeric grading are the systems most frequently used in Communication Disorders preparation programs. If grades have been specifically defined and the definitions are clearly understood and consistently used by all evaluators, then letter and number grading can be fair and objective, measuring a valid and reliable sample of academic and professional behavior. However, letter and number grading are not accepted by all institutions. Some use a binary system with *pass-fail* (P/F) or *satisfactory-unsatisfactory* (S/U) ratings. Binary evaluation can reduce learner pressure and is thought to encourage study for learning rather than study for high grades. This notion implies that learning for personal value and learning to obtain high grades are not compatible. However, some research (Gardner, 1961; Markle, 1964) has shown that standards and guidelines help individuals strive to attain the highest standard and that P/F or S/U systems have mediocrity as their highest standard (Schubert, 1978). Therefore, the binary systems tend to decrease learner effort. To ensure that a majority of students pass, programs are revised to accommodate the slowest learners, eventually leading to oversimplified, repetitious curriculum and practicum programs. With P/F or S/U evaluation, it is easy to identify learners who are doing unsatisfactory work and should therefore fail. It is impossible, however, to show the difference between marginally adequate learners and those who demonstrate superior achievement. Binary systems in Communication Disorders programs thus become discouraging to the good learners. Although binary methods may be less time-consuming, most supervisors who use them recognize the need for descriptive and qualitative measures of learner progress. These can be provided in narrative comments and/or through alphabetic or numeric grading. Alphabetic or numeric grading is a more systematic, complex method of evaluating than the binary method; when combined with narratives, it provides the most powerful and useful source of information about personnel competence.

To summarize, supervisors must consider carefully who and what is involved in the evaluation-feedback process and when, where, and how the process is to be executed. Supervision training programs should address supervisors' competence in this critical task, because it may ultimately have the strongest impact on the competence of the entire Communication Disorders profession.

SPECIAL CONSIDERATIONS

Five areas require special consideration for evaluation and grading in Communication Disorders: (a) marginal personnel, (b) minority language, multicultural personnel, (c) communication handicapped personnel, (d) supervising peers, and (e) generic supervision.

Marginal Personnel

Most evaluations of personnel, whether students or staff members, are completed without problems, especially if goals and objectives have been specified, if a well-written job description exists, and if a well-developed evaluation instrument is used. Some personnel, however, students as well as staff, are seriously lacking in knowledge, clinical and interpersonal skills, and dispositions; these are referred to as *marginal* students or professionals. It is helpful to be more precise than this when discussing marginal personnel, because the precision can help target specific areas that need to be developed. Having identified targets, supervisors can make a more productive remedial plan. Preservice and service clinical personnel can be described on eight levels of proficiency, presented in part A of Table 11-2 (see p. 280).

Once a person has been identified as belonging to one of the seven categories of competence, a remedial plan can be developed. Some guidelines for working with marginal personnel follow:

1. All personnel should be informed that standards exist and that evaluations will be used to ensure that they achieve and maintain those standards.
2. All evaluations should use instruments as reliable and valid as possible and be conducted by supervisors trained to evaluate.
3. When someone is identified as demonstrating characteristics of one of the marginal types, a competence committee should meet as quickly as possible with that person to discuss the area(s) of concern.
4. Mutually negotiated remedial plans should be developed, written, duplicated, and signed, with one copy for the marginal person, one for the committee chair, and one for the organization. The plan should specify the area(s) of deficit and the conditions of remediation (timetable, resources for remedial instruction, criteria, and consequences of not acquiring the competency).

5. The plan and consequences should be enforced.

The major difficulties in working with marginal personnel are two: the time commitment is generally excessive, and the marginal person may remain incompetent, even with significant remedial attention. Marginal personnel are at high risk for failing to attain professional competence. Supervisors should develop strong policies about marginal personnel and then follow and uphold those policies.

Nontraditional learners, such as minority language, multicultural personnel and those who manifest communication handicaps, also require special consideration.

Nontraditional Learners

Minority Language, Multicultural Personnel. Minority language, multicultural personnel in Communication Disorders clinical and supervision training programs and service delivery agencies have both advantages and disadvantages. Their background of knowledge is crucial in helping the Communication Disorders profession to provide quality services to non-English-speaking clients. To assure high-quality preparation for these personnel, as well as high-quality service delivery for non-English-speaking consumers, supervisors should modify the basic professional standards based on the language and cultural differences of the geographical area, at the same time not compromising the intent of the standards. They should also show sensitivity and respect to linguistic, nonlinguistic, and cultural differences among their clinical and supervision colleagues. With these two guidelines, supervisors, without being fluent in the minority language, should be able to evaluate the competence of Communication Disorders personnel (as well as the diagnostic or treatment status of minority language, multicultural clients) effectively and efficiently with fewer problems and conflicts. An identical tack can be followed with personnel who manifest some type of communication impairment.

Communication-Impaired Personnel. Advantages and disadvantages also exist for communication-impaired personnel working in the profession. They can often be an inspiration to the clients with whom they work. On the other hand, they may have difficulty with some clinical or supervision competencies if the communication problem is severe or hard to control. All Communication Disorders training programs and service delivery agencies should have a policy on how to modify the basic standards to accommodate speech-language pathologists and audiologists who may, for example, stutter or be language/learning disabled or hearing-impaired, without compromising the quality of clinical or supervision service rendered.

Minority language, multicultural and communication-impaired personnel can add richness to the profession. To maximize the potential benefits, supervisors must develop, implement, and maintain complete, clearly stated competence and evaluation/grading guidelines.

Evaluating and Grading Peers

Many opportunities exist for peer (or colleague) supervision and evaluation, which can benefit undergraduate and graduate preservice clinical and supervisor trainees as well as service-level clinicians and supervisors. This variation in supervision practice has advantages and disadvantages for the peer supervisee, peer supervisor, and staff supervisor. The primary benefits are that (a) peer supervisees may learn better because they feel more comfortable accepting assistance from a peer than from someone with real or perceived authority; (b) peer supervisors, especially clinicians or supervisor trainees, are closer to the problems encountered in the struggle toward competence and therefore may be more empathic toward supervisees (experienced supervisors may forget the struggle and focus more on the competencies than on the supervisees or the process); (c) peer supervision allows preservice trainees to develop objective evaluation, confrontation, and grading ability, making the transition to staff supervision smoother; and (d) staff supervisors can receive a different perspective on a supervisee's competence. Peer evaluation raises two primary difficulties: (a) the assumption that evaluation must be done by someone with superior status may hamper the process (in fact, with preparation, nearly anyone can evaluate); (b) peer supervisors may find it hard to separate the roles of friend and supervisor (they may find it difficult to say, in essence, "You fulfill my personal standards of what constitutes a friend but you do not meet our organization's standards for a Communication Disorders professional"). Peer supervision is one of the strongest reasons why Communication Disorders professionals should be competent in conflict communication and problem management strategies.

Generic Supervision

Generic supervision has advantages and disadvantages for Communication Disorders personnel. If speech-language pathologists and audiologists are supervised by someone other than a Communication Disorders supervisor, cross-disciplinary professional knowledge and clinical competence can enhance service delivery. The critical factor in assessment, of course, is the supervisors' knowledge and expertise in their own profession as well as in the other disciplines. The broader their knowledge and expertise, the more easily generic supervisors can evaluate experiences across disciplines in a meaningful manner. If Communication Disorders supervisors function as generic supervisors for other disciplines, they must be competent in speech-language pathology and/or audiology, competent in supervision strategies (especially strategies for assessment), and knowledgeable about the other disciplines. Although expert generic supervision demands wide knowledge, it can also be rewarding for both the supervisees and the supervisor.

SUMMARY

Thousands of people are involved in assessment processes in Communication Disorders each year and evaluation is a subject of increasing contention among personnel. A better understanding of the purpose and structure of evaluating mechanisms is a prerequisite for widespread improvement. Supervisors who pay attention to content are often vague about the process and vice versa. Supervisors must develop knowledge and skills in the areas of observation, communication, decision making, problem managing, clinical literacy, and technology. Information about policies and procedures, Matrix Management, and consequences will also prove helpful. If learning/performance goals and objectives are properly defined, they can be the basis of success for supervisees and supervisors alike. A comprehensive evaluation of personnel performance should guide improvement toward these goals, but supervisees often receive scant critical commentary on their progress.

The evaluation-feedback process, including grading, is another area for which supervisors should be prepared through their training. Alphabetic and numeric grading, unidimensional in nature (e.g., a grade of C translates to the single concept "average"), are the most commonly used forms of feedback for multidimensional phenomena such as clinical skills. Binary systems (e.g., pass/fail) have similar problems; both procedures are particularly susceptible to the charge of insufficient feedback to personnel. Alphabetic, numeric, and binary evaluation systems combined with narrative provide more complete feedback on which to develop future goals and objectives. A knowledge of the options for evaluation and feedback is the most direct route to improved assessment in Communication Disorders supervision.

The issues of assessment are further complicated and require still more knowledge for academically and clinically marginal personnel, minority language, multicultural personnel, and personnel with communication impairments, and for peer and generic supervision.

APPLICATIONS

Discussion Topics

1. When pass-fail grading has been used in clinical competence-based courses, it has often met with unsatisfactory results. Discuss why this is true and how the situation might be improved.
2. Discuss the advantages and disadvantages of feedback methods such as verbal, audiotaped, and written feedback. What effect does time have on feedback? What effect does reinforcement have (positive, negative, neutral)? What effect does nondirect (e.g., "bug-in-the-ear," audiotape) feedback have compared with direct and/or written feedback?
3. Discuss the notion that acquaintance with the supervisee affects clinical session evaluations.
4. Discuss reliability audits: Should they be done? How? How often? What standard of reliability should be set? What should happen if the reliability of a staff's assessment procedures does not meet the standard?
5. Discuss options for the supervisor in managing marginal students (both academic and clinical).

Laboratory Experiences

1. Establish the protocol for educational and clinical management of supervisees with communication disorders.
2. Grade a diagnostic report and discuss it with a colleague.
3. Evaluate a clinical session (in Speech-Language Pathology or Audiology) and give feedback to the supervisee. Discuss with a colleague.
4. Cosupervise with a colleague for a time and keep records of the experience.
5. Develop a clinical practicum competencies grading form.

Research Projects

1. Conduct a survey of Communication Disorders supervisors to learn about their preparation for the assessment process.

2. Conduct a comparative study of formal evaluation procedures and naturalistic evaluation procedures.

3. Conduct a survey to determine what practices exist for evaluating exceptional (marginal, minority language and multicultural, and communication-impaired) personnel.

4. Conduct a study to determine what types of information can and cannot be obtained from specific observation modes, including direct live (participant and nonparticipant), indirect live, videotape, closed circuit, audiotape, and lesson plan observation.

5. Conduct a survey to determine what percentage of Communication Disorders personnel are involved in generic supervision as supervisees or supervisors. What do they see as the advantages and disadvantages of generic supervision?

REFERENCES

American Speech and Hearing Association. (1976). *Comprehensive Assessment and Service Evaluation Information System (CASE).* Rockville, MD: Author.

American Speech-Language-Hearing Association. (1985). Clinical supervision in speech-language pathology and audiology (position statement). *Asha, 7*(6), 57–60.

Andersen, C. (1981). The effect of supervisor bias on the evaluation of student clinicians in speech-language pathology and audiology. *Dissertation Abstracts International, 41,* 4479B. (University Microfilms No. 81-12, 499)

Bales, R. (1950). *Interaction process analysis.* Chicago: University of Chicago Press.

Bess, F. (1987). Community-based speech-language-hearing clinic administration. In H. Oyer (Ed.), *Administration of programs in speech-language pathology and audiology* (pp. 84–99). Englewood Cliffs, NJ: Prentice-Hall.

Blodgett, E., Schmitt, J., & Scudder, R. (1987). Clinical session evaluation: The effect of familiarity with the supervisee. *The Clinical Supervisor, 5*(1), 33–43.

Blumberg, A. (1974). *Supervisors and teachers: A private cold war.* Berkeley, CA: McCutchan.

Boone, D., & Prescott, T. (1972). Content and sequence analysis of speech and hearing therapy. *Asha, 14,* 58–62.

Brasseur, J., & Anderson, J. (1983). Observed differences between direct, indirect, and direct/indirect videotaped supervisory conferences. *Journal of Speech and Hearing Research, 26,* 349–355.

Buckberry, E. (1980). Delayed written feedback: A supervisory approach to self-evaluation enhancement. *SUPERvision, 4*(1), 8–9.

Conover, H. (1974). *Conover Analysis System.* Unpublished manuscript, Ohio University, Athens.

Culatta, R., & Seltzer, H. (1977). Content and sequence analysis of the supervisory session: A report of clinical use. *Asha, 19,* 523–526.

Dublinske, S., & Grimes, J. (1971). *Program Planning Evaluation (PPE).* Unpublished materials from a New Mexico State University workshop, Las Cruces.

Edwards, D. (1980). Negative feedback as a positive interaction in supervisory conferences. *SUPERvision, 4*(1), 9-11.

Farmer, S. (1980). Interview Analysis System. *SUPERvision, 4*(4), 7.

Farmer, S. (1981). *Conversation Assessment Technique (CAT)*. Unpublished client-clinician interaction analysis system, New Mexico State University, Las Cruces.

Farmer, S. (1982). *The communicative disorders supervisory conference: An expanded perspective.* Unpublished manuscript, New Mexico State University, Las Cruces.

Farmer, S. (1983). *INREAL Training Evaluation Model (ITEM)—Interpersonal Communication Pacing (ICP).* Unpublished supervisor-supervisee interaction analysis system, New Mexico State University, Las Cruces.

Farmer, S. (1986). *Wholistic supervision.* Unpublished manuscript, New Mexico State University, Las Cruces.

Farmer, S. (1987). *Conversation Analysis System (CAS).* Unpublished client-clinician interaction analysis system, New Mexico State University, Las Cruces.

Flanders, N. (1965). *Interaction analysis in the classroom: A manual for observers.* Minneapolis: University of Minnesota.

Gardner, J. (1961). *Excellence.* New York: Harper & Row.

Geoffrey, V. (1973). *Report on supervisory practices in speech and hearing.* College Park: University of Maryland.

Ghitter, R. (1987). Relationship of interpersonal and background variables to supervisee clinical effectiveness. In S. Farmer (Ed.), *Clinical supervision: A coming of age. Proceedings of a national conference on supervision* (pp. 49-57). Las Cruces: New Mexico State University.

Hagler, P., & Holdgrafer, G. (1987). Effects of supervisory feedback on clinician and client discourse participation. In S. Farmer (Ed.), *Clinical supervision: A coming of age. Proceedings of a national conference on supervision* (pp. 106-112). Las Cruces: New Mexico State University.

Hunt, D. (1985). Some uses of the computer in teaching, training and testing: Student/learner self-assessment responding. In *Proceedings of the First Regional Conference on University Teaching: Teaching to Potential* (pp. 324-338). Las Cruces: New Mexico State University.

Kamara, C. (1987). The supervisor as a program manager. In S. Farmer (Ed.), *Clinical supervision: A coming of age. Proceedings of a national conference on supervision* (pp. 230-237). Las Cruces: New Mexico State University.

Klevans, D., & Volz, H. (1974). Development of a clinical evaluation procedure. *Asha, 9,* 489-491.

Laccinole, M., & Schill, M. (1982). Quantifying supervisory activities in speech-language pathology. *SUPERvision, 6*(1), 2-5.

Lashbrook, W., & Lashbrook, V. (1975). *Proana 5: A computer analysis of small group discussion.* Minneapolis, MN: Burgess.

Lougeay-Mottinger, J., Harris, M., Perlstein-Kaplan, K., & Felicetti, T. (1984). UTD competency based evaluation system. *Asha, 11,* 39-43.

Markel, G. (1981). Self-management in classrooms: Implications for mainstreaming. In P. Bates (Ed.), *Mainstreaming: Our current knowledge base* (pp. 161-183). Minneapolis: University of Minnesota.

Markle, S. (1964). *Good frames and bad: A grammar of frame writing.* New York: Wiley.

McCrea, E. (1980). Supervisee ability to self-explore and four facilitative dimensions of supervisor behavior in individual conferences in speech-language pathology. *Dissertation Abstracts International, 41,* 2134B. (University Microfilms No. 80-29, 239)

Mercaitis, P., & Peaper, R. (1984, November). *Supervisor ratings as a function of supervisor vs. clinical experience.* Paper presented at the annual convention of the American Speech-Language-Hearing Association, San Francisco.

Oratio, A. (1977). *Supervision in speech pathology: Handbook for supervisors and clinicians.* Baltimore, MD: University Park Press.

Oratio, A. (1979). *Pattern recognition.* Baltimore, MD: University Park Press.

Peaper, R., & Mercaitis, P. (1987). The nature of narrative written feedback provided to students. In S. Farmer (Ed.), *Clinical supervision: A coming of age. Proceedings of a national conference on supervision* (pp. 138-144). Las Cruces: New Mexico State University.

Sbaschnig, K., & Williams, C. (1983, November). *A reliability audit for supervisors.* Paper presented at the annual convention of the American Speech-Language-Hearing Association, Cincinnati, OH.

Sbaschnig, K., & Williams, C. (1984, November). *A reliability audit for externship supervisors.* Paper presented at the annual convention of the American Speech-Language-Hearing Association, San Francisco.

Schubert, G. (1978). *Introduction to clinical supervision in speech pathology.* St. Louis: Warren H. Green.

Schubert, G., Miner, A., & Till, J. (1973). *The Analysis of Behaviors of Clinicians (ABC) System.* Grand Forks: University of North Dakota.

Sergiovanni, T., & Starratt, R. (1979). *Supervision: Human perspectives.* New York: McGraw-Hill.

Shriberg, L., Bless, D., Carlson, K., Filley, F., Kwiatkowski, J., & Smith, M. (1976). *Grade point average, personality, and clinical competence.* Paper presented at the annual convention of the American Speech and Hearing Association, Houston, TX.

Shriberg, L., Filley, F., Hayes, D., Kwiatkowski, J., Schatz, J., Simmons, K., & Smith, M. (1975). The Wisconsin Procedure for Appraisal of Clinical Competence (W-PACC): Model and data. *Asha, 17,* 158-165.

Smith, K., & Anderson, J. (1982). Development and validation of an individual supervisory conference rating scale for use in speech-language pathology. *Journal of Speech and Hearing Research, 25,* 252-261.

Stuve, C. (1977). *The effect of supervisors' positive, negative, and neutral reinforcement on clinician performance, attitudes, and client performance.* Unpublished master's thesis, New Mexico State University, Las Cruces.

Thompson, C. (1988). *Observation modes and the attribution model in clinical supervision.* Unpublished master's thesis, New Mexico State University, Las Cruces.

Thorlacius, J. (1980). *Changes in supervisory behavior resulting from training in clinical supervision.* Paper presented at the annual meeting of the American Education Research Association, Boston. (EDRS No. ED 211 506, SP 019 343).

Underwood, J. (1979). *Underwood category system for analyzing supervisor-clinician behavior.* Unpublished manuscript, University of Northern Colorado, Greeley.

Weiss, R. (1983). *INREAL Training Evaluation Model (ITEM)* (revised). Unpublished interaction analysis system used in INREAL training, University of Colorado, Boulder.

Weller, R. (1971). *Verbal communication in instructional supervision.* New York: Teachers College Press, Columbia University.

PART FOUR
Research

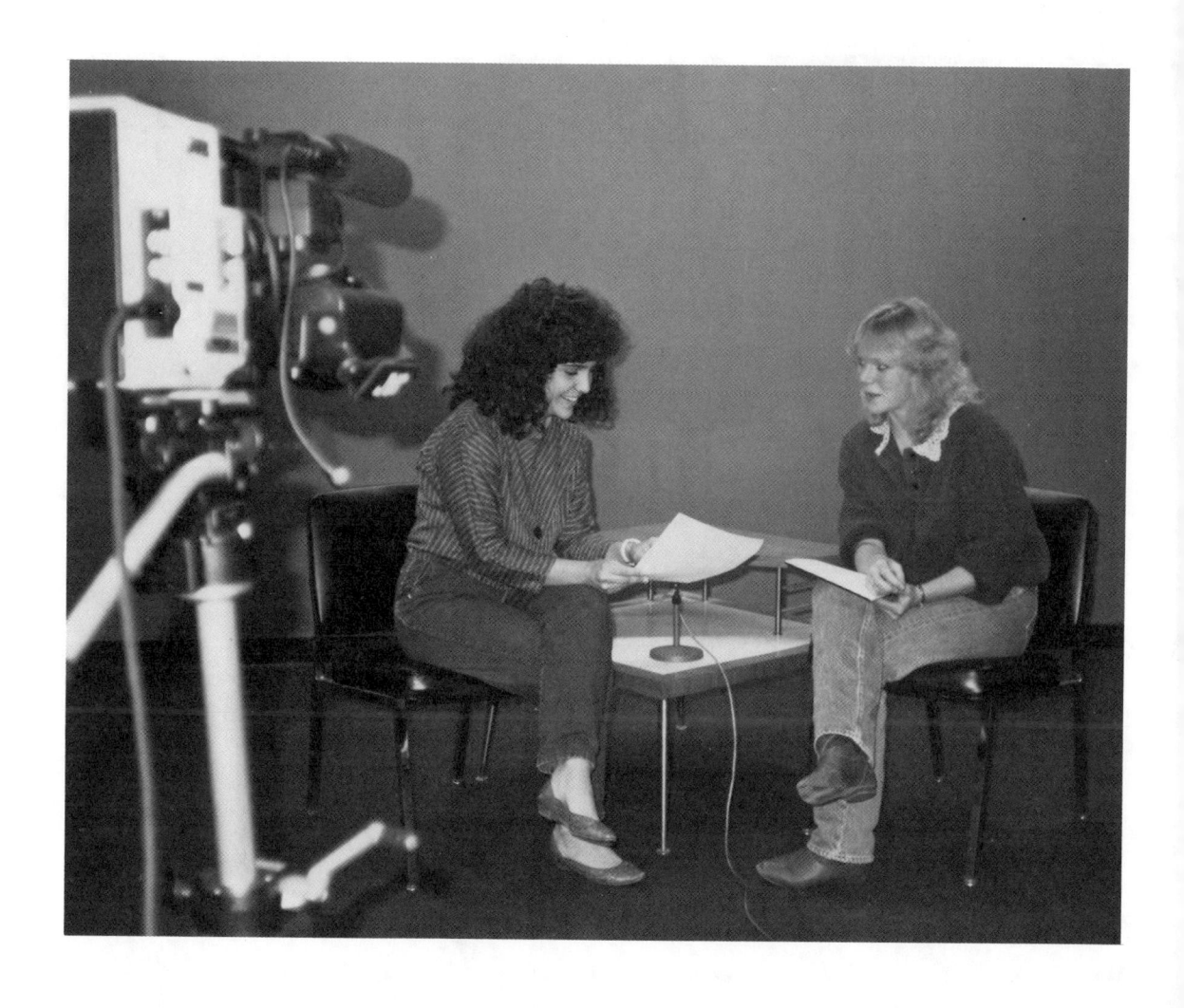

12
Research: Past, Present, Future

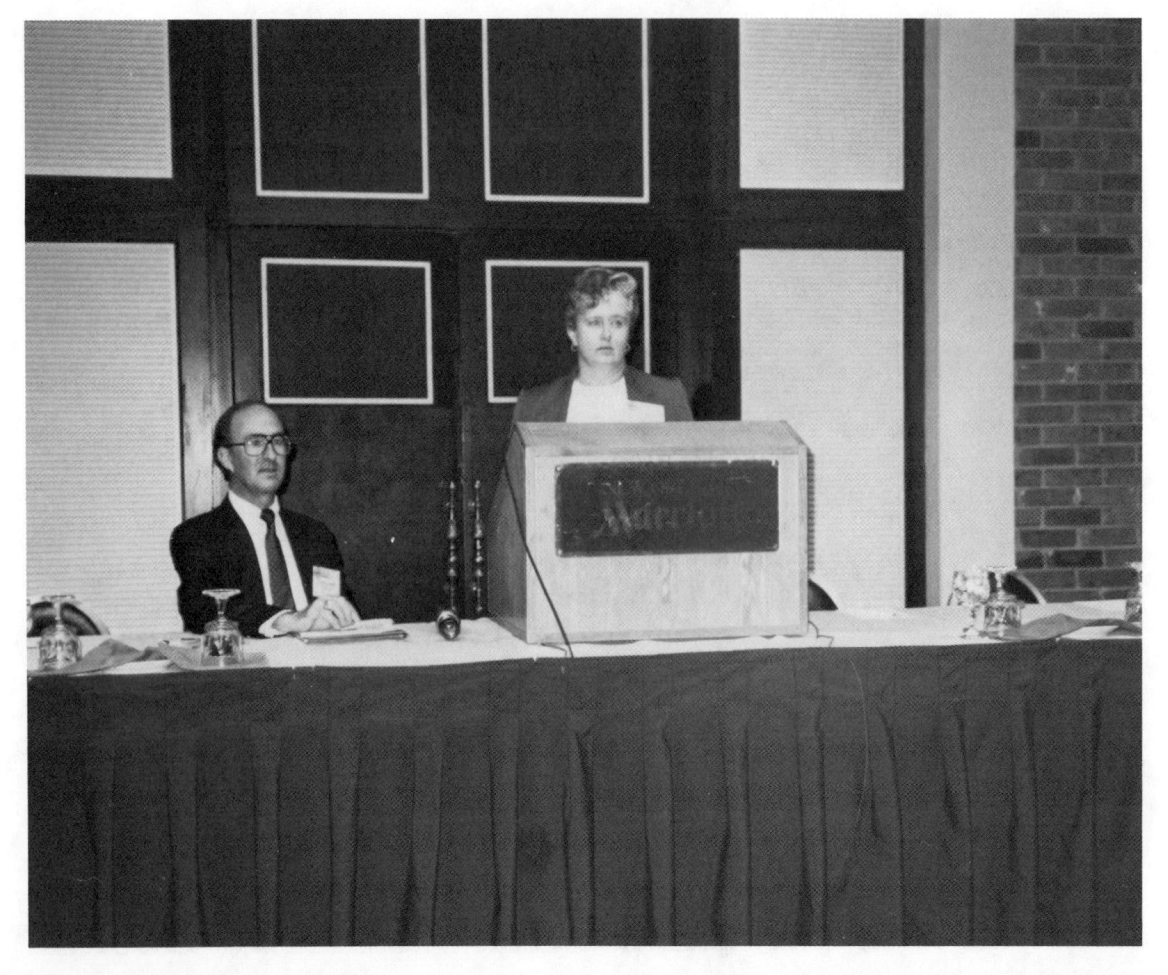

CRITICAL CONCEPTS

- ☐ *Two basic approaches to research exist: qualitative and quantitative.*
- ☐ *Methodological designs can be presented pictographically.*
- ☐ *Supervision research publications cluster into five areas: evaluation, supervisee perceptions of and expectations for supervision, interpersonal functioning in supervision, interpersonal conditions in supervisory conferences, and supervisory conferences.*
- ☐ *Researchers need to be aware of five research considerations: protection of human subjects, anonymity of data, tools for data collection, training of coders, and analysis of data.*
- ☐ *A strong need exists for preservice and service-level research.*

OUTLINE

INTRODUCTION

RESEARCH METHODOLOGY AND DESIGN
Qualitative Designs
Quantitative Designs

WHAT WE KNOW ABOUT THE SUPERVISORY PROCESS IN SPEECH-LANGUAGE PATHOLOGY AND AUDIOLOGY
Evaluation
Supervisee Perceptions of and Expectations for Supervision
Interpersonal Functioning in the Supervisory Process
Interpersonal Conditions in the Supervisory Conference
Supervisory Conferences

RESEARCH CONSIDERATIONS
Protection of Human Subjects
Anonymity of Data
Tools for Data Collection
Training of Coders and Reliable Data
Analysis of Data
Personal Growth Research

SUPERVISION RESEARCH AND THE FUTURE
PREAC Considerations
Supervisory Questions to be Answered

SUMMARY

APPLICATIONS

INTRODUCTION

Supervision, as a discipline, has come of age. Early discussions of supervision in the Speech-Language Pathology and Audiology literature expressed concern about the ability of clinicians to work independently given the generally low quality and quantity of supervision provided, at that time, in training programs. The volume of literature in supervision has gradually grown, with much of the early work devoted to opinions and theories about what supervision should be and only occasional, minimal descriptive data. Later work evolved to become increasingly research-oriented and enhanced in scholarly rigor.

Of critical importance has been the surge of interest in supervision since the 1960s. With the increased attention to supervision has come the

---

This chapter was contributed by Susann S. Dowling, University of Houston.

need to expand our knowledge about the phenomenon, and this has been done through substantial growth in supervision research.

The professional organization for supervisors, CUSPSPA, has helped to build interest in supervision and to encourage supervisory process research. Its network for research encourages the sharing of ideas, skills, bibliographies, and course syllabi. Most important, the organization serves as a means to establish and maintain nationwide contact among supervisors and supervision researchers.

The supervisor's five roles, Professional, Researcher, Educator, Administrator, and Clinician, have never been more important than now. The primary purpose of this chapter is to enhance your research ability, but research participation is also likely to make you a more well-rounded professional, a better educator and clinician, and a more efficient administrator.

The first section of this chapter describes the research that has been done in supervision and the statistical designs that have been used to analyze the data. The second section summarizes what is known about supervision as a result of that research. A third section is devoted to factors that must be considered in planning personal growth and scholarly research. Finally, considerations for future research are identified.

RESEARCH METHODOLOGY AND DESIGN

Supervisory research in speech-language pathology and audiology is diverse in scope and has used a variety of methodologies and statistical designs. Research has been both qualitative and quantitative. This section will give potential researchers a sense of the work done in the field, the types of questions asked, the research designs and statistics used to address the issues, and some strengths and weaknesses of the various approaches.

Qualitative Designs

When a new concept, process, or procedure is introduced in supervision, it generally appears in an expository scholarly article. Much of the early work in supervision fell into the category of new concepts introduced to stimulate discussion and appropriate action. Villareal (1964) and Kleffner (1964) both expressed concern about the importance of supervision and of supervisory qualifications. Similarly, in 1978, the ASHA Supervision Committee reported on the status of supervision in Speech-Language Pathology and Audiology. Each of these articles was primarily a call for action. But other kinds of thought pieces have been and continue to be published. For example, Ward and Webster (1965a) addressed the need to help clinicians enter into effective interpersonal relationships. Caracciolo, Rigrodsky, and Morrison (1978a) discussed the application of Rogerian theory to the supervisory process, and Pickering (1977) analyzed the communication concepts operating in the supervisory relationship. Thought articles, whether they call for action or present new concepts, continue to make valuable contributions to the supervisory literature.

Similarly, scholarly articles sometimes introduce new processes. These articles typically give a description of the approach, the author's impressions of its potential impact, and suggestions for implementation. The Boone and Prescott (1972) Content and Sequence Analysis of Speech and Hearing Therapy was introduced in this manner, as was the Culatta and Seltzer (1976) Content and Sequence Analysis of the Supervisory Session. Both instruments are observation systems designed to objectify the observation of behavior. The observer uses them to chart the frequency and sequence of defined categories of behavior, in treatment sessions and supervisory conferences, respectively. The articles introducing these systems gave examples of data to be collected and showed how to calculate ratios for the purpose of interpreting the findings.

The UTD (University of Texas at Dallas) Competency Based Evaluation System (Lougeay-Mottinger, Harris, Perlstein-Kaplan, & Felicetti, 1984), a clinical evaluation tool, and the Teaching Clinic, a peer-group method of supervision (Dowling, 1979b), were written to introduce new procedures to the field in a descriptive manner. Such new tools and concepts often provide the seeds for new research, as users gather outcome data when they implement the methods. One form of research in its broadest sense, then, is the descriptive thought article that introduces a new concept, process, or procedure.

Supervisory research may also have a qualitative focus. This type of research is often said to be sociological or phenomenological. Its purpose is to describe behavior in its natural state. The researcher observes, organizes, and interprets the behaviors. The data are descriptive and are given minimal statistical manipulation, if any. The design or layout of data varies depending on the types of questions asked.

Pickering's research (1984) is a prime example of qualitative methodology. She investigated supervisor and supervisee conference talk behavior in speech-language pathology supervisory conferences. The subjects in the study were 10 clinicians and 2 supervisors. The middle 10 to 15 minutes of each supervisory conference were audiotaped over a semester, a total of 84 taped segments. At the end of the semester, 40 of the segments were randomly selected, so that each of the 10 clinicians was represented by four tapes, one at the beginning of the semester, two in the middle, and one at the end. The researcher transcribed the tapes and analyzed them using seven *sensitizing concepts,* such as "Sharing aspects of one's humanness." The outcome of this research was a description and interpretation by the experimenter of the interpersonal climate of the supervisory conference. Although the intent was not quantitative, the research design shown in Figure 12-1 was used for data collection.

Qualitative research is a legitimate, viable approach to analyzing the supervisory process. Its strength is that it allows researchers to consider the process from a variety of philosophical view-

FIGURE 12-1
Qualitative design

	Supervisor 1					Supervisor 2			
Clinician	Tape 1	Tape 2	Tape 3	Tape 4	Tape 1	Tape 2	Tape 3	Tape 4
1	N=1	N=1	N=1	N=1	N=1	N=1	N=1	N=1
2	N=1	N=1	N=1	N=1	N=1	N=1	N=1	N=1
3	N=1	N=1	N=1	N=1	N=1	N=1	N=1	N=1
4	N=1	N=1	N=1	N=1	N=1	N=1	N=1	N=1
5	N=1	N=1	N=1	N=1	N=1	N=1	N=1	N=1

Dependent variables: 7 sensitizing concepts
Raw data: Conference talk behaviors
Statistic used: None

Source. "Interpersonal Communication in Speech-Language Pathology Supervisory Conferences: A Qualitative Study" by M. Pickering, 1984, *Journal of Speech and Hearing Disorders, 49,* pp. 189-195.

points and to integrate a wide range of information conceptually. A key advantage is ease of implementation. The method does not require knowledge of statistical techniques, although information about research design will maximize the quality of the collected data. This approach is an excellent resource for both accomplished and beginning researchers.

Qualitative research clearly also has limitations that potential researchers should consider before selecting it as a methodology. The data, once collected, may seem unwieldy and difficult to interpret. Although researchers organize the data according to selected criteria, such as the sensitizing concepts in the Pickering (1984) study, the information remains in its raw form and is not condensed quantitatively during the analysis. The generalizability of the data may also be limited. Finally, this type of research may be difficult to publish, as it is likely to come under attack from more quantitatively oriented researchers.

What kinds of questions could be addressed using a qualitative approach? The range of options is limitless; qualitative research can be used to describe any process in the clinical and supervisory environment. For example, if a researcher wants to explore types of behavior that occur in conferences on strategy development, a descriptive record of a sample of supervisor-supervisee statements about future planning could be made. The researcher would then be able to assess and describe the range of these behaviors. Qualitative, descriptive baseline data are needed in most cases before intervention is implemented to help supervisors predict the impact of specific supervisory tactics.

Quantitative Designs

Quantitative research approaches can be either nonparametric or parametric. If a researcher has decided against a qualitative approach for a particular question, then, nonparametric and parametric methodologies emerge as options. Nonparametric statistics allows the researcher to tabulate nominal, ordinal, and some interval data. Parametric statistics, such as the analysis of variance, is limited to interval or ratio level data. If the underlying assumptions about the research sample are met, parametric statistical methods are typically the more powerful (Siegel, 1956). A valuable research design resource is the text by Silverman (1977).

Nonparametric Procedures

Sign Test. An example of research using nonparametric statistics is a study by Sleight (1984 b) in which supervisors' self-evaluations were compared to evaluations by their supervisees. The supervisors rated themselves, and the supervisees completed a supervisor evaluation scale at the end of the term. The supervisors' mean scores per item for themselves were compared to those given by their supervisees using a nonparametric sign test. The design for the analysis appears in Figure 12-2.

Chi-Square. Chi-square, another nonparametric statistical method, has been used by several researchers, including Farmer (1984), Dowling and Bliss (1984), and Roberts and Naremore (1983), to answer the question of whether observed behaviors differed from those that were expected. Farmer (1984) compared untrained and trained coders' abilities to identify a supervisor's varying levels of verbal and nonverbal interpersonal communication pacing during the first 5 minutes of a supervisory conference. The four levels of verbal and nonverbal interpersonal communication pacing were presented on separate videotapes as follows: on Tape 1, the supervisor paced the clinician's verbal behavior but not the nonverbal; on Tape 2, the nonverbal behavior was paced but not the verbal; on Tape 3, both nonverbal and verbal behavior were paced; on Tape 4, neither nonverbal nor verbal behavior was paced. Half of the students viewing the tapes were trained to identify the verbal and nonverbal interpersonal communication pacing, and

FIGURE 12-2
Sign test design

Supervisor	Clinician
N = 8	N = 35

Dependent variables: 42 items from supervisor evaluation scale
Raw data: Supervisor, clinician ratings on supervisor scale
Statistic used: Sign Test

Source. "Supervisor Self-Evaluation in Communication Disorders" by C. Sleight, 1984b, *The Clinical Supervisor, 2,* 31-42.

half were not. The two groups of subjects, trained and untrained, were randomly assigned to view the four tapes. The data were assessed for differences between the untrained and trained observers' abilities to identify supervisor pacing. A two-by-two chi-square was used to analyze observed versus expected behavior for the two groups. The format for the analysis appears in Figure 12-3.

Nonparametric methods are important in the repertoire of the supervisory researcher because many data collection tools do not generate interval or ratio level data. Moreover, if sample sizes are small, nonparametrics are the methods of choice. Use of nonparametrics is likely to increase as single-subject designs are implemented in supervision research (see p. 338).

Parametric Methods. Parametric methods have been widely used in supervisory research. The examples that follow used correlation, a t-test, univariate analysis of variance, factor analysis, and multivariate analyses of variance. This list does not exhaust the range of parametric statistical methods. The appropriate method

FIGURE 12-3
Chi-square design

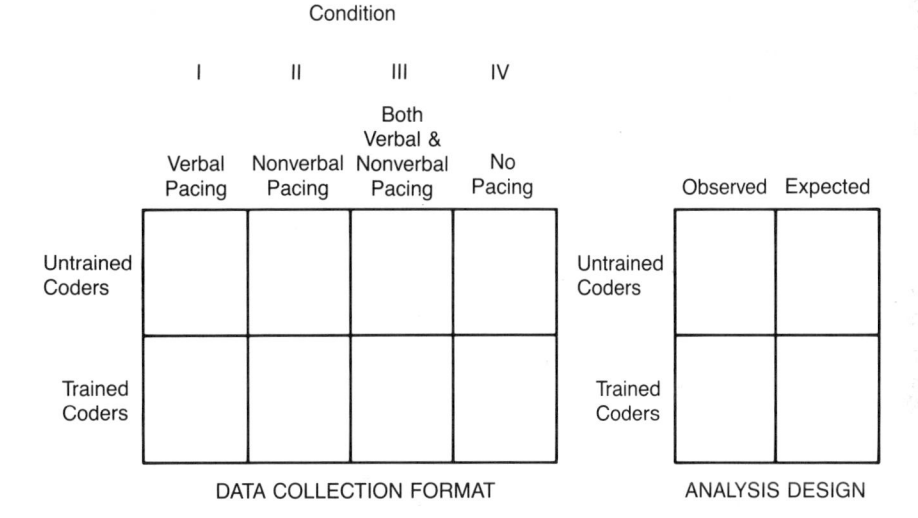

Condition

	I	II	III	IV		Observed	Expected
	Verbal Pacing	Nonverbal Pacing	Both Verbal & Nonverbal Pacing	No Pacing			
Untrained Coders					Untrained Coders		
Trained Coders					Trained Coders		

DATA COLLECTION FORMAT · · · · · · · · · · ANALYSIS DESIGN

Dependent variables: Ratings of the supervisor's verbal and nonverbal pacing behaviors
Raw data: Subjects completed Pacing Identification Form
Statistic used: Chi-square

Source. Supervisory Conferences in Communicative Disorders: Verbal and Nonverbal Interpersonal Communication Pacing by S. Farmer, 1984, doctoral dissertation, University of Colorado-Boulder.

depends on the type of data to be collected and the underlying research design.

Univariate analysis. A necessary decision within parametric statistics is whether to use a univariate or multivariate approach. *Univariate* means that the research has one or a limited number of dependent variables. With more than one dependent variable, univariate methods can still be used if the dependent variables are treated in the design layout as independent variables. Three or four dependent variables can be tested individually using a univariate statistic such as a t-test. The risk of this procedure lies in the increased probability of making a Type I alpha statistical error. This risk results from rejecting the null hypothesis inappropriately. In essence, the researcher says a finding is significant when in reality it is not.

If the research question involves several dependent variables, the researcher should proceed cautiously. A multivariate design may be selected to minimize the potential for alpha error, or a factor analysis can be used to reduce the number of variables. The researcher may need to study these topics in much greater depth. They are discussed in most statistics texts.

Correlational designs have been used successfully in supervisory research. They show the degree of relationship between variables. An example is the work of Smith and Anderson (1982b). This complex study assessed the perceived effectiveness of supervisory conferences in relation to the talk behaviors occurring in them, as measured by the M.O.S.A.I.C.S. observation system (Weller, 1971). The researcher conducted a factor analysis of the data from the Individual Conference Rating Scale (Smith, 1978), an 18-item conference evaluation scale that was used to rate the effectiveness of the conference. The factors identified were correlated to the actual talk behaviors during the conferences. One part of the study, as shown in Figure 12-4, correlated the direct and indirect factors that emerged from the factor analysis with each of the 42 M.O.S.A.I.C.S. categories from the perspective of the supervisee, supervisor, and trained raters.

Caracciolo, Rigrodsky, and Morrison (1978b)

	Supervisee	Supervisor	Trained Rater
Direct Variables	N=15	N=15	N=3
Indirect Variables	N=15	N=15	N=3

Dependent variables: 42 categories of M.O.S.A.I.C.S. observation system
Raw data: Conference effectiveness, data collected with the Individual Conference Rating Scale, and conference talk behaviors coded with the M.O.S.A.I.C.S. observation system
Statistic used: Correlation

Source. "Relationship of Perceived Effectiveness to Content in Supervisory Conferences in Speech-Language Pathology" By K. Smith and J. Anderson, 1982, *Journal of Speech and Hearing Research,* 25, pp. 243-251.

FIGURE 12-4
Correlational design

used t-tests and other statistical methods to consider graduate students' perceptions of the interpersonal conditions in the supervisory relationship. They evaluated four aspects of supervisor interpersonal functioning: level of regard, empathetic understanding, unconditionality of regard, and congruence. They measured 40 students' perceptions of the existence of these conditions at the beginning of a 9-week study, in the middle, and at the end. The students' mean perceptions or ratings for each of the four variables were compared from the beginning of the study to the end and from the middle to the end. T-tests were used to determine whether perceptions had changed at the designated intervals in the study. The design of the study appears in Figure 12-5.

T-tests were also used by Oratio (1978b) to compare supervisor and clinician perceptions of one therapy session. The session was rated both by the supervisor and by the graduate student clinicians immediately following the session. The items on the clinical evaluation scale were clustered into five categories: interpersonal relationship, technical skill, target behavior, client rapport, and therapy feedback. The mean rating for the clinicians in each of the five categories was compared to that of the supervisors using a product-moment correlation. T-tests were then used to determine whether the correlation coefficients differed significantly from zero, as demonstrated in Figure 12-6.

Analysis of variance (ANOVA) has also been used in supervisory research. Brasseur and Anderson (1983) wanted to know whether observers, supervisors, graduate students, and undergraduates with no clinical experience could identify direct and indirect supervisory styles in videotaped conferences. Videotapes of a direct, an indirect, and a combined direct/indirect supervisory conference were developed. Thirty supervisors, 30 graduate students, and 30

	Time 1	Time 2	Time 3
Level of Regard	N = 40	N = 40	N = 40
Empathetic Understanding	N = 40	N = 40	N = 40
Unconditional Regard	N = 40	N = 40	N = 40
Congruence	N = 40	N = 40	N = 40

Dependent variables: Level of regard, empathetic understanding, unconditionality of regard, and congruence
Raw data: Data collected from the Barrett-Lennard Relationship Inventory
Statistic used: t-test

Source: "Perceived Interpersonal Conditions and Professional Growth of Master's Level Speech-Language Pathology Students During the Supervisory Process" by G. Caracciolo, S. Rigrodsky, and E. Morrison, 1978, *Asha, 20,* pp. 467-477.

FIGURE 12-5
T-test design

	Supervisor Ratings	Clinician Ratings
Interpersonal Relationship	N = 45	N = 45
Technical Skill	N = 45	N = 45
Target Behavior	N = 45	N = 45
Client Rapport	N = 45	N = 45
Therapy Feedback	N = 45	N = 45

Dependent variables: x cluster scores from the 27-item clinical evaluation tool subdivided into five categories
Raw data: Supervisor and clinician self ratings of one therapy session
Statistic used: t-test, correlation

Source: "Comparative Perceptions of Therapeutic Effectiveness by Student Clinicians and Clinical Supervisors," by A. Oratio, 1978, *Asha, 20,* pp. 952–962.

FIGURE 12-6
T-test, correlational design

undergraduates were randomly assigned to view one of the three videotaped conference types. Thirty other individuals sampled to represent the above groups equally viewed all three. Each subject rated the conference using an 18-item Individual Supervisory Conference Rating Scale (Smith, 1978). A factor analysis of the data resulted in the emergence of four concepts: indirect statements, evaluation, suggestion, and suggestion/evaluation. As shown in Figure 12-7, a separate two-way analysis of variance was completed for each of the four concepts, comparing the observer (supervisor, graduate, or undergraduate) and the type of conference observed (direct, indirect, or direct/indirect).

Factor analysis. Factor analysis is generally used with research instruments such as clinical or supervisory rating scales and attitude surveys. These tools consist of multiple items that are intended to be the dependent variables in a study. It is often unclear at the outset which variables are relevant to the question at hand, and the researcher wishes to incorporate only the critical items. Also, on a practical level, large numbers of dependent variables require substantial increases in sample size (number of subjects) for adequate power (ability to reject the null hypothesis when it should be rejected) in the research design. Factor analysis allows the researcher to reduce the number of dependent variables by identifying a number of items that reflect one concept. Data from these items can then be grouped as one factor, substantially reducing the number of dependent variables. Remember that in the Brasseur and Anderson (1983) study, the 18-item rating scale used to observe videotaped conferences was reduced to 4 factors through factor analysis. A computer will be needed to complete such an analysis because of the complexity of the process.

Multivariate analysis. Multivariate analysis has been used in supervisory research in studies by Roberts and Naremore (1983) and Oratio, Sugarman, and Prass (1981). Multivariate analysis by definition incorporates more than one dependent variable. The same types of data collection

Conference Style

	Direct	Indirect	Direct/Indirect
Supervisors	N = 10	N = 10	N = 10
Graduate Students	N = 10	N = 10	N = 10
Undergraduate Students	N = 10	N = 10	N = 10

Dependent variables: Four direct/Indirect variables resulting from a factor analysis of the raw data
Raw data: Respondents' conference evaluations collected with the Individual Supervisory Conference Rating Scale
Statistic used: Analysis of variance (ANOVA)

Source. "Observed Differences Between Direct, Indirect, and Direct/Indirect Videotaped Supervisory Conferences" by J. Brasseur and J. Anderson, 1983, *Journal of Speech and Hearing Research, 26,* pp. 349–477.

FIGURE 12-7
Analysis of Variance (ANOVA) design

tools, observation systems, evaluation rating scales, and attitude surveys identified as likely candidates for factor analysis are typically used in multivariate research. In this case, however, all of the items are kept in the analysis as dependent measures.

Another example of a multivariate study is the Dowling, Sbaschnig, and Williams (1982) study that assessed the reliability and validity of the Culatta and Seltzer (1976) interaction analysis instrument, Content and Sequence Analysis of the Supervisory Session. In this study, three supervisors supervised each of four students who were all at different clock hour levels. The 12 supervisor-supervisee pairs audiotaped their conferences at three points during the term. Trained coders used the Culatta and Seltzer system to record the middle 5 minutes of each of the conferences. The supervisor/supervisee categories from the Culatta and Seltzer system were the dependent variables, and the independent variables were the supervisors, clock hour levels, and time. The goal was to determine whether the observation system could reliably assess the talk behaviors that occurred in the conferences. Because of the complexity of the design, Figure 12-8 represents the design at just one of the three data collection points.

Several examples have been presented of studies that used parametric statistics, ranging from correlational to multivariate analysis. Research using parametric analysis generally requires some background in statistics, although correlation, t-tests, and simple analysis of variance require minimal training. Researchers need greater sophistication for the more complex designs. With guidance, patience, and persistence, most univariate statistics can be calculated with a paper and pencil. Factor analysis falls somewhere between univariate and multivariate analysis in its complexity.

Research designs that use quantitative statistics are legitimate scholarly undertakings. Nonparametrics are easier to use and are appropriate

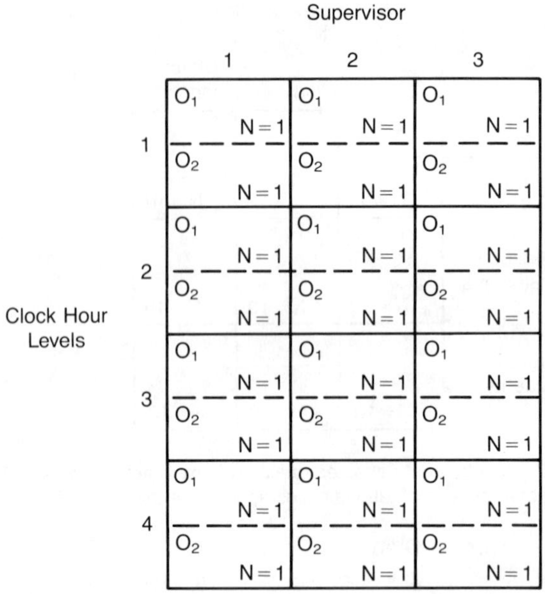

Supervisor

		1	2	3
Clock Hour Levels	1	O_1 N=1 / O_2 N=1	O_1 N=1 / O_2 N=1	O_1 N=1 / O_2 N=1
	2	O_1 N=1 / O_2 N=1	O_1 N=1 / O_2 N=1	O_1 N=1 / O_2 N=1
	3	O_1 N=1 / O_2 N=1	O_1 N=1 / O_2 N=1	O_1 N=1 / O_2 N=1
	4	O_1 N=1 / O_2 N=1	O_1 N=1 / O_2 N=1	O_1 N=1 / O_2 N=1

Dependent variables: Talk categories from the Culatta and Seltzer Supervisory Conference Analyses of the Supervisory Session
Raw data: Coded supervisor/supervisee conference talk behaviors
Statistic used: Multivariate analysis of variance (ANOVA)

Source. "Culatta and Seltzer Content and Sequence Analysis of the Supervisory Session: A Question of Reliability and Validity?" by S. Dowling, K. Sbaschnig, and C. Williams, 1982, *Journal of Communication Disorders, 15,* 353-362.

FIGURE 12-8
Multivariate Analysis of Variance (MANOVA) design

for nominal, ordinal, and some interval data. They are particularly helpful in studies using a limited number of subjects. Care must be taken to monitor scholarly rigor in designs involving nonparametrics, as this is often the area in which these designs are criticized when submitted for publication.

Parametric statistics typically require greater sophistication on the part of the researcher. Interval data or ratio level data are required for their use. Sample sizes necessary to test a hypothesis vary with the number of variables in the design and the statistic selected for the analysis. The greatest danger in using parametric statistics is misuse. For example, using a statistic when the underlying assumptions have not been met raises a serious question about the validity of the findings.

The information presented here about qualitative and quantitative research does not exhaust the possible methods of analysis approaches for supervisory research. For the beginning researcher, it is meant to provide a starting point for thought and planning.

WHAT WE KNOW ABOUT THE SUPERVISORY PROCESS IN SPEECH-LANGUAGE PATHOLOGY AND AUDIOLOGY

Evaluation

Evaluation of supervisee performance has been discussed extensively among practicing supervisors (see chapter 11). Multitudes of evaluation tools exist, ranging widely in types and quantity of items. Unfortunately, few of the tools have been validated empirically. The several studies that follow have considered evaluation of supervisees from a variety of viewpoints.

Schalk and Peroff (1972), in a study of supervisory reliability and consistency, asked 20 supervisors to rate the same videotape of articulation therapy on two occasions. Substantial intersupervisor variability was found; different supervisors tended to rate the videotape differently. Supervisors appeared to interpret the numbers on the rating scale variably, some tending to rate high or low. The supervisors were also found to be internally consistent, in that their second viewings produced results similar to the first.

Two studies have investigated whether the consistency of supervisors' ratings can be increased. Hagler and Fahey's (1982) intent was to reduce the variability of supervisors' ratings when they used the W-PACC (Shriberg, Filley, Hayes, Kwiatkowski, Schatz, Simmons, & Smith, 1975) to evaluate clinicians. Half of the 32 supervisors in the sample received information about typical ratings of clinical performance on the W-PACC (means and standard deviations of previous students' performance). The information was found to have no impact; variability of clinicians' ratings remained high.

Sbaschnig and Williams (1983) attempted to reduce supervisor variability both in supervisory conferences and in ratings of clinicians. Specific criteria for supervision were established. Supervisors were required to videotape each clinician twice per term, complete an evaluation observation checklist at least five times per term, hold a conference with the supervisee each week, write a summary of each conference, and end each conference by commenting on a strength of the supervisee. In addition, supervisors viewed, rated, and discussed three videotapes with the intent of reaching consensus on individual item ratings. The goal was to reduce variability of mean scores to less than .5 on the rating scale. The students supervised did perceive an increase in consistency among supervisors in that program.

Of serious concern were findings by Andersen (1981) that highlighted the susceptibility of supervisors to bias when evaluating supervisees. Fifty-two supervisors received fabricated clinician information about grade point average, earned clock hours, and evaluations of previous clinical and conference behavior. The supervisors then viewed a videotape of the clinician in therapy and were found to rate the clinician differently depending on the previously provided information. Grade point average and prior evaluations markedly influenced the supervisor's perceptions of performance.

Similarly, Roberts and Naremore (1983) found that supervisors approached imagined supervisory situations with preconceptions about what elements to observe, how to explain behavior, and general strategies for responding to a good or poor therapy session. In imagined sessions, the supervisors wanted more information about the clinician's background and about the session in general if the session was going poorly. More causal information was given for poor sessions, and supervisors thought they would be more likely to intervene if the session were poor. In general, supervisors tended to feel that clinicians in poor sessions were unlikely to change, citing underlying factors such as ability. Supervisors also perceived clinicians as primarily responsible for the success or failure of the clinical session.

The question of whether supervisees are accurate evaluators of their own behavior has also been considered, but results vary markedly. Oratio (1978b) had each of 21 beginning graduate students rate one of their own sessions from memory during the eighth week of a term and compared the ratings to those of their supervisors, completed while the session was being observed. He found that supervisors rated both client and clinician performance slightly higher than did the supervisees.

Dowling (1984) compared graduate students' own ratings, peer ratings, and supervisors' ratings of videotaped therapy segments. A 10-minute segment of each graduate student's therapy was rated by the student from memory; a videotape of that therapy was viewed and rated by the student, four peers, and three supervisors. All of the viewers rated the therapy similarly. Graduate students appeared to be accurate raters of both their own and their peers' clinical behavior.

Supervisee Perceptions of and Expectations for Supervision

Only a limited number of studies have addressed supervisees' perceptions of and expectations for supervision. An early study by Culatta, Colucci, and Wiggins (1975) compared 18 supervisors' expectations for 36 supervisees to those same clinicians' perceptions of those expectations. A marked gap existed. The supervisors' expectations for supervisees included pre-therapy conferences, a gradual transfer of client responsibility to supervisees, and a gradual decrease in the frequency of demonstration therapy by supervisors. Although the supervisees and supervisors were evaluating the same expectations for supervisor and supervisee behavior, there were considerable differences in how they evaluated the occurrence and frequency of occurrence of the behaviors. A serious breakdown in communication between supervisors and supervisees was documented in this research.

In a study by Dowling and Wittkopp (1982), students from six universities and at varying levels of clinical experience were assessed to determine their perceptions of the supervisory process. The major finding from this study was the variability of students' perceptions. The students used the supervisory experiences they had had as their model for supervision. Some had been observed in one out of three sessions, others in each session; both groups reported the patterns they had experienced as desirable. The respondents had little information about what should occur in the supervisory process, and their views were highly malleable. In related work, Larson (1982) determined that all supervisees expect and want to function actively in supervisory conferences. But Tihen (1984) found that clinicians' expectations for their supervisors varied with the level of clinical experience; more advanced clinicians had greater expectations for active involvement in the supervisory interaction.

In a study by Dowling (in press), students at three levels of clinical training (preclinical, undergraduate, and graduate) were asked to describe hypothetical typical and ideal conferences by completing a rating scale designed by Smith (1978) to evaluate supervisor and supervisee conference behavior. A significant gap was found between the two descriptions. Students expected typical conferences to be more direct and less positive than ideal conferences. Preclinical students had the most optimistic view of the supervisory process, followed by disillusionment after undergraduate clinical experience. By the time students had achieved graduate status, they reported a better feeling about typical conferences, even though they felt a substantial gap remained between typical and ideal.

Sleight (1985), using the Sleight Clinician Anxiety Test, compared an array of graduate students in regard to their confidence and anxiety about clinical practicum. Pre- and posttests were administered to a group of students prior to beginning practicum, to a second group involved only in observing treatment, and to a final group enrolled in their first clinical experience. Some of the students who were tested during their first clinical experience were tested again at the end of the second practicum and following a student teaching experience. Of the first three groups (preclinical, observation, first practicum), only those in practicum demonstrated significant differences in earlier and later measures. They showed decreased anxiety and increased confidence. A second practicum had no additional impact on confidence, but the student teaching experience substantially increased confidence.

Interpersonal Functioning in the Supervisory Process

Work in the interpersonal area has been based heavily on theories from disciplines other than speech-language pathology and audiology. A tool based on the work of Danish, D'Augelli, and Brock (1974) was used by Volz and Klevans (1979) to compare the verbal helping skills of new speech-language pathology graduate students to those of preclinical undergraduates. The two groups of students conducted peer interviews in which the interviewee discussed a personal problem. Helping skills were similar for the two groups, leading the researchers to believe that prior clinical experience alone (such as that of the graduate students) did not improve helping skills.

Volz, Klevans, Norton, and Putens (1978) identified a low level of helping skills in preclinical undergraduates and completed a series of studies to determine the strategies needed to teach these important skills. Students were assigned to three groups; one group was taught specific helping skills, another was taught role-learning principles, and the third was given information about clinical practice but none about interpersonal functioning. The helping skills group received both lecture information and structured practice in initial interactions, and the role-learning group practiced functioning in the prescribed roles. After training, each subject conducted an interview with a college-age role-played client concerned about an articulation problem. The three groups of students did not differ in their levels of helping skills. In a follow-up study, Klevans, Volz, and Friedman (1981) found that hands-on experience practicing helping skills was more effective than just training in how to use helping skills observation tools.

Dowling and Bliss (1984) explored cognitive complexity and rhetorical sensitivity, measures of interpersonal functioning in outstanding and failing clinicians. Cognitive complexity data were obtained by having subjects describe in writing someone they liked and someone they disliked; rhetorical sensitivity was sampled by means of a communication attitude survey. A cognitively complex, rhetorically sensitive person generally uses a more elaborated verbal code and can take the perspective of the listener and modify communication accordingly. Outstanding clinicians were expected to be superior on both measures. The findings did not substantiate the hypothesis; outstanding and failing clinicians could not be differentiated according to either of these parameters.

Farmer (1984) wanted to know whether trained and untrained coders differed in their ability to identify varying levels of verbal and nonverbal interpersonal communication pacing during the first 5 minutes of a supervisory conference. Pacing was defined as the supervisor's matching of the supervisee's verbal and/or nonverbal behavior. Four variations of pacing were presented, from no pacing to pacing of both verbal and nonverbal dimensions. Trained coders were significantly more proficient at identifying the exhibited pacing behaviors.

Interpersonal Conditions in the Supervisory Conference

A primary focus of research in speech-language pathology has been the interpersonal conditions existing in the supervisory conference. Caracciolo, Rigrodsky, and Morrison (1978b) examined graduate students' perceptions of those conditions and of their own professional growth during a 9-week study. Three tools were used. The Barrett-Lennard Relationship Inventory (1962) identified the students' perceptions of the supervisors' level of regard, unconditionality of regard, empathetic understanding, and congruence (Rogers, 1957). The Index of Adjustment and Values (Bills, Vance, & McClean, 1951) was used to measure changes in professional self-esteem, and a rating scale was used to judge clinical performance. A unique feature of this study was that the eight supervisors who took part were trained; they had completed an academic course in supervision and a supervision practicum. The 40 graduate clinicians felt that supervisors provided more positive than negative interpersonal conditions throughout the relationship. As a result of the facilitative interpersonal conditions, the gap between the clinicians' real and ideal professional selves narrowed, and professional self-esteem grew. The clinicians' self-ratings of clinical performance also improved throughout the study.

McCrea (1980) developed the McCrea Adapted Scales to assess interpersonal functioning in supervisory conferences. Based on the work of Carkhuff (1969), McCrea's study related supervisee self-exploration to the level of interpersonal facilitativeness provided by the supervisor in the conference. The supervisor's talk behaviors were observed for evidence of respect, empathic understanding, facilitative genuineness, and concreteness. The data indicated that supervisors assumed a static interpersonal set across conferences, providing conditions that were at best neutral. The levels of facilitative genuineness, concreteness, and respect were too low to stimulate supervisee self-exploration. McCrea felt that the supervisors exhibited underdeveloped interpersonal styles.

Pickering (1984) also examined interpersonal conditions in supervisory conferences. She analyzed forty 10-minute samples collected during the term from the middles of 2 supervisors' and 10 clinicians' audiotaped conferences. The tools for the qualitative analysis were sensitizing concepts derived from the work of Stewart and D'Angelo (1975) and three additional concepts evolved by the researcher. Two of the concepts were "Sharing aspects of one's humanness" and "Focusing on objective, cognitive issues." Pickering found that conferences were predominantly instructional, focused on the client and related progress. If interpersonal issues were addressed, they tended to involve the client and the discussion was solution-oriented. The relationship between the supervisor and the clinician was rarely discussed. Students tended to talk in cognitive, objective terms, although they did report past feelings more frequently than current feelings. Supervisors verbalized support and reinforced the clinicians during the conference, but tended not to reflect on feelings or interpret what clinicians had said. Supervisors rarely shared personal views during the conference. Pickering concluded that supervisors lacked skill in the interpersonal aspects of the conference.

Supervisory Conferences

The major focus of supervisory research has been the conference between supervisor and supervisee. Culatta and Seltzer (1976) pioneered the development of an observation system, the Content and Sequence Analysis of the Supervisory Session, to gather conference data. They found that supervisors dominated talk time, strategy development, and questioning in conferences, whereas supervisees provided the raw material for the conferences by giving information and observations about past events.

Culatta and Seltzer (1977) then used this tool as a feedback mechanism. Each of six supervisors verbally analyzed each of their conferences, with the researcher(s) listening passively. The researchers analyzed the first and last conferences of the term for each supervisor using the Content and Sequence Analysis of the Supervisory Session and found that supervisor behavior was static even though the supervisors had initially expressed a desire for change. Culatta and Seltzer felt that the analyses helped supervisors identify areas in need of change but were not sufficient to modify behavior.

Supervisor and supervisee ability to identify conference types was explored by Brasseur and Anderson (1983). (Refer to p. 323 for a description of the study design.) The supervisors and the two groups of supervisees (graduate and undergraduate) could readily distinguish between a direct conference and the remaining two conference types, indirect and direct/indirect. A conference that contained equal amounts of direct and indirect behavior was identified as indirect; degree of indirectness was not distinguished by the viewers. In addition, the scores of supervisors and supervisees, graduate or undergraduate, could not be differentiated, indicating that the three groups viewed the conferences similarly.

A final important finding from this study was the confirmation of the Individual Supervisory Conference Rating Scale (Smith, 1978) as a valid, reliable tool for identifying direct and indirect conference behaviors.

Smith and Anderson (1982b) investigated the relationship between the perceived effectiveness of conferences and the verbal interaction and content variables in those conferences. Fifteen supervisor/supervisee pairs audiotaped three conferences each during a 6-week period, for a total of 45 conferences. After each audiotaped conference, the supervisor and supervisee completed an Individual Conference Rating Scale indicating their perceptions of the conference. Individuals trained to use the M.O.S.A.I.C.S. (Weller, 1971) observation system then coded the verbal behaviors that occurred during 24 of the audiotaped conferences. Multiple findings were reported from this landmark study. In particular, direct and indirect supervisor behaviors and conference styles were defined. In indirect supervisory behavior, the supervisor used a supportive style, incorporated the supervisee's ideas into the conference, helped the supervisee set realistic client goals, and encouraged the supervisee to verbalize needs. In direct supervisory behavior, the supervisor used conference time to discuss clinician weaknesses and ways to improve materials, gave specific suggestions for therapy, and had a superior/subordinate relationship with the supervisee. During direct conferences, there were fewer questions and answers, minimal discussion of affect, less discussion of objectives, and a tendency to address methods and materials. Indirect conferences had more supervisee questions, more frequent discussions of affect, and a higher frequency of reflexive moves by the supervisor (reacting, responding, and summarizing).

Roberts and Smith (1982), in a post hoc analysis of the Smith (1978) data, considered the entirety of 45 conferences collected from 15 supervisor/supervisee pairs. The data were coded with the M.O.S.A.I.C.S. (Weller, 1971) observation system, and the dependent measures were five ratios calculated from that data. The ratios were initiatory/reflexive, analytic/evaluative, diagnostic/prescriptive, complex/simple, and participation/membership. Conferences were found to be static over time. The supervisors did more initiating in the conferences than did the supervisees, although the supervisors' behaviors fell equally into the categories of initiatory and reflexive. Thus, the supervisees responded predominately reflexively. The supervisors were reported to set the content and interaction patterns and guide the dialogue, and the supervisees passively followed that lead by responding, reacting, and in general participating less than the supervisors. Supervisors tended to give opinions and suggest tactics for future sessions, whereas supervisees reported facts about previous sessions. In interpreting the data, the authors felt that clinical supervision (colleagueship) was not occurring.

Kennedy (1981) studied the impact of written subjective and oral objective clinical feedback on subsequent conference talk behaviors. Each of the 18 supervisees was randomly assigned to one of the feedback conditions. The supervisory conferences were audiotaped, and two conferences per supervisee, a total of 36, were randomly selected. A 10-minute segment of each conference was coded with the M.O.S.A.I.C.S. (Weller, 1971) observation system. Kennedy found that both supervisor and supervisee talk behaviors in the conference were affected differently by the two types of feedback.

Cimorrell-Strong and Ensley (1982) examined conference talk behaviors to determine whether supervisee feedback to the supervisor would affect the content of conferences. The 16 supervisees were enrolled in a public school practicum. Nine supervisee/supervisor pairs were in the feedback condition, and seven were not. After each conference the supervisees in the feedback condition evaluated their supervisors in writing. All conferences were audiotaped during the 6-week study, and a 5-minute segment of each conference was coded using the Culatta and Seltzer (1976) Content and Sequence Analysis of the Supervisory Conference. Feedback to supervisors about their behavior had no impact on conference talk; the behaviors did not change. All conferences were dominated by supervisor talk, although supervisees in the feedback condition did ask more questions. Supervisors in the nonfeedback condition were more likely to provide bad evaluations.

The impact of conference type, direct or indirect, on subsequent supervisee clinical behavior was examined by Nilsen (1983). Ten supervisors and 31 supervisees participated in the study; all conferences were audiotaped, as were the therapy sessions preceding and following the conferences. The conferences were analyzed with the Blumberg (1980) observation system to determine the percentage of direct and indirect statements used by the supervisor. During the conferences, specific supervisee behaviors were targeted for change in subsequent sessions. After each conference, supervisees rated their perceptions of the supervisors' verbal style. Of the 31 conferences, only 5 were indirect conferences. If supervisors perceived that change was needed, they tended to use a direct style. An indirect style was used when there was no perceived need for behavioral change. Changes in supervisee clinical behavior were noted after direct conferences; although it could not be documented statistically, the researcher felt that even greater changes occurred after conferences that were a combination of direct and indirect. Interestingly, supervisees tended to perceive supervisor talk behavior as indirect even when it was primarily direct. The highest percentage of change of supervisee clinical behaviors occurred when the conference was on the day of the observation and the supervisee received a written observation checklist during the conference.

Shapiro (1985b) also studied the influence of specific conditions in the supervisory conference on subsequent therapy behavior. He studied the commitments made by 64 clinicians during 384 individual conferences collected from 12 universities and the outcomes of those commitments. Two clinician experience levels were represented in the study. Commitments were alternately verbal and written. The verbal and written agreements were presented in a counterbalanced order. The commitments were further classified by type (content). Shapiro found that the average number of commitments kept was affected by the type of commitment, oral or written, and by the order of the treatment conditions. The experience level of the clinician combined with the factor of oral or written commitment was also found to be significant.

Peaper (1984) analyzed supervisees' perceptions of conferences, and the impact of supervisees' planning of the conference agenda on those perceptions. Peaper developed a form to measure the perceived value of the conference. The 19 supervisees evaluated the conference at the outset of the study. The experimental group, 9 supervisees, developed the agendas for the seven remaining conferences with their supervisor. At the end of the study, all supervisees again completed a conference evaluation form. The only significant finding was that the supervisees who had planned the conference agendas felt they were able to set the tone of the meetings and had more opportunity to control the flow of the conference.

The talk behaviors in group supervisory conferences (Teaching Clinics) have been compared to conventional one-on-one conferences. In a study by Dowling and Shank (1981), two matched groups of five graduate clinicians and two supervisors each participated alternately in conventional and Teaching Clinic supervision for 4 weeks during an 8-week study. Conferences were videotaped at 2-week intervals and were sampled and coded with the Culatta and Seltzer (1976) Sequence and Content Analysis of the Supervisory Session. The talk behaviors in conventional and Teaching Clinic conferences could not be differentiated, indicating that the two methods elicited similar conference talk behaviors.

Later research by Dowling, Sbaschnig, and Williams (1982) indicated that the Culatta and Seltzer (1976) Content and Sequence Analysis of the Supervisory Session was neither valid nor reliable as a research tool. As a result, the data from the Dowling and Shank (1981) study were reanalyzed using the M.O.S.A.I.C.S. (Weller, 1971) observation system. The Teaching Clinic and conventional conferences were found to be significantly different. General and interpretive statements, explanations, and discussions of objectives occurred more frequently in conventional conferences. The conventional conferences appeared to be more indirect than the Teaching Clinic conferences (Dowling, 1983b).

In the Teaching Clinic conferences alone (Dowling, 1983a), supervisor, peer, and supervisee talk behavior could not be differentiated, indicating equality of verbal participation. The supervisors dominated in the categories of structuring and soliciting, but supervisees controlled strategy development. Objectives were discussed in the Teaching Clinics, and evaluation was minimal.

In a later study (Dowling, 1987), four groups of graduate students, 24 in all, participated in a total of 19 Teaching Clinics in conjunction with practicum. The Individual Conference Rating Scale developed by Smith (1978) and modified by Brasseur and Anderson (1983) was used to evaluate the conferences. Each supervisee completed two 18-item conference rating scales at the end of each Teaching Clinic, one to describe supervisor behavior and the other for that of peers. Peer and supervisor behaviors were perceived as significantly different; peers were thought to provide more suggestions, and supervisors were seen to function as teachers and superiors. Supervisors, even in this group process, tended to set the tone for each conference, as supervisees mirrored the type and quantity of the supervisors' verbal behaviors. The number of Teaching Clinics in which a group participated did affect the perceptions of both peers and supervisors, as did the clinician group in which a supervisee participated. Notably, an individual's role in the Teaching Clinic did not alter his or her perceptions of either peers or supervisors. The role of demonstration clinician was not as stressful as expected; assuming this function had no impact on the supervisee's perceptions of others' behavior.

The literature reported in this section has been drawn almost exclusively from published research and doctoral dissertations. A substantial body of information, presented as convention papers, also exists in unpublished form. Supervisory process research is steadily growing. Even now, what is known remains overshadowed by what is unknown. The section that follows is intended for readers whose interest is growing and for those contemplating research projects in supervision.

RESEARCH CONSIDERATIONS

In the planning and implementation stages of a project, a researcher needs to take great care to incorporate safeguards that protect and enhance the quality of collected data and of the study itself. Considerations such as the protection of human subjects, use of research tools, coder training, and data analysis are of utmost importance to research quality.

Protection of Human Subjects

The protection of human subjects is a critical issue. Subjects should be alerted to risks and/or benefits of participation in a study and should know that the researcher has taken every precaution to protect them. For example, they need to know whether information obtained from the study will be released and in what form. They need to know what they will be asked to do if they choose to participate and how much of their time it will take. The researcher, in all cases, needs to distribute release forms describing the study, subject involvement, and risks and benefits; depending on the risk involved, the subjects must agree in writing to participate in the study. Subjects must be able to refuse involvement knowing that their refusal will not have negative consequences for them. Participants must also be aware that they may choose to withdraw from a study at any time without penalty. It is in the researchers' and the subjects' best interests to keep signed release forms on file after the completion of the study.

Anonymity of Data

A component of human subject protection may also be used to enhance overall study quality. Subject anonymity, the assignment of a number or letter to an individual, reduces the possibility of data contamination due to a researcher's or coder's knowledge about the person involved. Behavior of known individuals may be interpreted differently. Similarly, each subject group needs to remain anonymous to avoid unintentional bias. If the researcher hypothesizes that a treatment will have a given outcome, he or she may unconsciously skew the posttreatment data in the direction predicted. Similarly, the data segments need to be in random order for data coding. This prevents, for example, the coding of all pretreatment data at one time, again with the intent of insuring anonymity and avoiding bias. For the same reasons, the researcher typically cannot be one of the subjects studied. Each of these anonymity measures requires added experimenter control but is essential for high-quality publishable research.

Tools for Data Collection

The selection of an appropriate data collection tool is often an arduous task because a limited number of reliable, valid tools is available. Indeed, an instrument may not exist to collect the exact data desired. Researchers often develop their own tools to gather data, but unless a researcher validates the tool before data collection and then assesses the reliability of data collected, the value of the results is questionable and the study is often unpublishable. It is not sufficient to have a group of individuals develop a tool, even though it is discussed at length, without further validation. Field testing, input from experts, and statistical assessment of validity and reliability must be conducted before data collection. Studies that can serve as resources and examples of the assessment of validity and reliability are Smith and Anderson (1982a), Brasseur and Anderson (1983), Casey (1980), and Dowling, Sbaschnig, and Williams (1982).

Training of Coders and Reliable Data

Many data collection tools require the experimenter to train others to code the data. Generally researchers should avoid coding their own data if any value judgments must be made. Knowledge of the test hypothesis opens the door to unintentional data contamination.

The first aspect of coder training is an exposure to the tool and then practice in coding data similar to those that will be collected in the study. Intercoder agreement with a criterion or expert coder is typically the first level of agreement established. The level of agreement considered acceptable is to some extent determined by the ambiguity of the system being used. After the establishment of intercoder agreement, intracoder consistency is assessed. Once an acceptable level of agreement has been established, actual data coding may begin. During coding of the real data, agreement should be sampled periodically. If agreement drops significantly, data coding may need to stop until agreement is re-established. After checking the various forms of coder agreement, the researcher should analyze the overall reliability of the data. A more extensive discussion of coder training and reliability can be found in Dowling (1979).

Analysis of Data

A final but important factor in research rigor is the selection of the appropriate statistic to analyze the data. Care must be taken to ensure that the data meet the conditions necessary for use of a given statistic. As noted in the section on research designs, take care to avoid repeated t-tests, one-way ANOVAs, or other univariate measures when multivariate analysis is more appropriate. The danger is a Type 1 alpha error, saying a finding is significant when in reality it is a function of chance alone. Similarly, the research design needs as much power as possible (the ability to reject the null hypothesis when it is false). Power can be calculated before data collection on the basis of pilot data. Problems with power tend to arise from two interrelated sources: design factors and number of subjects. The simpler or fewer variables in the design and the more subjects available, the greater the power or ability to identify a significant difference when it exists. Drawing a picture of the design often helps clarify the independent and dependent variables in the researcher's mind (see Figures 12-1 through 12-8). It may also be helpful to talk to a statistical consultant during the design phase of the study.

Personal Growth Research

The preceding section has been for experimenters who are interested in doing research for publication. Research can also be conducted for purposes of personal growth. Supervisors in the field or in training often want to observe and improve their own supervisory behavior but are intimidated by formal research. Supervisors desiring personal growth continually pose questions and seek answers. The questioning and data collection procedures for this kind of research are very similar to those already described, although the tools used are likely to be more informal. Issues such as coder agreement and statistical treatment are of less or minimal importance. Audiotape and videotape are valuable research tools for personal growth, particularly if objective data are collected and analyzed from the recorded interactions. Feedback from supervisees may also be an important source of research information for a supervisor's development. Personal growth research, while less formal, is the foundation of quality supervision. Often, supervisors involved in personal growth inquiry later move toward more formal research endeavors.

SUPERVISION RESEARCH AND THE FUTURE

PREAC Considerations

Table 12-1 lists the supervisory research that has been published since 1960, arranged by type of publication and according to the components of the PREAC model of supervisor roles (Professional, Researcher, Educator, Administrator, and Clinician). The research is further categorized by research approach (thought paper, qualitative analysis, single-subject, quantitative analysis, or questionnaire). The major research has been in the area of the Educator role, the predominant approach has been the thought paper, and a majority of the publications have appeared in *Asha*. An impressive number of publications fall into the quantitative analysis category.

Areas needing additional research are readily identifiable. For example, the supervisor's evolution as a Professional sorely needs work, as do the roles of Researcher, Administrator, and Clinician. The publications represent well the past emphasis on the clinical education role of the Communication Disorders supervisor.

Also evident from Table 12-1 is the lack of single-subject and qualitative studies. Future researchers can direct their efforts toward the sparsely represented areas of inquiry and in-

TABLE 12-1
Five types of Communication Disorders supervision publications, categorized by publication type and supervision roles

Type of Study	Author/Date	Type of Publication	P	R	E	A	C
Single-Subject	Ingrisano (1979)	Dissertation			X		
Quantitative Analysis	Johnson (1970)	Dissertation			X		
	Hall (1971)	Dissertation			X		
	Underwood (1973)	Dissertation			X		
	Kaplan & Dreyer (1974)	J. of Comm. Dis.			X		
	Culatta, Colucci, & Wiggins (1975)	Asha			X		
	Schubert & Laird (1975)	JNSSHA			X		
	Oratio (1976)	J. of Comm. Dis.			X		
	Schubert & Nelson (1976)	JNSSHA			X		
	Volz (1976)	Dissertation			X		
	Culatta & Seltzer (1977)	Asha			X		
	Dowling (1977)	Dissertation			X		
	Goodwin (1977)	Dissertation			X		
	Brookshire, Nicholas, Krueger, & Redmond (1978)	JSHD			X		
	Caracciolo, Rigrodsky, & Morrison (1978a)	Asha			X		
	Oratio (1978a)	Acta Symbolica			X		
	Oratio (1978b)	Asha			X		
	Smith (1978)	Dissertation			X		
	Volz, Klevans, Norton, & Putens (1978)	JSHD			X		
	Dowling (1979a)	Asha			X		
	Dowling (1979b)	JNSSHA			X		
	Oratio (1979)	Asha			X	X	
	Brasseur (1980)	Dissertation			X		
	Casey (1980)	Dissertation			X		
	McCrea (1980)	Dissertation			X		
	Andersen (1981)	Dissertation			X		
	Anderson (1981)	Asha	X	X	X		
	Dowling (1981)	JNSSHA			X		
	Dowling & Shank (1981)	J. of Comm. Dis.			X		
	Kennedy (1981)	Dissertation			X		
	Klevans, Volz, & Friedman (1981)	JSHD			X		
	Oratio, Sugarman, & Prass (1981)	J. of Comm. Dis.			X		
	Cimorell-Strong & Ensley (1982)	Asha			X		
	Dowling, Sbaschnig, & Williams (1982)	J. of Comm. Dis.			X		
	Dowling & Wittkopp (1982)	J. of Comm. Dis			X		
	Larson (1982)	Dissertation			X		
	Roberts (1982)	Dissertation			X		

TABLE 12-1
continued

Type of Study	Author/Date	Type of Publication	P	R	E	A	C
	Roberts & Smith (1982)	*JSHR*			X		
	Smith & Anderson (1982a)	*JSHR*		X			
	Smith & Anderson (1982b)	*JSHR*			X		
	Brasseur & Anderson (1983)	*JSHR*			X		
	Dowling (1983a)	*The Clin. Super.*			X		
	Dowling (1983b)	*J. of Comm. Dis.*			X		
	Nilsen (1983)	Dissertation			X		
	Roberts & Naremore (1983)	*JSHR*			X		
	Crichton & Oratio (1984)	*Asha*			X		
	Dowling (1984)	*The Clin. Super.*			X		
	Dowling & Bliss (1984)	*J. of Comm. Dis.*			X		
	Farmer (1984)	Dissertation			X		
	Peaper (1984)	*The Clin. Super.*			X		
	Peaper & Wener (1984)	*Asha*			X		
	Sleight (1984b)	*The Clin. Super.*			X		
	Tihen (1984)	Dissertation			X		
	Tufts (1984)	Dissertation			X		
	Dowling (1985)	*The Clin. Super.*			X		
	Runyan & Seal (1985)	*The Clin. Super.*			X		
	Shapiro (1985b)	Dissertation			X		
	Sleight (1985)	*The Clin. Super.*			X		
	Dowling (1986)	*The Clin. Super.*			X		
	Hagler (1986)	Dissertation			X		
	Blodgett, Schmitt, & Scudder (1987)	*The Clin. Super.*			X		
	Dowling (1987)	*J. of Comm. Dis.*			X		
	Larson & Kallail (1987)	*The Clin. Super.*				X	
	Mercaitis & Peaper (1987)	*The Clin. Super.*			X		
	Roberts & McCready (1987)	*JSHR*			X		
	Dowling (in press)	*The Clin. Super.*			X		
Questionnaire	Black, Miller, Anderson, & Coates (1961)	*JSHD*, MS #7				X	X
	Rees & Smith (1967)	*Asha*				X	X
	Rees & Smith (1968)	*Asha*				X	X
	Stace & Drexler (1969)	*Asha*				X	X
	Ryan (1970)	*Asha*				X	
	Anderson (1972)	*LSHSS*	X				
	Anderson (1973)	*Asha*	X				
	Schubert & Aitchison (1975)	*Asha*	X				
	ASHA (1981)	*Asha*	X				
	Peaper & Wener (1984)	*Asha*			X		
Thought Paper	ASHA (1961)	*JSHD*, MS #8	X			X	
	Perkins (1962)	*Asha*	X				
	Halfond (1964)	*Asha*	X		X		
	O'Neil & Peterson (1964)	*Asha*	X		X		
	Van Riper (1965)	*Asha*			X		

TABLE 12-1
continued

Type of Study	Author/Date	Type of Publication	P	R	E	A	C
	Ward & Webster (1965a)	*Asha*			X		
	Ward & Webster (1965b)	*Asha*			X		
	Brooks & Hannah (1966)	*JSHD*			X		
	Erickson & Van Riper (1967)	*Asha*			X		X
	Miner (1967)	*Asha*	X		X		
	Mowrer (1969)	*JSHD*			X		
	ASHA (1970)	*Asha*	X			X	
	Caracciolo, Rigrodsky, & Morrison (1978b)	*Asha*			X		
	Andrews (1971)	*Asha*	X		X	X	
	ASHA (1972)	*LSHSS*	X			X	
	Boone & Prescott (1972)	*Asha*			X		
	ASHA (1973)	Manual	X			X	
	O'Toole (1973)	*LSHSS*			X		
	ASHA (1973-1974)	Manual	X			X	
	Anderson (1974)	*Asha*	X			X	
	Klevens & Volz (1974)	*Asha*			X		
	Prescott & Tesauro (1974)	*JSHD*			X		
	Schubert (1974)	*Asha*	X		X	X	X
	Bernthal & Beukelman (1975)	*JNSSHA*			X		
	Shriberg, Filley, Hayes, Kwiatkowski, Schatz, Simmons, & Smith (1975)	*Asha*			X		
	Culatta & Harris (1976)	*Asha*			X		
	Culatta & Seltzer (1976)	*Asha*			X		
	Willbrand & Tibbitts (1976)	*LSHSS*	X			X	
	ASHA (1977)	*Asha*	X		X	X	
	Baldes, Goings, Herbold, Jeffrey, Wheeler, & Freilinger (1977)	*LSHSS*	X		X		
	Gerstman (1977)	*Asha*			X		
	Monnin & Peters (1977)	*LSHSS*			X		
	Pickering (1977)	*Asha*			X		
	ASHA (1978a)	*Asha*	X				
	ASHA (1978b)	*Asha*					X
	Caracciolo, Rigrodsky, & Morrison (1978a)	*Asha*			X		
	Caracciolo, Rigrodsky, & Morrison (1978b)	*Asha*			X		
	Dowling (1979a)	*JNSSHA*			X		
	Dowling (1979b)	*Asha*			X		
	Oratio (1979)	*Asha*		X	X		
	Culatta & Helmick (1980)	*Asha*	X				
	Culatta & Helmick (1981)	*Asha*	X				
	Dowling (1981)	*JNSSHA*		X			
	Irwin (1981a)	*J. of Comm. Dis.*			X		
	Irwin (1981b)	*J. of Comm. Dis.*			X		
	ASHA (1982a)	*Asha*	X				

TABLE 12-1
continued

Type of Study	Author/Date	Type of Publication	P	R	E	A	C
	ASHA (1982b)	*Asha*	X				
	Adair (1983)	*Sem. in Sp/Lang.*				X	
	Battin (1983)	*Sem. in Sp/Hrng.*				X	
	ASHA (1984)	*Asha*	X	X	X	X	X
	Crichton & Oratio (1984)	*Asha*				X	
	Lougeay-Mottinger, Harris, Perlstein-Kaplan, & Felicetti (1984)	*Asha*				X	
	Sleight (1984a)	*Asha*	X				
	ASHA (1985)	*Asha*	X	X	X	X	X
	O'Neill (1985)	*Asha*	X		X	X	
	Shapiro (1985a)	*JNSSHA*	X	X	X	X	X
	Farmer (1986)	*The Clin. Super.*			X		
	ASHA (1986)	Manual				X	
	Bess (1987)	Book chapter				X	
	Doehring (1987)	Book chapter		X			
	Engnoth (1987)	Book chapter	X				
	Farmer (1987a)	*The Clin. Super.*			X		
	Farmer (1987b)	*The Clin. Super.*			X		
	Gavett (1987)	Book chapter				X	
	Griffith (1987)	Book chapter	X			X	
	Hardick & Oyer (1987)	Book chapter	X			X	
	McCready, Shapiro, & Kennedy (1987)	Book chapter		X			
	Oyer (1987)	Book chapter	X			X	
	Rassi (1987)	Book chapter			X	X	
	Sedge (1987)	Book chapter	X			X	
	Terrio, Haas, & O'Sullivan (1987)	*Asha*	X				
	Ulrich (1987)	Book chapter	X				
	Farmer (1988)	*The Clin. Super.*			X		
	Strike & Gillam (1988)	Book chapter		X			
Qualitative Analysis	Hatten (1966)	Dissertation			X		
	Irwin & Nickles (1970)	*Asha*			X		
	Engnoth (1974)	Dissertation			X		
	Irwin (1975)	*Human Comm.*			X		
	Pickering (1979)	Dissertation			X		
	Pickering (1984)	*JSHD*			X		
	Gunter (1985)	*Australian JHCD*			X		
Books	Oratio (1977)	Speech-Language			X		
	Rassi (1978)	Audiology			X		
	Schubert (1978)	Speech-Language			X		
	Monnin & Peters (1981)	Speech-Language			X	X	
	Crago & Pickering (1987)	Spch.-Lang./Aud.	X	X	X	X	
	Anderson (1988)	Spch.-Lang./Aud.	X	X	X	X	
	Farmer & Farmer (1989)	Spch.-Lang./Aud.	X	X	X	X	X

*P = Professional, R = Researcher, E = Educator, A = Administrator, and C = Clinician.

crease the publications in professional journals other than *Asha*.

Two other sparsely represented areas not discernable from the table are Audiology supervision and nonverbal behavior in supervision.

Single-Subject Designs. Interest in single-subject designs as vehicles for supervisory research is likely to increase. Research intended for publication as well as for personal growth is well suited to this type of design. A baseline of behavior is observed and then a specific treatment is applied, followed by removal and then reapplication of the treatment (Strike & Gillam, 1988). A subject's behavior is observed in each of these conditions. With just one or a limited number of subjects, important research questions become answerable. The design allows each subject to serve as his or her own control, eliminating the need for matched subjects. Therefore, problems relating to sample size and matched controls are reduced. A safe prediction, then, is that single-subject research will increase markedly in the future.

Two other sparsely represented areas are audiology supervision and nonverbal communication. As an increasing number of audiologists become interested in supervision, the gap in audiology-related research is likely to be filled. Nonverbal communication may present a more difficult problem; research in this area has just begun. Farmer (1984) studied the impact of various aspects of the supervisor's nonverbal behavior on conferences. But numerous issues have not begun to be addressed, such as the use of space and of specific body movements in conferences. A more sophisticated nonverbal issue, paralinguistics, has not been considered. Unfortunately, the required knowledge of real time analyzers, sonographs, and advanced computer equipment may delay research in paralinguistics (S. Farmer, personal communication, May 17, 1987).

Researcher Identification. The PREAC model facilitates the scrutiny of completed work but does not clarify who will be doing supervisory research in the future or how. One likely trend for the future is increased networking among supervisors for research and professional growth purposes. In this process, CUSPSPA is likely to play an increasing role; it already serves as a vital nationwide linkage for those interested in supervision.

CUSPSPA's established Network and Research Net have particular potential to further cooperative research among supervisors. Mentoring to foster and refine research skills is on the increase and will be critical for the continued evolution of supervisory process research. Researcher interest profiles and listings of resources for syllabi and research consultation already exist. Use of the Network and Research Net systems in the future is limited only by the imagination. For example, several researchers could analyze the same set of video or audiotapes but for different purposes. A variety of individuals might consider an issue comprehensively by coordinating their efforts. Videotape libraries, typescripts, and coding centers could be developed. Computer bulletin boards for supervisors, cooperative writing via a modem, and computer communication among supervisors have all become possible. Given the vast range of opportunities, the future for cooperative research endeavors is unlimited.

The remaining concern is who will do the research. There is and always will be a core of individuals, usually in academia, who will be actively involved in this endeavor. But this is not enough. The problem needs to be considered in the broader context of supervision as a profession and career. A major concern to supervisors (ASHA, 1978a) is low status, low salaries, and lack of job security. The issue of status and that of who should be doing research are inextricably entwined.

For supervisors to be granted equal status in an academic environment by administrators and those who primarily teach and do research, they must engage in scholarly activity. Two factors make this activity difficult for supervisors: workload and rewards. Supervisors' workloads typically preclude anything but direct clinical education. Supervisors are also undermined as potential researchers by promotion/salary increment criteria. Rarely is a supervisor required to do research to earn a promotion or a raise in salary. Supervisors therefore approach the task of research with twofold discouragement from their environment. Supervisors must nevertheless be aware that unless they engage in research the long-term problems of status, job security, and salary will not correct themselves. Supervisors need to stress the importance of a research component, with appropriate release time, in their job descriptions. Similar problems of doing supervision research are prevalent in other supervision worksites.

The answer to the question of who should be doing research is clearly anyone interested in becoming a supervisor or who currently is one. Leaving research to academics is not enough. Research for practicing supervisors may start with personal growth endeavors. After additional coursework or continuing education, or linkage with a researcher through the CUSPSPA Research Net, these same individuals may later choose to pursue research for publication.

Supervisory Questions to be Answered

As was noted at the start of this chapter, supervision research is in its infancy. The questions have just begun to be asked. The opportunity for interested readers to contribute to the profession is ripe and waiting. Additional research tools need to be developed and validated. More information is needed about conferences, in particular the impact of conference style and content on outcomes. Of special importance is the effect of supervisory training on subsequent supervisor/supervisee interpersonal and conference behaviors. The effect of training supervisees to participate in supervision is unknown. Factors that enhance the quality of supervision and the supervisee's satisfaction with the process also need to be clarified. Some specific questions of relevance for the immediate future follow:

1. How might single-subject design strategies be used to assess specific interventions designed to alter supervisor behaviors in conferences?
2. Does supervision make a difference?
3. Do modifications in the supervisors' behavior improve (a) the perceived quality of conferences, (b) clinicians' conference and therapy behavior, and (c) clients' learning?
4. What can be done to enhance supervisees' ability to interact effectively in supervisory conferences, as measured by (a) supervisee satisfaction with the process, (b) professional growth, and (c) development of self-supervisory behavior?
5. Which aspects of supervisor and supervisee behavior are critical to effectiveness of the supervisory conferences?
6. What types of data collection tools need to be developed and validated?

An example of the establishment of a research procedure follows. If a researcher were interested in the question, "What impact does the supervisor's question type have on the supervisee's perception of conference effectiveness?" the problem could be addressed in at least two ways.

For personal growth research, a supervisor could consistently use open-ended questions with some supervisees and closed-ended questions with others. The supervisor would informally observe the results or ask for feedback from the supervisees. The supervisees might also be asked to judge each conference as effective/noneffective.

For scholarly research, supervisors might be randomly assigned to two groups. One group would be trained to ask closed-ended questions, the other open-ended questions. The number of questions asked per conference could also be a variable in the study. After each conference, the supervisee would complete a validated, reliable conference evaluation form or would verbally describe perceptions of conference effectiveness, to be coded in a manner developed and validated by the researcher. Conference audiotapes could also be coded with an observation system to determine effectiveness.

SUMMARY

An array of topics has been addressed in the preceding pages. An introduction to supervision research opened the discussion. The next section examined various specific statistical designs for research. The outcomes of studies were then presented by topic. The next section considered planning strategies for research, then the future of supervision research. The application material that follows provides further opportunities to explore the concerns of this chapter.

APPLICATIONS

Discussion Topics

1. Discuss the advantages and disadvantages of qualitative or quantitative designs.
2. Discuss supervisees' perceptions of supervision conferences. What additional research is needed in this area?
3. Discuss ways to teach effective interpersonal clinical and/or supervisory skills.
4. Discuss what kinds of research questions could be answered using a chi-square analysis approach, a measure of the difference between expected and observed behavior.
5. Discuss the available types of research tools. Determine whether analysis using each tool would be qualitative or quantitative and, if quantitative, whether it would be a univariate or multivariate analysis.

Laboratory Experiences

1. View a videotape of a supervisory conference. Determine whether the conference was direct or indirect according to the criteria reported by Smith and Anderson (1982b).
2. Select and analyze a supervisory research study. Determine whether the study was qualitative or quantitative and then identify its independent and dependent variables.
3. List the ways in which research will enhance your own professional development.
4. Role-play a supervisory conference with a peer. Assess the interpersonal effectiveness of that conference in relation to positive regard, unconditionality of regard, empathy, psychological contact, and clinician self-exploration.
5. Observe a therapy session and collect objective data to facilitate problem-managing in the supervisory conference.

Research Projects

1. Design a research study for personal growth to identify your STYLE in supervisory conferences.

2. Develop a training procedure to foster active supervisee participation in conferences.

3. Design a study to determine whether a supervisor's use of direct or indirect questions in the conference alters the supervisee's perception of the value of the conference.

4. Develop guidelines for supervisee self-evaluation following a therapy session.

5. Design a pilot study to assess whether supervisory training influences the occurrence of supervisee strategy development in conferences.

REFERENCES

Adair, M. (1983). Accountability in hospitals. *Seminars in Speech and Language, 4,* 159-169.

American Speech and Hearing Association. (1961). F. Darley (Ed.), Public school speech and hearing services. *Journal of Speech and Hearing Disorders* (Monograph Supplement 8).

American Speech and Hearing Association. (1970). Report of Committee on Supportive Personnel. Guidelines on the role, training, and supervision of the communication aide. *Asha, 12* 78-80.

American Speech and Hearing Association. (1972). Supervision in the schools. Report of task force on supervision. *Language, Speech and Hearing Services in the Schools, 3,* 4-10.

American Speech and Hearing Association. (1973). *Essentials of program planning, development, management, and evaluation.* W. Healey, Project Director. Washington, DC: Author.

American Speech and Hearing Association. (1973-1974). *Program supervision guidelines for comprehensive language, speech and hearing services in the schools.* Rockville, MD: Author.

American Speech and Hearing Association. (1977). Report of the Committee on the Clinical Fellowship Year. Models for Clinical Fellowship Year Experiences. *Asha, 19,* 624-642.

American Speech and Hearing Association. (1978a). Current status of supervision of speech-language pathology and audiology. Report of Committee on Supervision of Speech Pathology and Audiology. *Asha, 20,* 478-486.

American Speech and Hearing Association (1978b). Principles underlying the requirements for the Certificate of Clinical Competence adopted. *Asha, 20,* 331-333.

American Speech-Language-Hearing Association. (1981). Employment and utilization of supportive personnel in audiology and speech-language pathology. *Asha, 23,* 165-169.

American Speech-Language-Hearing Association. (1982a). Committee on Supervision in Speech-Language Pathology and Audiology. Minimum qualifications for supervisors and suggested competencies for effective clinical supervision. *Asha, 24* 339-342.

American Speech-Language-Hearing Association. (1982b). Suggested competencies for effective supervision. *Asha, 24,* 1021-1023.

American Speech-Language-Hearing Association. (1984). Committee on Supervision in Speech-Language-Pathology and Audiology. Clinical supervision in speech-language pathology and audiology (draft form). *Asha, 5,* 45–48.

American Speech-Language-Hearing Association. (1985). Clinical supervision in speech-language pathology and audiology (position statement). *Asha, 7*(6), 57–60.

American Speech-Language-Hearing Association. (1986). *Planning and development of quality services in the schools.* Rockville, MD: Author.

Andersen, C. (1981). The effect of supervisor bias on the evaluation of student clinicians in speech-language pathology and audiology. *Dissertation Abstracts International, 41,* 4479B. (University Microfilms No. 81-12, 499)

Anderson, J. (1972). Status of supervision in speech, hearing and language programs in schools. *Language, Speech and Hearing Services in the Schools, 3,* 12–23.

Anderson, J. (1973). Status of college and university programs of practicum in the schools. *Asha, 15,* 60–65.

Anderson, J. (1974). Supervision of school speech, hearing, and language programs: An emerging role. *Asha, 16,* 7–10.

Anderson, J. (1981). Training of supervisors in speech-language pathology and audiology. *Asha, 23,* 77–82.

Anderson, J. (1988). *The supervisory process in speech-language pathology and audiology.* San Diego: Little, Brown/College-Hill Press.

Andrews, J. (1971). Operationally written therapy goals in supervised clinical practicum. *Asha, 13,* 358–387.

Baldes, R., Goings, R., Herbold, D., Jeffrey, R., Wheeler, G., & Freilinger, J. (1977). Supervision of student speech clinicians. *Language, Speech and Hearing Services in the Schools, 8,* 76–84.

Barrett-Lennard, G. (1962). Dimensions of therapist response as causal factors in therapeutic change. *Psychological Monographs, 76,* 1–36.

Battin, R. (1983). Clinical accountability: Private practice. *Seminars in Speech and Hearing, 4,* 147–159.

Bernthal, J., & Beukelman, D. (1975). Self-evaluation by the student clinician. *Journal of National Student Speech and Hearing Association, 3,* 39–44.

Bess, F. (1987). Community-based speech-language-hearing clinical administration. In H. Oyer (Ed.), *Administration of programs in speech-language pathology and audiology* (pp. 84–100). Englewood Cliffs, NJ: Prentice-Hall.

Bills, R., Vance, E., & McClean, O. (1951). An index of adjustment and values. *Journal of Consulting Psychology, 15,* 257–261.

Black, M., Miller, E., Anderson, J., & Coates, N. (1961). Supervision of speech and hearing programs. *Journal of Speech and Hearing Disorders (Monograph Supplement) 7,* 22–32.

Blodgett, E., Schmitt, J., & Scudder, R. (1987). Clinical session evaluation: The effect of familiarity with the supervisee. *The Clinical Supervisor, 5,* 33–43.

Blumberg, A. (1980). *Supervisors and teachers: A private cold war* (2nd ed.). Berkeley, CA: McCutchan.

Boone, D., & Prescott, T. (1972). Content and sequence analysis of speech and hearing therapy. *Asha, 14,* 58–62.

Brasseur, J. (1980). The observed differences between direct, indirect, and direct/indirect videotaped supervisory conferences by speech-language pathology supervisors, graduate students, and undergraduate students. *Dissertation Abstracts International, 41,* 2131B. (University Microfilms No. 80-29, 212)

Brasseur, J., & Anderson, J. (1983). Observed differences between direct, indirect, and direct/indirect videotaped supervisory conferences. *Journal of Speech and Hearing Research, 26,* 349-477.

Brooks, R., & Hannah, E. (1966). A tool for clinical supervision. *Journal of Speech and Hearing Disorders, 31,* 383-387.

Brookshire, R., Nicholas, L., Krueger, K., & Redmond, K. (1978). Sampling of speech pathology treatment activities: An evaluation of momentary and interval sampling procedures. *Journal of Speech and Hearing Disorders, 21,* 652-666.

Caracciolo, G., Rigrodsky, S., & Morrison, E. (1978a). A Rogerian orientation to the speech-language pathology supervisory relationship. *Asha, 20,* 286-291.

Caracciolo, G., Rigrodsky, S., & Morrison, E. (1978b). Perceived interpersonal conditions and professional growth of master's level speech-language pathology students during the supervisory process. *Asha, 20,* 467-477.

Carkhuff, R. (1969). *Helping and human relations: A primer for lay and professional helpers* (Vol. 1). New York: Holt, Rinehart & Winston.

Casey, P. (1980). The validity of using small segments for analyzing supervisory conferences with McCrea's Adapted System. *Dissertation Abstracts International, 41,* 1729B. (University Microfilms No. 80-24, 566)

Cimorell-Strong, J., & Ensley, K. (1982). Effects of student clinician feedback on the supervisory conference. *Asha, 24,* 23-29.

Crago, M., & Pickering, M. (Eds.) (1987). *Supervision in human communication disorders: Perspectives on a process.* San Diego: Little, Brown/College-Hill Press.

Crichton, L., & Oratio, A. (1984). Retrospective study: Speech-language pathologists' clinical fellowship training. *Asha, 26,* 39-43.

Culatta, R., Colucci, S., & Wiggins, E. (1975). Clinical supervisors and trainees: Two views of a process. *Asha, 17,* 152-157.

Culatta, R., & Harris, A. (1976). A competency-based system for the initial training of speech pathologists. *Asha, 18,* 733-738.

Culatta, R., & Helmick, J. (1980). Clinical supervision: The state of the art. Part I. *Asha, 22,* 985-993.

Culatta, R., & Helmick, J. (1981). Clinical supervision: The state of the art. Part II. *Asha, 23,* 21-31.

Culatta, R., & Seltzer, H. (1976). Content and sequence analysis of the supervisory session. *Asha, 18,* 8-12.

Culatta, R., & Seltzer, H. (1977). Content and sequence analysis of the supervisory session: A report of clinical use. *Asha, 19,* 523-526.

Danish, S., D'Augelli, A., & Brock, G. (1974). *Helping skills verbal response system.* Unpublished manuscript, Pennsylvania State University, University Park.

Doehring, D. (1987). Research on human communication disorders. In M. Crago & M. Pickering (Eds.), *Supervision in communication disorders:*

Perspectives on a process (pp. 81–107). San Diego: Little, Brown/College-Hill Press.

Dowling, S. (1977). A comparison to determine the effects of two supervisory styles, conventional and teaching clinics, in the training of speech pathologists. *Dissertation Abstracts International, 37,* 889B. (University Microfilms No. 77-01, 883)

Dowling, S. (1979a). Developing student self-supervisory skills in clinical training. *Journal of National Student Speech and Hearing Association, 7,* 37–41.

Dowling, S. (1979b). The teaching clinic: A supervisory alternative. *Asha, 21,* 646–649.

Dowling, S. (1981). Observational analysis: Procedures for training coders and data collection. *Journal of National Student Speech and Hearing Association, 9,* 82–88.

Dowling, S. (1983a). An analysis of conventional and teaching clinic supervision. *The Clinical Supervisor, 1,* 15–29.

Dowling, S. (1983b). Teaching clinic conference participant interaction. *Journal of Communication Disorders, 16,* 385–387.

Dowling, S. (1984). Clinical evaluation: A comparison of self, self with videotape, peers and supervisors. *The Clinical Supervisor, 2,* 9–17.

Dowling, S. (1985). Clinical performance characteristics of failing, average and outstanding clinicians. *The Clinical Supervisor, 3,* 49–55.

Dowling, S. (1986). Supervisory training: Impetus for clinical supervision. *The Clinical Supervisor 4,* 27–35.

Dowling, S. (1987). Teaching clinic conferences: Perceptions of supervisor and peer behavior. *Journal of Communication Disorders, 20,* 119–128.

Dowling, S. (in press). Typical, ideal conferences: perceptions as a function of training. *The Clinical Supervisor.*

Dowling, S., & Bliss, L. (1984). Cognitive complexity, rhetorical sensitivity: Contributing factors in clinical skill? *Journal of Communication Disorders, 17,* 9–17.

Dowling, S., Sbaschnig, K., & Williams, C. (1982). Culatta and Seltzer content and sequence analysis of the supervisory session: A question of reliability and validity? *Journal of Communication Disorders, 15,* 353–362.

Dowling, S., & Shank, K. (1981). A comparison of the effects of two supervisory styles, conventional and teaching clinic, in the training of speech and language pathologists. *Journal of Communication Disorders, 14,* 51–58.

Dowling, S., & Wittkopp, J. (1982). Students' perceived supervisory needs. *Journal of Communication Disorders, 15,* 319–328.

Engnoth, G. (1974). A comparison of three approaches to supervision of speech clinicians in training. *Dissertation Abstracts International, 34,* 6261B. (University Microfilms No. 74-12, 552)

Engnoth, C. (1987). Public school speech-language-hearing administration. In H. Oyer (Ed.), *Administration of programs in speech-language pathology and audiology* (pp. 54–84). Englewood Cliffs, NJ: Prentice-Hall.

Erickson, R., & Van Riper, C. (1967). Demonstration therapy. *Asha, 9,* 33–35.

Farmer, S. (1984). Supervisory conferences in communicative disorders: Verbal and nonverbal interpersonal communication pacing. *Dissertation Abstracts International, 44,* 2715B. (University Microfilms No. 84-00, 891)

Farmer, S. (1986). Relationship development in supervisory conferences: A tripartite view of the process. *The Clinical Supervisor, 3,* 5-21.

Farmer, S. (1987a). Visual literacy and the clinical supervisor. *The Clinical Supervisor, 5*(1), 45-71.

Farmer, S. (1987b). Conflict management and clinical supervision. *The Clinical Supervisor, 5*(3), 5-27.

Farmer, S. (1988). Communication competence in clinical education/supervision: Critical notions. *The Clinical Supervisor, 6,* 29-47.

Gavett, E. (1987). Career development: An issue for the master's degree supervisor. In M. Crago & M. Pickering (Eds.), *Supervision in human communication disorders: Perspectives on a process* (pp. 55-79). San Diego: Little, Brown/College-Hill Press.

Gerstman, H. (1977). Supervisory relationships: Experiences in dynamic communication. *Asha, 19,* 527-529.

Goodwin, W. (1977). The frequency of occurrence of specified therapy behaviors of student speech clinicians following three conditions of supervisory conferences. *Dissertation Abstracts International, 37,* 3889B. (University Microfilms No. 77-01, 892)

Griffith, T. (1987). Administration of community hospital speech-language-hearing programs. In H. Oyer (Ed.), *Administration of programs in speech-language pathology and audiology.* (pp. 100-128). Englewood Cliffs, NJ: Prentice-Hall.

Gunter, C. (1985). Clinical reports in speech-language pathology: Nature of supervisory feedback. *Australian Journal of Human Communication Disorders, 13,* 37-51.

Hagler, P. (1986). *Effects of feedback on supervisor talk.* Doctoral dissertation, Indiana University.

Hagler, P., & Fahey, R. (1982, November). *Effect of providing supervisors with normative statistics before student evaluation.* Paper presented at the annual convention of the American Speech-Language-Hearing Association, Toronto, Ontario, Canada.

Halfond, M. (1964). Clinical supervision: Stepchild in training. *Asha, 6,* 441-444.

Hall, A. (1971). The effectiveness of videotape recordings as an adjunct to supervision of clinical practicum by speech pathologists. *Dissertation Abstracts International, 32,* 612B. (University Microfilms No. 71-18, 014)

Hardick, E., & Oyer, H. (1987). Administration of speech-language-hearing programs within the university setting. In H. Oyer (Ed.), *Administration of programs in speech-language pathology and audiology* (pp. 36-54). Englewood Cliffs, NJ: Prentice-Hall.

Hatten, J. (1966). A descriptive and analytical investigation of speech therapy supervisors-therapist conferences. *Dissertation Abstracts, 26,* 5595-5596. (University Microfilms No. 71-18, 014)

Ingrisano, D. (1979). An experiment in clinical process reactivity. *Dissertation Abstracts International, 40,* 3231B. (University Microfilms No. 79-00, 395)

Irwin, R. (1975). Microcounseling interviewing skills of supervisors of speech clinicians. *Human Communication, 4,* 5-9.

Irwin, R. (1981a). Training speech pathologists through microtherapy. *Journal of Communication Disorders, 14,* 93-103.

Irwin, R. (1981b). Video self-confrontation in speech pathology. *Journal of Communication Disorders, 14,* 235–243.

Irwin, R., & Nickles, A. (1970). The use of audiovisual films in supervised observation. *Asha, 31,* 363–367.

Johnson, T. (1970). The development of a multidimensional scoring system for observing the clinical process in speech pathology. *Dissertation Abstracts International, 30,* 5735B–5736B. (University Microfilms No. 70–11, 036)

Kaplan, N., & Dreyer, D. (1974). The effect of self-awareness training on student speech pathologist-client relationships. *Journal of Communication Disorders, 7,* 329–342.

Kennedy, K. (1981). The effect of two methods of supervisor preconference written feedback on the verbal behavior of participants in individual speech pathology supervisory conferences. *Dissertation Abstracts International, 42,* 2071A. (University Microfilms No. 81–23, 492)

Kleffner, F. (Ed.). (1964). *Seminar on guidelines for the internship year.* Washington, DC: American Speech and Hearing Association.

Klevans, D., & Volz, H. (1974). Development of a clinical evaluation procedure. *Asha, 9,* 489–491.

Klevans, D., Volz, H., & Friedman, R. (1981). A comparison of experiential and observational approaches for enhancing the interpersonal communication skills of speech-language pathology students. *Journal of Speech and Hearing Disorders, 46,* 208–213.

Larson, L. (1982). Perceived supervisory needs and expectations of experienced vs. inexperienced student clinicians. *Dissertation Abstracts International, 42,* 4758B. (University Microfilms No. 82–11, 183)

Larson, L., & Kallail, K. (1987). A consumer satisfaction survey for a university speech-language-hearing center. *The Clinical Supervisor, 5*(3), 29–43.

Lougeay-Mottinger, J., Harris, M., Perlstein-Kaplan, K., & Felicetti, T. (1984). UTD competency based evaluation system. *Asha, 11,* 39–43.

McCrea, E. (1980). Supervisee ability to self-explore and four facilitative dimensions of supervisor behavior in individual conferences in speech-language pathology. *Dissertation Abstracts International, 41,* 2134B. (University Microfilms No. 80–29, 239)

McCready, V., Shapiro, D., & Kennedy, K. (1987). Identifying hidden dynamics in supervision: Four scenarios. In M. Crago & M. Pickering (Eds.), *Supervision in human communication disorders: Perspectives on a process.* San Diego: Little, Brown/College-Hill Press.

Mercaitis, P., & Peaper, R. (1987). Factors influencing supervision evaluation by students in speech-language pathology. *The Clinical Supervisor, 5*(2), 39–53.

Miner, A. (1967). A symposium: Improving supervision of clinical practicum. *Asha, 9,* 471–481.

Monnin, L., & Peters, K. (1977). Problem solving supervised experiences in the schools. *Language, Speech and Hearing Services in the Schools, 8,* 99–106.

Monnin, L., & Peters, K. (1981). *Clinical practice for speech pathologists in the schools.* Springfield, IL: Charles C. Thomas.

Mowrer, D. (1969). Evaluating speech therapy through precision recording. *Journal of Speech and Hearing Disorders, 34,* 239–244.

Nilsen, J. (1983). Supervisor's use of direct/indirect verbal conference style and alteration of clinician behavior. *Dissertation Abstracts International, 42,* 3935B. (University Microfilms No. 83-09, 991)

O'Neill, J. (1985). The clinical supervisor: Proctor or accountant? *Asha, 27,* 23-24.

O'Neill, J., & Peterson, H. (1964). The use of closed circuit television in a clinical speech training program. *Asha, 6,* 445-447.

Oratio, A. (1976). A factor-analytic study of criteria for evaluating student clinicians in speech pathology. *Journal of Communication Disorders, 9,* 199-210.

Oratio, A. (1977). *Supervision in speech pathology: A handbook for supervisors and clinicians.* Baltimore, MD: University Park Press.

Oratio, A. (1978a). Interrelationship between interpersonal and technical skills of student clinicians in speech therapy. *Acta Symbolica, 7,* 29-41.

Oratio, A. (1978b). Comparative perceptions of therapeutic effectiveness by student clinicians and clinical supervisors. *Asha, 20,* 959-962.

Oratio, A. (1979). Computer assisted interaction analysis in speech-language pathology and audiology. *Asha, 21,* 179-184.

Oratio, A., Sugarman, M., & Prass, M. (1981). A multivariate analysis of clinical perceptions of supervisory effectiveness. *Journal of Communication Disorders, 14,* 31-42.

O'Toole, T. (1973). Supervision of the clinical trainee. *Language, Speech and Hearing Services in the Schools, 4*(3), 132-139.

Oyer, H. (Ed.). (1987). *Administration of programs in speech-language pathology and audiology.* Englewood Cliffs, NJ: Prentice-Hall.

Peaper, R. (1984). An analysis of student perceptions of the supervisory conference and student developed agendas for that conference. *The Clinical Supervisor, 2,* 55-64.

Peaper, R., & Wener, D. (1984). A comparison of clinical plans and reports. *Asha, 26,* 37-41.

Perkins, W. (1962). Our profession: What is it? *Asha, 4,* 339-344.

Pickering, M. (1977). An examination of concepts operative in the supervisory process and relationship. *Asha, 19,* 607-610.

Pickering, M. (1979). Interpersonal communication in speech-language pathology clinical practicum: A descriptive humanistic perspective. *Dissertation Abstracts International, 40,* 2140B. (University Microfilms No. 79-23, 892)

Pickering, M. (1984). Interpersonal communication in speech-language pathology supervisory conferences: A qualitative study. *Journal of Speech and Hearing Disorders, 49,* 189-195.

Prescott, T., & Tesauro, P. (1974). A method for quantification and description of clinical interactions with aurally handicapped children. *Journal of Speech and Hearing Disorders, 39,* 235-243.

Rassi, J. (1978). *Supervision in audiology.* Baltimore, MD: University Park Press.

Rassi, J. (1987). The uniqueness of audiology supervision. In M. Crago & M. Pickering (Eds.), *Supervision in human communication disorders: Perspectives on a process* (pp. 31-54). San Diego: Little, Brown/College-Hill Press.

Rees, M., & Smith, J. (1967). Supervised school experience for student clinicians. *Asha, 9,* 251-257.

Rees, M., & Smith, J. (1968). Some recommendations for supervised school experience for student clinicians. *Asha, 10,* 93–103.

Roberts, J. (1982). An attributional model of supervisors' decision-making behavior in speech-language pathology. *Dissertation Abstracts International, 42,* 2794B. (University Microfilms No. 81-28, 040)

Roberts, J., & McCready, V. (1987). Different clinical perspectives of good and poor therapy sessions. *Journal of Speech and Hearing Research, 30,* 335–342.

Roberts, J., & Naremore, R. (1983). An attributional model of supervisors' decision-making behavior in speech-language pathology. *Journal of Speech and Hearing Research, 6,* 537–549.

Roberts, J., & Smith, K. (1982). Supervisor-supervisee role differences and consistency of behavior in supervisory conferences. *Journal of Speech and Hearing Research, 25,* 428–434.

Rogers, C. (1957). The necessary and sufficient conditions for therapeutic personality change. *Journal of Consulting Psychology, 21,* 95–103.

Runyan, S., & Seal, B. (1985). A comparison of supervisors' ratings while observing a language remediation session. *The Clinical Supervisor, 3,* 61–75.

Ryan, B. (1970). The use of videotape recording (VTR) in university speech pathology and audiology training centers. *Asha, 12,* 555–556.

Sbaschnig, K., & Williams, C. (1983, November). *A reliability audit for supervisors.* Paper presented at the annual convention of the American Speech-Language-Hearing Association, Cincinnati, OH.

Schalk, M., & Peroff, L. (1972, November). *Consistency and reliability of supervisory evaluations at university training centers.* Paper presented at the annual convention of the American Speech and Hearing Association, San Francisco.

Schubert, G. (1974). Suggested minimum requirements for clinical supervisors. *Asha, 16,* 305.

Schubert, G. (1978). *Introduction to clinical supervision.* St. Louis: W. H. Green.

Schubert, G., & Aitchison, C. (1975). A profile of clinical supervisors in college and university speech and hearing training programs. *Asha, 17,* 440–447.

Schubert, G., & Laird, B. (1975). The length of time necessary to obtain a representative sample of clinician-client interaction. *Journal of National Student Speech and Hearing Association, 3,* 26–32.

Schubert, G., & Nelson, J. (1976). An analysis of verbal behavior occurring in speech pathology supervisory conferences. *Journal of National Student Speech and Hearing Association, 4,* 17–26.

Sedge, R. (1987). Administration of a military-based program of speech-language pathology and audiology. In H. Oyer (Ed.), *Administration of programs in speech-language pathology and audiology* (pp. 129–157). Englewood Cliffs, NJ: Prentice-Hall.

Shapiro, D. (1985a). Clinical supervision: A process in progress. *Journal of National Student Speech-Language-Hearing Association, 13,* 89–108.

Shapiro, D. (1985b). An experimental and descriptive analysis of supervisee's commitments and follow through behaviors as one measure of supervisory effectiveness in speech-language pathology and audiology. *Dissertation Abstracts International, 45,* 2889B. (University Microfilms No. 84-26, 682)

Shriberg, L., Filley, F., Hayes, D., Kwiatkowski, J., Schatz, J., Simmons, K., & Smith, M. (1975). The Wisconsin Procedure for Appraisal of Clinical Competence (W-PACC): Model and data. *Asha, 17,* 158–165.

Siegel, S. (1956). *Non-parametric statistics.* New York: McGraw-Hill.

Silverman, F. (1977). *Research design in speech pathology and audiology.* Englewood Cliffs, NJ: Prentice-Hall.

Sleight, C. (1984a). Games people play in clinical supervision. *Asha, 26,* 27–29.

Sleight, C. (1984b). Supervisor self-evaluation in communication disorders. *The Clinical Supervisor, 2,* 31–42.

Sleight, C. (1985). Confidence and anxiety in student clinicians. *The Clinical Supervisor, 3,* 25–48.

Smith, K. (1978). Identification of perceived effectiveness components in the individual supervisory conference in speech pathology and an evaluation of the relationship between ratings and content in the conferences. *Dissertation Abstracts International, 39,* 680B. (University Microfilms No. 78-13, 175)

Smith, K., & Anderson, J. (1982a). Development and validation of an individual supervisory conference rating scale for use in speech-language pathology. *Journal of Speech and Hearing Research, 25,* 252–261.

Smith, K., & Anderson, J. (1982b). Relationship of perceived effectiveness to content in supervisory conferences in speech-language pathology. *Journal of Speech and Hearing Research, 25,* 243–251.

Stace, A., & Drexler, A. (1969). Special training for supervisors of student clinicians: What private speech and hearing centers do and think about training their supervisors. *Asha, 11,* 318–320.

Stewart, J., & D'Angelo, G. (1975). *Together: Communicating interpersonally.* Reading, MA: Addison-Wesley.

Strike, C., & Gillam, R. (1988). Toward practical research in supervision. In J. Anderson, *The supervisory process in speech-language pathology and audiology* (pp. 273–298). San Diego: Little, Brown/College-Hill Press.

Terrio, L., Haas, W., & O'Sullivan, M. (1987). Profiling applications in audiological supervision. *Asha, 29,* 25–28.

Tihen, L. (1984). Expectations of student speech/language clinicians during their clinical practicum. *Dissertation Abstracts International, 44,* 3048B. (University Microfilms No. 84-01, 620)

Tufts, L. (1984). A content analysis of supervisory conferences in communicative disorders and the relationship of the content analysis system to the clinical experience of supervisees. *Dissertation Abstracts International, 44,* 3048B. (University Microfilms No. 84-01, 588)

Ulrich, S. (1987). Supervision: A developing specialty. In M. Crago & M. Pickering (Eds.), *Supervision in human communication disorders: Perspectives on a process* (pp. 3–29). San Diego: Little, Brown/College-Hill Press.

Underwood, J. (1973). Interaction analysis between the supervisor and the speech and hearing clinician. *Dissertation Abstracts International, 34,* 2995B. (University Microfilms No. 73-29, 608)

Van Riper, C. (1965). Supervision of clinical practice. *Asha, 7,* 75–77.

Villareal, J. (Ed.). (1964). *Seminar on guidelines for supervision of clinical practicum.* Washington, DC: American Speech and Hearing Association.

Volz, H. (1976). The effects on clinical performance, client progress, and client satisfaction of two programs to enhance the helping skills of undergraduate students in speech pathology (doctoral dissertation, Pennsylvania State University, 1975). *Dissertation Abstracts International, 37,* 716B.

Volz, H., & Klevans, D. (1979). *Verbal helping skills of graduate students in speech pathology.* Paper presented at the annual convention of the American Speech-Language-Hearing Association, Atlanta.

Volz, V., Klevans, D., Norton, S., & Putens, D. (1978). Interpersonal communication skills of speech-language pathology undergraduates: The effects of training. *Journal of Speech and Hearing Disorders, 43,* 524–542.

Ward, L., & Webster, E. (1965a). The training of clinical personnel: I. Issues in conceptualization. *Asha, 7,* 38–40.

Ward, L., & Webster, E. (1965b). The training of clinical personnel: II. A concept of clinical preparation. *Asha, 7,* 103–107.

Weller, R. (1971). *Verbal communication in instructional supervision.* New York: Teachers College Press, Columbia University.

Willbrand, M., & Tibbits, D. (1976). Compensation for supervisors of clinical practicum in public school settings. *Language, Speech and Hearing Services in the Schools, 7,* 128–131.

Appendix A Competencies for Effective Clinical Supervision

1.0 TASK: ESTABLISHING AND MAINTAINING AN EFFECTIVE WORKING RELATIONSHIP WITH THE SUPERVISEE

Competencies required:
1.1 Ability to facilitate an understanding of the clinical and supervisory processes
1.2 Ability to organize and provide information regarding the logical sequences of supervisory interaction—that is, joint setting of goals and objectives, data collection and analysis, evaluation
1.3 Ability to interact from a contemporary perspective with the supervisee in both the clinical and supervisory process
1.4 Ability to apply learning principles in the supervisory process
1.5 Ability to apply skills of interpersonal communication in the supervisory process
1.6 Ability to facilitate independent thinking and problem solving by the supervisee
1.7 Ability to maintain a professional and supportive relationship that allows both supervisor and supervisee growth
1.8 Ability to interact with the supervisee objectively
1.9 Ability to establish joint communications regarding expectations and responsibilities in the clinical and supervisory processes

2.0 TASK: ASSISTING THE SUPERVISEE IN DEVELOPING CLINICAL GOALS AND OBJECTIVES

Competencies required:
2.1 Ability to assist the supervisee in planning effective client goals and objectives
2.2 Ability to plan, with the supervisee, effective goals and objectives for clinical and professional growth
2.3 Ability to assist the supervisee in using observation and assessment in preparation of client goals and objectives
2.4 Ability to assist the supervisee in using self-analysis and previous evaluation in preparation of goals

and objectives for professional growth

2.5 Ability to assist the supervisee in assigning priorities to clinical goals and objectives

2.6 Ability to assist the supervisee in assigning priorities to goals and objectives for professional growth

3.0 TASK: ASSISTING THE SUPERVISEE IN DEVELOPING AND REFINING ASSESSMENT SKILLS

Competencies required:

3.1 Ability to share current research findings and evaluation procedures in communication disorders

3.2 Ability to facilitate an integration of research findings in client assessment

3.3 Ability to assist the supervisee in providing rationale for assessment procedures

3.4 Ability to assist supervisee in communicating assessment procedures and rationale

3.5 Ability to assist the supervisee in integrating findings and observations to make appropriate recommendations

3.6 Ability to facilitate the supervisee's independent planning of assessment

4.0 TASK: ASSISTING THE SUPERVISEE IN DEVELOPING AND REFINING MANAGEMENT SKILLS

Competencies required:

4.1 Ability to share current research findings and management procedures in communication disorders

4.2 Ability to facilitate an integration of research findings in client management

4.3 Ability to assist the supervisee in providing rationale for treatment procedures

4.4 Ability to assist the supervisee in identifying appropriate sequences for client change

4.5 Ability to assist the supervisee in adjusting steps in the progression toward a goal

4.6 Ability to assist the supervisee in the description and measurement of client and clinician change

4.7 Ability to assist the supervisee in documenting client and clinician change

4.8 Ability to assist the supervisee in integrating documented client and clinician change to evaluate progress and specify future recommendations

5.0 TASK: DEMONSTRATING FOR AND PARTICIPATING WITH THE SUPERVISEE IN THE CLINICAL PROCESS

Competencies required:

5.1 Ability to determine jointly when demonstration is appropriate

5.2 Ability to demonstrate or participate in an effective client-clinician relationship

5.3 Ability to demonstrate a variety of clinical techniques and participate with the supervisee in clinical management

5.4 Ability to demonstrate or use jointly the specific materials and equipment of the profession

5.5 Ability to demonstrate or participate jointly in counseling of clients or family/guardians of clients

6.0 TASK: ASSISTING THE SUPERVISEE IN OBSERVING AND ANALYZING ASSESSMENT AND TREATMENT SESSIONS

Competencies required:

6.1 Ability to assist the supervisee in learning a variety of data collection procedures
6.2 Ability to assist the supervisee in selecting and executing data collection procedures
6.3 Ability to assist the supervisee in accurately recording data
6.4 Ability to assist the supervisee in analyzing and interpreting data objectively
6.5 Ability to assist the supervisee in revising plans for client management based on data obtained

7.0 TASK: ASSISTING THE SUPERVISEE IN DEVELOPMENT AND MAINTENANCE OF CLINICAL AND SUPERVISORY RECORDS

Competencies required:

7.1 Ability to assist the supervisee in applying recordkeeping systems to supervisory and clinical processes
7.2 Ability to assist the supervisee in effectively documenting supervisory and clinically related interactions
7.3 Ability to assist the supervisee in organizing records to facilitate easy retrieval of information concerning clinical and supervisory interactions
7.4 Ability to assist the supervisee in establishing and following policies and procedures to protect the confidentiality of clinical and supervisory records
7.5 Ability to share information regarding documentation requirements of various accrediting and regulatory agencies and third-party funding sources

8.0 TASK: INTERACTING WITH THE SUPERVISEE IN PLANNING, EXECUTING, AND ANALYZING SUPERVISORY CONFERENCES

Competencies required:

8.1 Ability to determine with the supervisee when a conference should be scheduled
8.2 Ability to assist the supervisee in planning a supervisory conference agenda
8.3 Ability to involve the supervisee in jointly establishing a conference agenda
8.4 Ability to involve the supervisee in joint discussion of previously identified clinical or supervisory data or issues
8.5 Ability to interact with the supervisee in a manner that facilitates the supervisee's self-exploration and problem solving
8.6 Ability to adjust conference content based on supervisee's level of training and experience
8.7 Ability to encourage and maintain supervisee motivation for continuing self-growth
8.8 Ability to assist the supervisee in making commitments or changes in clinical behavior
8.9 Ability to involve the supervisee in ongoing analysis of supervisory interactions

9.0 TASK: ASSISTING THE SUPERVISEE IN EVALUATION OF CLINICAL PERFORMANCE

Competencies required:

9.1 Ability to assist the supervisee in the use of clinical evaluation tools
9.2 Ability to assist the supervisee in the description and measurement of his/her progress and achievement
9.3 Ability to assist the supervisee in developing skills of self-evaluation
9.4 Ability to evaluate clinical skills with the supervisee for purposes of grade assignment, completing of Clinical Fellowship Year, professional advancement, and so on

10.0 TASK: ASSISTING THE SUPERVISEE IN DEVELOPING SKILLS OF VERBAL REPORTING, WRITING, AND EDITING

Competencies required:

10.1 Ability to assist the supervisee in identifying appropriate information to be included in a verbal or written report
10.2 Ability to assist the supervisee in presenting information in a logical, concise, and sequential manner
10.3 Ability to assist the supervisee in using appropriate professional terminology and style in verbal and written reporting
10.4 Ability to assist the supervisee in adapting verbal and written reports to the work environment and communication situation
10.5 Ability to alter and edit a report as appropriate while preserving the supervisee's writing style

11.0 TASK: SHARING INFORMATION REGARDING ETHICAL, LEGAL, REGULATORY, AND REIMBURSEMENT ASPECTS OF THE PROFESSION

Competencies required:

11.1 Ability to communicate to the supervisee a knowledge of professional codes of ethics (e.g., ASHA, state licensing boards, and so on)
11.2 Ability to communicate to the supervisee an understanding of legal and regulatory documents and their impact on the practice of the profession (licensure, PL 94–142, Medicare, Medicaid, and so on)
11.3 Ability to communicate to the supervisee an understanding of reimbursement policies and procedures of the work setting
11.4 Ability to communicate a knowledge of supervisee rights and appeal procedures specific to the work setting

12.0 TASK: MODELING AND FACILITATING PROFESSIONAL CONDUCT

Competencies required:

12.1 Ability to assume responsibility
12.2 Ability to analyze, evaluate, and modify own behavior
12.3 Ability to demonstrate ethical and legal conduct
12.4 Ability to meet and respect deadlines
12.5 Ability to maintain professional protocols (respect for confidentiality, etc.)
12.6 Ability to provide current information regarding professional

standards (PSB, ESB, licensure, teacher certification, etc.)

12.7 Ability to communicate information regarding fees, billing procedures, and third-party reimbursement

12.8 Ability to demonstrate familiarity with professional issues

12.9 Ability to demonstrate continued professional growth

13.0 TASK: DEMONSTRATING RESEARCH SKILLS IN THE CLINICAL OR SUPERVISORY PROCESS

Competencies required:

13.1 Ability to read, interpret, and apply clinical and supervisory research

13.2 Ability to formulate clinical or supervisory research questions

13.3 Ability to investigate clinical or supervisory research questions

13.4 Ability to support and refute clinical or supervisory research findings

13.5 Ability to report results of clinical or supervisory research and disseminate as appropriate (e.g., in-service, conferences, publications)

American Speech-Language-Hearing Association. (1985). Clinical supervision in speech-language pathology and audiology (position statement). Asha, 7, 57-60.

Appendix B Characteristics of Communication Disorders Supervision STYLES

STYLE I

Key descriptors: Directing, Training, Informing, Telling, Ordering

Purpose:

- Emphasis on cognitive development (information and skill)
- Emphasis on teaching or instructing

Inquiry mode: Realist

Decision style: Supervisor makes decisions

Leadership Styles: Directive, Challenger, Instructor

Philosophical orientation: Essentialism

Psychological orientation: Behaviorism

General Orientation:

- Supervisor seldom gets supervisees' ideas or opinions in problem management
- Supervision is goal and task oriented
- Goals and tasks are set by supervisor
- Concern for performance lies primarily with supervisor
- Concern for control lies with supervisor
- Emphasis is on work, with little overt concern for relations
- Emphasis is on organizing, initiating, directing, completing, and evaluating
- Well-defined sequential plans and procedures are set for all aspects of supervision
- Supervision is supervisor centered
- Supervisee deficits, rather than strengths, are emphasized
- Inductive reasoning is stressed

Uses:

- For crisis intervention
- With marginal supervisees (academic and clinical)
- With shy, reticent, nonassertive clinicians
- With supervisees who have low decision making responsibilities, such as aides
- For time or cost efficiency
- With beginning clinicians
- Often used inappropriately by supervisors with minimal or no training in supervision

Results:

- Generates minimal cooperative teamwork
- Supervisees have little or no influence on goals, methods, and work activities

APPENDIX B CHARACTERISTICS OF COMMUNICATION DISORDERS SUPERVISION STYLES

- Supervisors tend to set only average goals
- Efficiency in operations results from arranging conditions of work so that human elements interfere as little as possible

If used inappropriately (i.e. if differential supervision is not used):

- Provides some supervisees with relatively little learning
- Attitudes may be hostile and counter to organization's goals
- Supervisees may be dissatisfied with membership in the organization, with supervision, and with their own achievements
- Supervisor's decision making may lower supervisees' motivation to implement the decision
- Supervisees may overtly accept goals but covertly strongly resist them

Process:

- Pedagogical
- Bottom-up (data-driven, nonexperiential) information processing stressed
- Convergent thinking used ("correct" or "right" methods stressed)
- Majority of decisions made by supervisor
- Decisions made one-on-one; discourages teamwork
- Exclusion (problem management without collaboration)
- Review and evaluation completed by supervisor
- Emphasis on observation of words and behavior

Communication:

- Interpersonal communication style: Driver
- Conflict communication style: Competitive
- Organizational communication:
    Very little communication aimed at achieving organization's objectives
    Flow of information is downward
    Supervisors share minimum information with supervisees
    Supervisees tend to view supervisor interaction with great suspicion
    Upward communication is very inadequate
    Supervisees may feel no responsibility for initiating upward communication
    Upward communication tends to be inaccurate
    Supervisor does majority of talking
    Supervisor criticizes a great deal
    Supervisor does little asking, accepting, or encouraging of supervisees' feelings, ideas, opinions, or suggestions

Relationships:

- Supervisees do not feel at all free to discuss aspects of their work
- Supervisees exhibit subservient attitudes toward supervisors
- Supervisor and supervisee have no knowledge or understanding of each other's problems; perceptions of each other are often in error
- Little personal interaction occurs
- Observation/evaluation done to determine worth

Population:

- Used with both audiologists and speech-language pathologists
- Used primarily with supervisees in Readiness State 1 (unable and unwilling or insecure) and Readiness State 2 (unable but willing or confident)

STYLE II

Key descriptors: Administering, Controlling, Monitoring, Managing, Regulating

Purpose:

- Emphasis on cognitive development; some affective interest (dispositions and competence)
- Emphasis on teaching or instructing

Inquiry mode: Analyst

Decision style: Supervisor makes decisions

Leadership styles: Administrative, Analyst

Philosophical orientation: Essentialism

Psychological orientation: Behaviorism

General orientation:

- Supervisor sometimes gets supervisees' ideas and opinions in problem management
- Goal and task orientation is low
- Goals and tasks are set by supervisor; supervisees may or may not have opportunity to comment
- Concern for performance lies primarily with supervisor
- Concern for control lies with supervisor
- Supervisor shows little overt concern for relations or work
- Emphasis is on examining, measuring, administering, controlling, maintaining
- Supervision tends to operate on intuition and chance; supervisor has great freedom
- Supervision is supervisor centered, maybe client centered
- Supervisee deficits, rather than strengths, are emphasized
- Inductive reasoning is stressed

Uses:

- For time or cost efficiency
- With nontraditional personnel
- With supervisees who have low decision making responsibilities, such as aides
- May be misused by laissez-faire or burned-out supervisors

Results:

- Generates relatively little cooperative teamwork
- Supervisees have virtually no influence on goals, methods, work activities
- Supervisors have moderate to somewhat more than moderate influence
- Supervisors tend to set high goals for supervisees and organization
- Exerting minimum effort to get required work done is appropriate to sustain organization membership

If used inappropriately (i.e., if differential supervision is not used):

- Provides some supervisees with relatively little learning
- Attitudes are sometimes hostile and counter to organization's goals
- Supervisees range from dissatisfaction to moderate satisfaction with membership in the organization, supervision, and their own achievements
- Supervisor's decision making may lower supervisees' motivation to implement the decisions
- Supervisees overtly accept goals but covertly resist them

Process:

- Pedagogical
- Bottom-up information processing stressed
- Convergent thinking used
- Some decisions made by supervisee but usually checked by supervisor
- One-on-one decisions; supervisee occasionally consulted; poor for teamwork
- Exclusion (problem management without collaboration)
- Review and evaluation generally completed by supervisor

APPENDIX B   CHARACTERISTICS OF COMMUNICATION DISORDERS SUPERVISION STYLES   359

- Emphasis on observation of words and behavior

Communication:

- Interpersonal communication style: Analytical
- Conflict communication style: Avoiding
- Organizational communication:
    - Little communication aimed at achieving organization's objectives
    - Flow of information is mostly downward
    - Supervisors share only information they feel supervisees need
    - Supervisees view interaction with mixed acceptance and suspicion
    - Upward communication is very limited
    - Supervisees feel relatively little responsibility for initiating accurate upward communication; usually communicate filtered information, and only when requested; supervisees may "yes" the supervisor
    - Upward communication tends to be what the supervisor wants to hear
    - Adequacy and accuracy of horizontal communication are fairly poor
    - Supervisor does majority of talking; supervisee is passive
    - Supervisor criticizes a great deal
    - Supervisor does little asking, accepting, or encouraging of supervisees' feelings, ideas, opinions, or suggestions

Relationships:

- Supervisees tend to have subservient confidence or trust in supervisors
- Supervisees may not feel very free to discuss aspects of their work
- Supervisees show subservient attitudes toward supervisors
- Supervisor and supervisee have some knowledge or understanding of each other's problems; perceptions are often in error
- Little interaction

- Observation/evaluation done to monitor and sometimes to guide

Population:

- Used with audiologists and speech-language pathologists
- Used primarily with supervisees in Readiness State 2 (unable but willing or confident)

STYLE III

Key descriptors: Advising, Mentoring, Coaching, Consulting, Participating

Purpose:

- Emphasis on affective development (relationships and dispositions)
- Emphasis on learning through genuine communication

Inquiry mode: Idealist

Decision style: Supervisor and supervisee make decisions together, or supervisee makes decisions with supervisor encouragement

Leadership styles: Consultive, Motivator, Developer

Philosophical orientation: Existentialism

Psychological orientation: Humanism

General orientation:

- Supervisor usually gets and tries to use supervisees' ideas and opinions
- Supervision is goal and task directed
- Goals and tasks are established jointly by supervisor and supervisee
- Concern for performance lies with both supervisor and supervisee
- No overt supervisor or supervisee concern for control is shown

- Emphasis is on relations, with little overt concern for work
- Emphasis is on listening, accepting, trusting, advising, and encouraging
- Mentoring and coaching occur; emphasis is on feelings and big-picture planning
- Supervision is supervisee or client centered
- Supervisee strengths, rather than deficits, are emphasized
- Deductive reasoning is stressed

Uses:

- For developing networking and linkages
- For supervising peers
- For developing confidence, risk-taking, and creativity in supervisees
- With outgoing, assertive clinicians
- With supervisees who are capable of moderate decision making
- For developing supervisee dispositions
- For establishing affiliation, acceptance, security

Results:

- Helps many supervisees to learn about themselves
- Generates attitudes that are usually favorable and supportive of organization's goals
- Leaves supervisees generally satisfied with membership in the organization, with supervision, and with their own achievements
- Generates a moderate amount of cooperative teamwork
- Gives supervisees moderate influence on goals, methods, and work activities
- Gives supervisors moderate influence over supervisees
- Decision making contributes somewhat to motivation to implement ideas
- Supervisees overtly accept goals but occasionally covertly resist them
- Supervisors tend to seek very high goals
- Thoughtful attention to need of people for satisfying relationships leads to a comfortable, friendly organization atmosphere and work tempo

Process:

- Andragogical
- Top-down (experiential) information processing stressed
- Divergent thinking used (multiple solutions method)
- Broad policy decisions made by supervisor; specific decisions made jointly
- Decisions made jointly one-on-one; partially encourages teamwork
- Inclusion (problem management with collaboration)
- Review and evaluation completed jointly by supervisor and supervisee
- Emphasis on intuition and understanding

Communication:

- Interpersonal communication style: Amiable
- Conflict communication style: Accommodation
- Organizational communication:
    Quite a bit of communication aimed at achieving organization's objectives
    Flow of information is downward and upward (vertical)
    Supervisors share needed information and answer most questions
    Supervisees tend to accept supervisor interaction or do not openly question it
    Some upward communication exists
    Supervisees feel some responsibility for upward communication
    Upward communication tends to be what supervisor wants to hear; other information may be limited or cautiously given
    Adequacy and accuracy of horizontal communication are fair to good
    Supervisor and supervisee do balanced talking

APPENDIX B   CHARACTERISTICS OF COMMUNICATION DISORDERS SUPERVISION STYLES

Supervisor does little direct criticizing; more extending and reflecting

Supervisor does much asking, listening, accepting, and encouraging of supervisees' feelings, ideas, opinions, and suggestions

Relationships:

- Supervisors and supervisees have substantial mutual confidence or trust
- Supervisors are generally supportive of supervisees
- Supervisees feel quite free to discuss aspects of their work
- Supervisees exhibit cooperative, reasonably favorable attitudes toward supervisors
- Supervisors and supervisees know and understand each other quite well; perceptions are moderately accurate
- Moderate personal interaction, often with fair amount of confidence/trust
- Observation/evaluation done for monitoring, guidance; some use of self-guidance
- Supervisors tend not to be defensive

Population:

- Used with both audiologists and speech-language pathologists
- Used primarily with supervisees in Readiness State 3 (able but unwilling or insecure)

STYLE IV

Key descriptors: Collaborating, Transacting, Negotiating, Integrating, Unifying

Purpose:

- Emphasis on cognitive and affective development (professional competence)
- Emphasis on learning through instruction and genuine communication

Inquiry mode(s): Synthesist and Pragmatist

Decision style: Decisions are negotiated between supervisor and supervisee

Leadership styles: Collaborative, Catalyst, Inspirer

Philosophical orientation: Experimentalism

Psychological orientation: Cognitivism

General orientation:

- Supervisor always gets supervisees' ideas and opinions and uses them
- Supervision is goal and task directed
- Goals and tasks are established jointly by supervisor and supervisee
- Concern for performance lies with both supervisor and supervisee
- No overt supervisor or supervisee concern for control is shown
- Emphasis is on relations and work
- Emphasis is on interacting, motivating, integrating, participating, innovating
- Well-defined plans and procedures are set; strong concern for two-way communication is shown
- Supervision is supervisee or client centered
- Supervisee strengths, rather than deficits, are emphasized
- Deductive reasoning is stressed

Uses:

- For advanced clinicians, CFY clinicians, peers
- For clinicians who don't have opportunities to watch colleagues work
- With outgoing, assertive clinicians
- With supervisees who are capable of independent decision making
- For improving morale problems
- For meeting needs of others
- For developing networks and linkages

- For establishing affiliation, acceptance, security

Results:

- Provides supervisees with academic information and learning about self
- Generates attitudes that are strongly favorable and supportive of organization's goals
- Supervisees have relatively high satisfaction with membership in the organization, with supervision, and with their own achievements
- Generates a very substantial amount of cooperative teamwork
- Supervisees have a great deal of influence on goals, methods, and work
- Supervisors have substantial, but indirect, influence over supervisees
- Decision making contributes substantially to motivation to implement ideas
- Goals are fully accepted, both overtly and covertly
- Supervisors tend to seek extremely high goals
- Work accomplishment is from committed people; interdependence through a "common stake" leads to relationships of trust and respect

Process:

- Andragogical
- Top-down information processing stressed
- Divergent thinking used
- Rewards and involvement used for motivation
- Decision making widely done throughout organization
- Decisions largely made on group pattern; encourages teamwork
- Inclusion (problem management with collaboration)
- Review and evaluation completed jointly by supervisor and supervisee
- Emphasis on intuition and understanding

Communication:

- Much communication with both individuals and groups
- Flow of information is downward, upward, and horizontal
- Supervisors seek to give all relevant needed and wanted information
- Supervisor interaction generally accepted; candidly questioned, if not
- A great deal of upward communication exists
- Supervisees feel considerable responsibility for upward communication
- Upward communication tends to be accurate and freely given
- Adequacy and accuracy of horizontal communication are good to excellent
- Strong forces exist to obtain complete and accurate information
- Supervisor and supervisee do balanced talking
- Supervisor does little direct criticizing; more extending and reflecting
- Supervisor does much asking, listening, accepting, and encouraging of supervisees' feelings, ideas, opinions, and suggestions

Relationships:

- Supervisors and supervisees have complete mutual confidence or trust
- Supervisors display supportive behavior fully and in all situations
- Supervisees feel completely free to discuss aspects of their work
- Supervisees exhibit cooperative, favorable attitudes toward supervisors and organization
- Supervisors and supervisees know and understand each other very well; perceptions are usually quite accurate
- Extensive, friendly personal interaction; high degree of confidence and trust
- Observation/evaluation done for self-guidance or coordinated problem management
- Supervisors tend not to be defensive

APPENDIX B CHARACTERISTICS OF COMMUNICATION DISORDERS SUPERVISION STYLES

Population:

- Used with audiologists and speech-language pathologists
- Used primarily with supervisees in Readiness State 4 (able and willing or confident)

Note. These four STYLES of Communication Disorders supervision were developed by synthesizing information from the following sources:

Blake, R., & Mouton, J. (1964). *The managerial grid.* Houston: Gulf.

Blumberg, A. (1974). *Supervisors and teachers: A private cold war.* Berkeley, CA: McCutchan.

Dobson, R., Dobson, J., & Kessinger, J. (1980). *Staff development: A humanistic approach.* Lanham, MD: University Press of America.

Farmer, S. (1984). Supervisory conferences in communicative disorders: Verbal and nonverbal interpersonal communication pacing. *Dissertation Abstracts International, 44, 2715B.* (University Microfilms No. 84-00, 891)

Harrison, A., & Bramson, R. (1982). *The art of thinking.* New York: Anchor/Doubleday.

Hersey, P., & Blanchard, K. (1982). *Management of organizational behavior: Utilizing human resources* (4th ed.). Englewood Cliffs, NJ: Prentice-Hall.

Kilmann, R., & Thomas, K. (1975). Interpersonal conflict: Handling behavior as reflections of Jungian personality dimensions. *Psychological Reports, 37,* 971-980.

Knapp, M. (1978). *Social intercourse: From greeting to goodbye.* Boston: Allyn & Bacon.

Likert, R. (1967). *The human organization: Its management and value.* New York: McGraw-Hill.

Price, J. (1984). *Personal Inventory.* Shawnee Mission, KA: G. H.

Reddin, W. (1970). *Managerial effectiveness.* New York: McGraw-Hill.

Sergiovanni, J., & Elliot, D. (1975). *Educational and organizational leadership in elementary schools.* Englewood Cliffs, NJ: Prentice-Hall.

Wonder, J., & Donovan, P. (1984). *Whole-brain thinking.* New York: Random House/Ballantine.

Glossary

Algorithms Guaranteed paths to productive outcomes.

Andragogy Adult learning based on equal responsibilities of the teacher and learner; a concept used in Communication Disorders supervision STYLES III and IV (see Appendix B).

Artifacts analysis A method of naturalistic evaluation where supervisors examine materials and environments used by the personnel being evaluated in order to discover and understand personal and professional patterns.

ASHA The American Speech-Language-Hearing Association. It is the national governing body for speech-language pathologists and audiologists.

Biases Positive and negative personal preferences that affect supervisors' observation consciously and unconsciously.

Bottom up–top down information processing A cognitive psychology theory of attention in learning. Bottom-up learning is data driven; top-down learning is conceptually, experientially driven. The concept is used in the four STYLES of Communication Disorders supervision; bottom-up processing (intensity of stimulus) predominates in STYLES I and II, top-down processing (personal biases) predominates in STYLES III and IV (see Appendix B).

Categorical supervisor A speech-language pathologist or audiologist who supervises in his or her area(s) of ASHA certification.

Channels of communication The means through which symbols (language) are exchanged between and among people: watching/moving, listening/talking, and reading/writing.

Chi-square A test for differences among several multiple-choice categories.

Clinical education The teaching and training of Communication Disorders clinicians. It is the primary domain of supervision for most supervisors.

Clinical Fellowship Year (CFY) To become certified by ASHA, a speech-language pathologist or audiologist completes a required period of employment after the master's degree. During this time the clinical fellow is supervised by a speech-language pathologist or audiologist holding the Certificate of Clinical Competence (CCC).

Clinical literacy Having the knowledge, skills, and dispositions to read, interpret, and produce written clinical material.

Clinical reporting The use of clinical literacy and communication competence in the oral and written transmission of clinical information.

Clinical supervisor A supervisor who works in college and university training programs where the emphasis is on developing student clinical competence.

Closed circuit television (CCTV) A television system dedicated to a specific, closed environment such as one building. Signals are transmitted only within the system.

Cognitive styles Preferences of sensory modality (auditory, visual, haptic, taste, smell), context (e.g., alone, in a group), and environment (e.g., heat, light, noise) for obtaining information. The concept also includes aptitudes for learning: perceptual processing, language, scientific and creative thinking, formal reasoning, eye/hand coordination, artistry, writing, and socialness.

Commission on Accreditation of Rehabilitation Facilities (CARF) The federal agency exclusively devoted to establishing standards for rehabilitation agencies and accrediting institutions and agencies that meet those standards.

Committee on Supervision of Speech-Language Pathology and Audiology An ASHA committee established in 1974 for the purpose of studying supervision in Speech-Language Pathology and Audiology.

Communication competence Having and using the knowledge of who can say, write, or sign what, in what way, where and when, by what means, and to whom.

Concepts the ideas and issues studied and written about in the general body of supervision literature, as well as in the literature specific to supervision in Communication Disorders; one third of the Trigonal Model of Communication Disorders supervision.

Connoisseurship The skills and dispositions of appreciation, inference, disclosure, and description associated with high-quality supervision.

Constituents The people who may be involved in supervision, including supervisors, supervisees, clients/patients, parents, family, or significant others, and ancillary personnel; one third of the Trigonal Model of Communication Disorders supervision.

Contexts The worksites where supervisors are employed, including college and university clinics, schools, medical settings, community speech-language and hearing centers, and businesses; one third of the Trigonal Model of Communication Disorders supervision.

Continuous communication Communication in which messages blend together to create meaning.

Convergent thinking Logical induction or deduction (formal logic process), usually used because a relatively complete set of facts is available; associated with vertical thinking.

Council on Professional Standards An ASHA board that formulates, implements, maintains, and monitors overall standards and procedures of the organization.

Creativity a fluent (smooth and rapid) and flexible (divergent, adaptable, inclusive) process used to develop novel and useful outcomes to a problem.

CUSPSPA The Council of University Supervisors of Practicum in Speech-Language Pathology and Audiology, which evolved in 1974 from the Council of University Supervisors of Practicum in the Schools. The purpose of CUSPSPA is to unify through a network those persons interested in supervision in Communication Disorders.

Data base A collection of information that can be organized, reorganized, managed, and maintained by electronic means.

Decision axis A horizontal line that represents information gathered over a long time and organized in relation to the two poles of a decision.

Dependent variable That which is being measured in a research study.

Differential supervision The process of matching a supervisor's modes of action (STYLES) to the needs, abilities, and willingness of supervisees.

Discrete communication Communication in which all messages are clearly different from each other.

Discursive communication Communication in which all speakers and listeners share approximately the same background knowledge.

Divergent thinking Fluent, flexible, and elaborate thinking, often implying creativity; associated with lateral thinking.

Editing The revising, refining, altering, or adapting of written material for clarity, accuracy, completeness, correctness, or to meet publication standards; may be done by the writer (self-editing) or by another reader.

Education Standards Board (ESB) An ASHA committee of the Council of Professional Standards that formulates, implements, maintains, and monitors the standards and procedures of educational training programs.

Evaluation Arriving at a judgment or decision about a person's or program's work based on data from observing, testing (measuring), and grading.

Field supervisor A supervisor who is generally employed as a clinician or staff supervisor in a setting such as a school or hospital, but also supervises student clinicians who are completing off-campus practicum assignments in affiliation with a college or university Communication Disorders program.

Formula writing An approach to clinical reporting in which a standard report format (organization, sequence, vocabulary, style) is determined, with a skeletal form containing slots (syntactic positions) for fillers (semantic data).

Generic supervisor A supervisor from one discipline who is responsible for overseeing the work of staff members in other disciplines.

Guided observation A technique in which an experienced observer directs an inexperienced observer's attention to specific features of a situation as a way of teaching new observational strategies.

Heuristics Methods of deriving and evaluating potential productive outcomes to problems; planning and creativity are two examples.

Hypothesis An assumption or prediction that becomes the basis of a research project. The research intent is to test the accuracy of the hypothesis.

Independent variable A condition controlled or manipulated by the researcher to determine its impact on the dependent variable.

Inquiry modes Styles of thinking or organizing world experiences and knowledge; Synthesist, Idealist, Pragmatist, Analyst, and Realist are examples.

INREAL INter-REActive Learning. An educational philosophy based on the premise that learning occurs through shared, genuine communication rather than instruction. Supervisors use nonverbal and verbal Reactive Language strategies such as Silence, Observation, Understanding, Listening (S.O.U.L.); Reaction Time Latency (RTL); Mirroring (M); Self Talk (ST); Parallel Talk (PT); Verbal Monitoring and Reflecting (VM & R); Expansion (E); and Modeling (MD) to join supervisees' worlds of knowledge and to negotiate contextual meaning that results in mutual learning.

Interpersonal communication pacing (ICP) A supervisor's verbal matching and/or nonverbal mirroring of the communication behavior of supervisees in order to establish rapport and facilitate interaction and learning.

Interval data Data that reflect equal distance between data points and have an arbitrarily assigned zero. Because the intervals are equal, these data can be added and subtracted. Personality test scores are an example.

Intuitive communication Communication that is transacted without the conscious use of logic (e.g., emotions).

Joint Commission on Accreditation of Hospitals (JCAH) The agency responsible for establishing and monitoring standards for and offering accreditation to four types of medical institutions: (a) acute care general hospitals; (b) long-term care facilities; (c) psychiatric and substance-abuse facilities and programs; and (d) ambulatory health care organizations.

Lateral thinking Intuitive, divergent, creative, low-probability thinking.

Leadership styles Behavioral characteristics that reflect traits of different kinds of leaders. The styles are used to accomplish tasks as well as to meet the relationship needs and concerns of members of a group or organization.

Linear communication Logical, rational negotiated meaning.

Macrofocus A broad-focus observation strategy that yields low agreement between observers, high degrees of inference, many opportunities and much information for generalizing, a high degree of subjectivity, and a fairly complete picture of the total therapeutic process; cf. *microfocus*.

Marginal personnel People who lack the knowledge, skills, and/or dispositions to perform the required tasks within a specific discipline.

Matrix management The use of a geometic configuration composed of a vertical and a horizontal axis (e.g., a two-by-two quadrant matrix) to define varying degrees of opposite conditions (e.g., unilateral-bilateral or direct-indirect supervision styles), or to combine two conditions (e.g., question-asking behavior + use of supervisee's ideas) for the purpose of matching an appropriate condition to the requirements of a given supervision situation.

Maximax A problem management strategy of maximizing the maximum gain. Usually also increases risk.

Microfocus A narrow-focus observation strategy that yields high agreement between observers, low degrees of inference, little information from which generalizations can be made, a low degree of subjectivity, and a partial picture of the therapeutic process; cf. *macrofocus*.

Minimax A problem management strategy of minimizing the maximum risk; usually also lowers the potential gain.

Modes of observation Forms or types of observation, including medium (e.g., live, videotape, CCTV, audiotape), location, and protocol.

Naturalistic evaluation A process of evaluation used to discover and understand, rather than to determine; videotaping, connoisseurship, artifacts analysis, and portfolio development are methods of naturalistic evaluation.

Nominal data Data that can be classified only. Gender and type of hearing loss are examples of nominal data.

Nondiscursive communication Communication in which components of the message are not common to speakers and listeners.

Nonparametric statistics A method used to make inferences or generalizations from collected data; the prerequisite assumptions are more flexible than for parametric statistics.

Nontraditional communication Three types of nontraditional communication are important in supervision: (a) the communication patterns of a different or varied linguistic system (nonstandard American English); (b) the communication patterns of minority language, multicultural populations; and (c) the communication patterns of adult learners.

Null hypothesis A formal hypothesis worded negatively (e.g., "There will *not* be a change...").

Observation competence The ability to apply observational knowledge and skills to all dimensions of behavior.

On-campus supervisor A supervisor who works in a college or university training program clinic.

Ordinal data Data that can be ranked according to a given value or property but for which the amount of difference between ranks is unknown. An example would be the degree of directness in a supervision conference. Variations in directness could be put in sequential order, but it would be unknown whether one level differed more or less than another.

Parametric statistics An approach that allows the researcher to make inferences or generalizations from collected data. Specified assumptions about the research population, such as sample size and homogeneity, must be met as a prerequisite for using this group of statistics.

Pedagogy A mode of teaching in which the teacher assumes full responsibility for the teaching-learning process; a concept used in Communication Disorders supervision STYLES I and II (see Appendix B).

Pentagonal Model of Communication Disorders supervision A model unique to Communication Disorders supervision that involves the interaction of the Constituents, Concepts, and Contexts components of the supervision process within the Professional, Research, Educational, Administrative, and Clinical domains.

Philosophical belief systems Orientations to living that structure thinking about personal values, choices, and decisions; the guiding forces behind personal approaches to teaching and learning. Essentialism, experimentalism, and existentialism are examples.

Planning A heuristic operator used to structure in advance actions that will change the current state, or status quo, into some other future state.

Portfolio development A form of naturalistic evaluation where a file or collection of materials, records, photographs, audio- and videocassettes, and other artifacts is developed to represent the person's performance.

PREAC The acronym for the five domains and associated roles in which Communication Disorders supervisors act: Professional, Research, Educational, Administrative, and Clinical.

Preparation The combination of education (internally controlled learning) and training (externally controlled learning).

Primary supervisor A supervisor whose job is full-time clinical education.

Probability Relative frequency with which an event occurs or is likely to occur (objective probability); how strongly one believes something will occur or happen (subjective probability).

Problems A situation requiring decision making or choice making without all the necessary information available.

Problem managing The ongoing process of creating an outcome (or outcomes) to a problem. The assumption in problem managing is that problems are ongoing rather than episodic; therefore, outcomes will be revised or the problem will be redefined and will require continuous management.

Problem solving The process of finding a solution to a problem. The assumption in problem solving is that once a solution is found the problem no longer exists. Problem solving carries a connotation of finality that problem managing does not.

Process A series of actions or operations marked by gradual, continuous, transactive changes that lead to a particular result.

Professional Services Board (PSB) An ASHA committee of the Council on Professional Standards that formulates, implements, maintains, and monitors standards and procedures for service delivery agencies.

Program management Supervision tasks relating to administration or coordination of programs.

Psychological belief system The implementation counterparts of philosophical belief systems. Behaviorism, cognitivism, and humanism are examples.

Qualitative research A data collection and analysis process in which numerical data are

GLOSSARY

neither gathered nor manipulated. Thoughtful analysis is completed for a specified theoretical orientation.

Quantitative research Scientific inquiry based on data collection and manipulation as the means to answer a given question.

Ratio data Similar to interval data except that an absolute zero exists. Reaction time latency is an example.

Reasoning The use of formal logic (rules for analyzing a situation, position, or statement to determine internal consistency) and natural discourse (the communication exchange involved in the process of comprehending a problem).

Recording systems Organized procedures for written documentation of occurrences and behaviors.

Research Critical and exhaustive examination and/or experimentation to discover new facts and their appropriate interpretation or to revise accepted ideas in light of new information.

Research design An organizational plan used to assign subjects to specific conditions in order to collect and then analyze data to answer a research question.

Risk Exposure to the chance of loss.

Roles Characteristics and tasks of specific jobs in which a supervisor is involved in the Communication Disorders supervision process. The Communication Disorders supervisor may be involved in five roles: Professional, Researcher, Educator (academic and clinical), Administrator, and Clinician.

Schemata Cognitive data structures used to store concepts; every kind of concept requires schemata to represent it.

Secondary supervisor A supervisor whose job involves part-time clinical education and part-time administration, academic teaching, clinical service delivery, and/or research.

Signal detection theory A part of information theory that explains whether a target condition is present or not.

Sign test A test for plus or minus change in related measures. Results of the sign test indicate whether or not an apparent change is actually significant.

Spreadsheet A computer program in which a user can enter, modify, and manipulate data organized in a rectangular array of rows and columns (table).

Staff supervisor A supervisor who works in service delivery sites where the focus is on monitoring and maintaining professional staff competence.

States of nature Environmental conditions.

Strand A bipolar dimension of supervisory behavior (e.g., direct-indirect communication pattern).

Styles Specific dimensions of focus in the Communication Disorders supervision process. Common styles referred to in the literature include *unilateral-bilateral* (quantity of talk from each participant), *direct-indirect* (quality of talk), *task-oriented–person-oriented*, *communicative-instructive* (intent of the communication), *supervisor-oriented, supervisee-oriented, client-oriented,* and so forth.

STYLES Distinctive, characteristic, identifiable aggregates of behavior in connection with people and their relationships, tasks and their products, and the process of supervision. There are four basic STYLES of Communication Disorders supervision (see Appendix B).

SUPERNET Acronym for Supervision of University Practicum: Education and Research NETwork. The purpose of SUPERNET is to coordinate supervision research and help organize professional groups of supervisors at the state, regional, and local levels.

Supervision A necessary, artistic/scientific and changing process composed of three components (Constituents, Concepts, and Contexts) that interact within the Professional, Research, Educational, Administrative, and Clinical domains of speech-language pathology and audiology to assure initial and continuing training of competent professionals who can provide quality services for education or health care consumers. Supervisors, who are specialists in the Communication Disorders profession, require training to meet the standards of quality set by the ASHA Committee on Supervision.

Supervision competence The combination of supervisory skills and dispositions.

a. Supervision skill is developed or acquired excellence in performing technical acts associated with Communication Disorders supervision, as measured by some set of performance criteria.

b. Supervision dispositions are internalized, integrated skills. A supervisor's learned technical skill has become a disposition if the supervisor tends to use it in appropriate supervision situations.

Supervision forms Dyadic (two-person) and group supervision.

Supervision types Combinations of the four supervision STYLES with the two supervision forms to create eight different ways of doing Communication Disorders supervision. They are used for differential supervision.

Supervisees Communication Disorders students, trainees, or clinicians who are the recipients of supervisors' efforts.

Supervisors People who engage in professional, research, education, administration, and clinical activities in a variety of settings in order to meet the goal of supervision.

Syllogism A three-step argument consisting of two premises, both assumed to be true, and a conclusion that follows from the premises (e.g., "All As are Bs; all Bs are Cs; therefore, all Cs are As").

Syntality The behavioral tendencies of a group taken as a unit that correspond to the personality traits of an individual; an individual has a characteristic personality whereas a group has a characteristic syntality.

System A group of entities and the dynamic relations among them.

Systematic observation A thorough, regular method of observing occurrences and behaviors

Telecommunication Electronic communication involving machines (or people and machines) that uses existing telephone, radio, and television systems. Voice, text, photographs and other images, and handwriting are among the signals that can be sent and received via telecommunication.

Transactional mutuality The making of meaning through negotiated interactions.

Trigonal Model of Communication Disorders supervision The combination of Constituents, Concepts, and Contexts of supervision into a theoretical triangular form.

t-test A test for the difference between two mean scores from the same group of subjects.

Type 1 alpha statistical error The erroneous appearance of a statistically significant result because of small sample size, discarding irregular scores, or a too liberal probability level.

Uncertainty A decision situation in which each possible action has more than one possible outcome, depending on the states of nature, with each state having an unknown probability.

Utility Usefulness; satisfaction with a given outcome.

Value The monetary payoff of an action, dependent upon mathematics or objective probability.

Variance A measure of the amount of spread or variation in scores. A small amount of variance means subjects' scores were similar, with minimal differences among them.

Vertical thinking Analytical, logical, sequential, high-probability thinking.

Video discs A secondary memory system used for storing visual information in electronic equipment.

Video resume A presentation of one's professional experience and abilities on videotape.

Visual literacy The knowledge, skills, and dispositions for recording, interpreting, integrating, utilizing, and reporting visual experiences.

Word processing A category of computer application that allows electronic entry, modification, editing, and printing of text.

Author Index

Abrahamson, J., 267
Abrell, R., 57, 68
Acheson, K., 58
Adair, M., 337t
Adams, J., 218, 219, 221
Aitchison, C., 335t
Alter, K., 255
American Speech-Language-Hearing Association, 5, 6, 7, 9, 19, 20, 22, 24, 74, 78, 88, 89, 127, 156, 157, 230, 231, 279, 296, 316, 335t, 336t, 337t, 338
Andersen, C., 302, 325, 334t
Anderson, J., 5, 6, 18, 24, 137, 157, 172, 175, 230, 298t, 300, 320, 320f, 321, 322, 323f, 328, 329, 331, 332, 334t, 336t, 337t
Andrews, J., 336t
Apple Computer, Inc., 226
Attridge, C., 137

Backus, O., 5
Baldes, R., 336t
Bales, R., 138, 141, 298t
Bandler, R., 105, 106, 117
Barbour, C., 64
Barnes, K., 20
Barrett-Lennard, G., 327
Bash, M., 210
Battin, R., 230, 331t
Baugh, L., 239
Beavin, J., 56, 103
Behrmann, M., 172, 268

Belenky, M., 107, 109
Bennet, C., 255
Berger, C., 114, 125
Berlin, L., 118
Berne, E., 132
Bernstein, B., 104
Bernthal, J., 6, 336t
Bertalanffy, L. von, 56, 207
Bess, F., 284, 337t
Beukelman, D., 336t
Bierwisch, M., 96
Billings, B., 230
Bills, R., 327
Black, M., 335t
Blake, R., 33, 59
Blanchard, K., 47, 58
Blank, M., 118
Bless, D., 302
Bliss, L., 318, 327, 335t
Block, J. 45
Blodgett, E., 302, 335t
Blumberg, A., 59, 64, 111, 124, 137, 298t, 330
Boase, P., 98, 120, 217, 219, 222
Bobrow, D., 213
Boehm, A., 156
Boone, D., 58, 298t, 316, 336t
Borker, R., 108, 109
Bourne, L., 45, 207, 208, 211
Boyer, E., 175
Bramson, R., 33, 38, 44
Brandt, D., 123

t = table; f = figure

Brasseur, J., 47, 124, 298t, 300, 321, 322, 323f, 328, 331, 332, 334t, 335t
Brinkerhoff, R., 25
Broadbent, M., 119
Brock, G., 327
Broffman, S., 230
Brooks, R., 336t
Brookshire, R., 334t
Bross, I., 188, 197
Buchheimer, A., 106, 119
Buckberry, E., 67, 71, 295
Burks, D., 106

Calabrese, R., 114, 125
Camp, B., 210
Caracciolo, G., 316, 320, 321f, 327, 334t, 336t
Carkuff, R., 328
Carlson, K., 302
Carlson, R., 106
Carnell, C., 230
Carreras, N., 118
Cartwright, C., 156
Cartwright, G., 156
Casey, P., 125, 332, 334t
Cazden, C., 117
Chabon, S., 230
Chapman, R., 254
Cimorell-Strong, J., 329, 334t
Clinchy, B., 107
Coates, N., 335t
Cogan, M., 57, 58, 64, 124
Colucci, S., 326, 334t
Condon, W., 106, 119
Conger, J., 214
Conover, H., 139, 254, 298t
Conture, E., 5
Cornett, B., 230
Corvey, S., 32, 47, 215
Coulter, D., 56, 207
Council of University Supervisors of Practicum in Speech-Language Pathology and Audiology (CUSPSPA), 18
Crago, M., 6, 57, 60, 337t
Craig, C., 31, 32
Crichton, L., 74, 335t, 337t
Culatta, R., 124, 137, 142, 298t, 316, 323, 326, 328, 330, 331, 334t, 336t
Compata, J., 125
Cunningham, R., 111, 113
Currier, R., 267

D'Angelo, G., 101, 328
D'Augelli, A., 327
Danish, S., 327
Davis, K., 138
Daynes, R., 267
deBono, E., 208, 209, 210, 212, 218, 221, 222
Delamont, S., 156
Deutsch, M., 131
deVille, J., 39
Dewar, D., 68, 71
Dewey, J., 219, 222
Diedrich, W., 190
Dimmer, J., 220, 222
Dobson, J., 26, 27, 29, 44, 47
Dobson, R., 26, 27, 29, 44, 47
Dodd, D., 213
Doehring, D., 337t
Donovan, P., 44, 218
Dowling, S., 25, 46, 64, 70, 124, 156, 317, 318, 323, 324f, 325, 326, 327, 330, 331, 332, 334t, 335t, 336t
Drexler, A., 335t
Dreyer, D., 334t
Dublinske, S., 20, 296
Duffy, F., 57
Duke, J., 131
Dunlop, R., 267
Dyer, W., 217

Eadie, W., 106
Edwards, D., 300
Egan, G., 133, 192, 194
Ekstrand, B., 45, 207, 208, 211
Elliot, E., 59
Elliott, L., 257, 259
Emerick, L., 122, 230
English, R., 230
Engnoth, G., 337t
Ensley, K., 329, 334t
Epstein, C., 218
Erhardt, H., 32, 47, 215
Erickson, F., 105, 119
Erickson, R., 336t

Faber, H., 117
Fagin, R., 56
Fahey, R., 325
Falvey, N., 257, 259
Farmer, J., 58, 59, 64, 219, 220, 222, 266, 267, 337t

AUTHOR INDEX

Farmer, S., 6, 7, 18, 25, 32, 39, 47, 48, 58, 59, 64, 66, 68, 70, 71, 99, 105, 114, 115, 118, 119, 123, 125, 127, 133, 134, 139, 157, 160, 161, 162, 163, 219, 220, 222, 255, 266, 267, 292, 298t, 300, 318, 319f, 327, 335t, 337t, 338
Faucett, R., 170
Fear, R., 122
Fein, D., 74
Feldhusen, J., 217, 219
Felicetti, T., 299t, 317, 337t
Ferber, A., 97
Festinger, L., 75
Filley, A., 134
Filley, F., 58, 279, 299t, 300, 302, 325, 336t
Fisch, R., 74, 135
Fitch, J., 254
Flanders, N., 59, 298t
Flower, R., 5, 59, 64, 230, 232
Fox, D., 230
Frankel, J., 113
Frazer, G., 197
Freilinger, J., 336t
French, J., 131
Friedman, R., 156, 327, 334t
Fuller, R., 267

Gagne, R., 190
Gall, M., 58
Gardner, J., 303
Garrett, E., 190
Gavett, E., 44, 337t
Gazda, G., 117
Geoffrey, V., 301
George, A., 75
Gershaw, N., 218
Gerstman, H., 336t
Ghitter, R., 303
Gibbs, D., 120
Gillam, R., 337t, 338
Gilligan, C., 107, 109
Ginott, H., 117
Gleason, J., 105, 107
Goebel, M., 266
Goings, R., 336t
Goldberg, S., 165
Goldberger, N., 107
Goldhaber, G., 121, 139
Goldhammer, R., 57, 124
Goldman, R., 68, 71

Goldstein, A., 218
Golper, L., 156
Gonzales, D., 156
Goodwin, W., 334t
Gordon, M., 156
Gordon, T., 117
Gordon, W., 217, 219, 221
Goss, B., 98, 99, 138
Greene, J., 32, 33, 44, 47
Greif, E., 107
Grice, H., 107, 114, 213
Griffith, T., 337t
Grijalva, L., 156
Grimes, J., 20, 296
Grinder, J., 105, 106, 117
Guilford, J., 212
Guinty, C., 156
Gunter, C., 337t

Haas, R., 337t
Haas, W., 106, 119
Hagler, P., 169, 295, 325, 335t
Halfond, M., 5, 335t
Hall, A., 56, 334t
Hall, D., 44
Hall, G., 74, 75
Halliday, M., 96, 118
Hannah, E., 336t
Hanson, M., 230
Harden, R.J., 257
Harden, R.W., 257
Hardick, E., 337t
Hargrave, J., 230
Harris, A., 336t
Harris, M., 157, 299t, 317, 337t
Harris, R., 156
Harris, T., 132
Harrison, A., 33, 39, 44
Harryman, E., 237
Hart, R., 106
Harvey, J., 157
Hasan, R., 118
Hatten, J., 5, 337t
Hawes, L., 133
Hayes, D., 58, 279, 299t, 300, 325, 336t
Hayes, W., 122, 230
Healey, W., 244
Hebalk, B., 58
Helmick, J., 336t
Helsila, M., 139

Herbert, J., 137
Herbold, D., 336t
Hersey, P., 47, 58
Holdgrafer, G., 169, 295
Holloway, J., 254, 255
Hood, S., 252
Horii, Y., 266
Howe, L., 218
Hubbell, R., 96, 103
Hull, R., 46
Hunt, D., 300
Hunter, M., 57
Hutchinson, B., 230
Hyman, C., 74

Idol, L., 57
Ingham, H., 135
Ingrisano, D., 58, 334t
INREAL staff, 68
Irwin, R., 67, 70, 124, 159, 336t, 337t

Jackson, C., 257, 266, 267
Jackson, D., 56, 103
Jackson, P., 212
Jaggar, A., 156
Janis, I., 121
Jeffrey, R., 336t
Johnson, K., 125
Johnson, T., 334t
Jones, S., 244
Joos, M., 104

Kadushin, A., 132
Kagan, J., 214
Kallail, K., 335t
Kamara, A., 257, 259
Kamara, C., 257, 259, 277
Kaplan, N., 334t
Katz, L., 64
Katz, N., 128
Katz, R., 256
Kay Electronics Corporation, 266
Keen, P., 215
Kendon, A., 97, 106, 118, 119
Kennedy, K., 135, 329, 334t, 337t
Kessinger, J., 26, 27, 29, 44, 47
Kiefer, F., 96
Kilmann, R., 42, 44, 129, 130
Kirschenbaum, H., 218
Kirtley, D., 5
Kleffner, F., 5, 74, 316

Klein, P., 218
Klevans, D., 115, 156, 165, 298t, 327, 334t, 336t
Knapp, M., 42, 44, 97, 102, 105, 129, 130, 165
Knepflar, K., 230, 231
Knowles, M., 29, 58, 127
Kolb, D., 32, 47
Konarska, K., 253
Kopra, L., 267
Kopra, M., 267
Kramer, C., 107
Kramer, J., 170
Kramer, W., 46
Krescheck, J., 237
Krueger, K., 334t
Kunze, L., 156
Kwiatkowski, J., 58, 279, 299t, 300, 302, 325, 336t

Laccinole, M., 292
LaFrance, M., 106, 119
Laird, B., 334t
Lakoff, R., 107, 108
Lane, V., 139, 266
Langellier, K., 18, 45, 107, 108, 109
Larkin, J., 211
Larson, L., 326, 334t, 335t
Lashbrook, V., 138, 255, 299t
Lashbrook, W., 138, 255, 299t
Lawrence, J., 230
Lawyer, J., 128
Lefferts, R., 234
Lewis, D., 32, 33, 44, 47
Lightfoot, R., 170
Lillywhite, R., 230
Lissner, R., 252, 255
Lombardino, L., 252
Long, L., 106, 119
Loucks, S., 74, 75
Lougeay-Mottinger, J., 157, 299t, 317, 337t
Luft, J., 135, 136
Lynch, J., 107, 108
Lyngby, A., 74
Lyon, M., 220, 222

MacLearie, E., 5
McCaulley, M., 31, 44, 47
McClean, O., 327
McCormick, L., 68, 71
McCrea, E., 125, 137, 299t, 328, 334t
McCready, V., 135, 163, 335t, 337t

AUTHOR INDEX

McKenny, J., 215
McMahon, J., 156
Mager, R., 236, 244
Mahaffey, R., 252
Maltz, D., 108, 109
Markel, G., 302
Markle, S., 303
Matecum, T., 125
Mawdsley, B., 57, 58, 137, 157
Mayer, R., 206
Mayo, C., 106, 119
Mazlish, E., 117
Mecham, M., 230
Meitus, T., 230, 232
Mercaitis, P., 157, 300, 302, 335t
Mercer, A., 115
Mervis, C., 211
Messal, S., 257, 259
Messick, S., 212
Michalak, D., 64, 124, 127
Middleton, G., 230
Milisen, R., 5
Miller, E., 335t
Miller, J., 254
Miller, L., 105
Miller, L.R., 252
Miller, Lynda, 206, 207
Miner, A., 5, 299t, 336t
Molyneaux, D., 139, 266
Monnin, L., 6, 336t, 337t
Moore, M., 230
Mordecai, D., 254, 255
Mornout, C., 46
Morrison, E., 316, 320, 321f, 327, 334t, 336t
Mosher, R., 124
Mountain View College, 44
Mouton, J., 33, 59
Mowrer, D., 336t
Mueller, P., 257
Muma, J., 105
Mussen, P., 214
Myers, G., 75, 98
Myers, I., 31, 44, 47
Myers, M., 75, 98

Naremore, R., 318, 322, 325, 335t
Natalle, E., 18, 45, 107, 108, 109
Neidecker, E., 230, 232, 236, 244
Nelson, J., 124, 334t
Nesbit, E. 220, 222

Nevin, A., 57
Newlove, B., 74
Nicholas, L., 334t
Nickles, A., 159, 337t
Nicolosi, L., 237
Nielsen, D., 197
Nilsen, J., 330, 335t
Norman, D., 213
Norris, M., 257
Norton, R., 39, 44, 105
Norton, S., 327, 334t

Oas, D., 25
Ogston, W., 106, 119
Olsen, H., 64
Olson, R., 212, 214, 219, 221
O'Neill, J., 335t, 337t
Oratio, A., 6, 57, 59, 74, 137, 255, 299t, 321, 322f, 325, 334t, 335t, 337t
Ortman, K., 217
Osborn, A., 218
O'Sullivan, M., 337t
O'Toole, T., 336t
Oyer, H., 232, 337t

Palin, M., 254, 255
Palmer, C., 254, 255
Pannbacker, M., 230
Paolucci-Whitcomb, P., 57
Parks, M., 98
Patterson, C., 210
Pea, R., 210
Peaper, R., 157, 301, 302, 330, 335t
Penner, K., 257, 259
Perkins, W., 335t
Perlstein-Kaplan, K., 299t, 317, 337t
Peroff, L., 325
Perry, W., 109
Peters, K., 6, 336t, 337t
Peters, T., 257
Peterson, H., 252, 335t
Pickering, M., 6, 24, 118, 124, 125, 316, 317, 317f, 318, 328, 336t, 337t
Pines, D., 20
Prass, M., 322, 334t
Prather, E., 59
Prescott, T., 58, 298t, 316, 336t
Price, J., 39, 41, 44
Puett, V., 230
Purpel, D., 124
Putens, D., 327, 334t

Raiffa, H., 194, 199
Rapoport, A., 132
Rassi, J., 6, 19, 78, 157, 230, 337t
Rathmel, B., 58
Raths, J., 64
Raven, B., 131
Reddin, W., 39, 64
Redmond, K., 334t
Rees, M., 5, 335t
Rigrodsky, S., 316, 320, 321f, 327, 334t, 336t
Robbins, S., 4
Roberts, J., 6, 111, 113, 124, 142, 163, 318, 322, 325, 329, 334t, 335t
Roberts, R., 210
Rogers, C., 327
Rogers, R., 76
Rosch, E., 211
Rose, S., 118
Rowe, M., 102
Rowen, B., 156
Rumelhart, D., 213
Runyan, S., 157, 335t
Rushakoff, G., 252, 257, 259, 266, 267
Rutherford, W., 75
Ryan, B., 335t

Sacks, H., 107
Sanders, K., 230
Sbaschnig, K., 125, 300, 323, 324f, 325, 331, 332, 334t
Schalk, M., 325
Schatz, J., 58, 279, 299t, 300, 325, 336t
Scheflen, A., 119
Schegloff, E., 107
Scherer, K., 97
Schill, M., 292
Schmitt, J., 120, 302, 335t
Schmitz, H., 230
Schubert, G., 6, 20, 74, 115, 124, 165, 168, 173, 175, 230, 299t, 304, 334t, 335t, 336t, 337t
Schultz, M., 191
Schwartz, A., 252
Scudder, R., 156, 302, 335t
Seal, B., 157, 335t
Searle, J., 96, 114
Sedge, R., 337t
Seltzer, H., 124, 137, 142, 298t, 316, 323, 328, 330, 331, 336t
Sergiovanni, T., 56, 59, 60, 135, 289
Shank, K., 330, 331, 334t

Shapiro, D., 135, 330, 335t, 337t
Shepard, N., 197
Shewan, C., 18
Shriberg, L., 58, 279, 299t, 300, 302, 325, 336t
Shultz, J., 105, 119
Siegel, G., 117
Siegel, S., 318
Siegle, D., 46
Silbar, J., 253
Silverman, F., 318
Simmons, K., 58, 279, 299t, 300, 325, 336t
Simon, A., 175
Simon, C., 142
Simon, S., 218
Sleight, C., 31, 32, 132, 318, 319f, 326, 335t, 337t
Smith, D., 133
Smith, D. D., 215
Smith, J., 5, 335t
Smith, K., 6, 111, 113, 124, 137, 142, 157, 299t, 300, 320, 320f, 322, 326, 329, 331, 332, 334t, 335t
Smith, M., 58, 279, 299t, 300, 302, 325, 336t
Smith-Burke, M., 156
Solomon, B., 46
Sperloff, G., 123
Spradlin, J., 117
Sprafkin, R., 218
Stace, A., 335t
Stallings, J., 156
Starkweather, C., 59
Starratt, R., 56, 59, 60, 135, 289
Stevens, L., 105
Stewart, J., 101, 128, 328
Stillman, R., 157
Strike, C., 337t, 338
Strunk, W., 237
Stubbs, M., 156
Stuve, C., 302
Sugarman, M., 322, 334t
Sziraki, D., 125

Tarule, J., 107
Tepper, D., 106, 119
Terrio, L., 337t
Tesauro, P., 336t
Thomas, K., 42, 44, 129, 130
Thompson, C., 220, 222, 303
Thompson, J., 165
Thorlacius, J., 299t

AUTHOR INDEX

Tibbets, D., 336t
Tidwell, A., 170
Tihen, L., 326, 335t
Till, J., 299t
Tufts, L., 335t
Turner, R., 197
Turton, L., 5

Ulrich, S., 6, 18, 337t
Underwood, J., 125, 137, 299t, 334t

Van Hattum, R., 4
Van Riper, C., 335t, 336t
Vance, E., 327
Vaughn, G., 170
Vegely, A., 257, 259
Villareal, J., 316
Vinson, B., 257, 259
Volz, H., 115, 165, 298t, 327, 334t, 336t

Ward, L., 59, 316, 336t
Ward, S., 106
Wasinger, J., 217
Watzlawick, P., 56, 74, 103, 135
Weakland, J., 74, 135
Webster, E., 123
Webster, E. J., 59, 316, 336t
Weinberg, B., 230
Weinberg, R., 156, 232

Weiner, F., 254, 255
Weiss, R., 47, 115, 299t
Weller, R., 124, 137, 255, 299t, 320, 329, 331
Wener, D., 335t
Wertzberger, D., 220, 222
Wheeler, G., 336t
White, E., 237
White, H., 67, 71
White, R., 213
Whitman, R., 98, 120, 217, 219, 222
Wiener, F., 230
Wiggins, E., 326, 334t
Wiio, O., 139
Willbrand, M., 336t
Williams, C., 300, 323, 324f, 325, 331, 332, 334t
Wilmot, J., 128, 131, 132, 134
Wilmot, W., 128, 131, 132, 134
Wing, P., 230
Winkelgren, W., 206
Winston, P., 268
Wittkopp, J., 46, 326, 334t
Wonder, J., 44, 218
Wood, B., 97

Yager, E., 127
Yarbrough, E., 114, 129, 130

Zollman, D., 267

Subject Index

ABC Leadership Style, 39, 40–41t, 43–44t
Accuracy of verbal behavior, 168
Acrolect style of communication, 105
Action descriptors, 177
Actor-observer bias, 302
Administrator Role (Administrative Domain), 7, 8, 20, 23t, 48, 85–89, 86–87t, 96, 121, 144t, 157, 184, 217, 221–222t, 230, 254, 255, 264, 276, 283, 316, 334–337t
AI (Artificial Intelligence), 267
Algorithms, 208
Alternative actions in decision making, 185, 189, 198
American Academy of Speech Correction, 3
Analysis of Behaviors of Clinicians (ABC) System (Schubert), 299t
Analyst inquiry mode, 37t, 63f
Andragogy learning style, 29–30, 127–128
Anecdotal records (logs and journals), 234
ANOVA (Analysis of Variance), 321, 323f
Anthropological/ethnological descriptions, 176
Appleworks, 254, 255
Art of Thinking, 33
Artifacts analysis, 289
ASHA (American Speech-Language-Hearing Association), 3, 19, 20, 74, 127, 156, 157, 173, 220, 276, 300
Assessment, 275
   consequences, 286
   evaluating and grading peers, 305
   generic supervision, 306

   in PREAC domains, 283
   marginal personnel, 304–305
   Matrix Management, 283–286
   nontraditional learners, 305
   policies and procedures, 277, 278t
   purpose of, 277
   preparation for, 276
ASSIST-M, 58
Assumptions in observation, 164
Assumptions of supervision, 7–9
Atmosphere (ambiance), 166
Attention, 214
Attitudes conveyed by verbal behavior, 168
Attribution Theory, 45–46, 162–163
Audiology supervision, 78, 338
Audiotape recording, 170–171, 329
Axioms of communication, 97–98

Barrett-Lennard Relationship Inventory, 321f, 327
Basolect style of communication, 105
Behaviorism, 27, 63f
Behaviorist/Associationist theory of problem managing, 207
Biases, 162–163, 276, 302–303, 325
Bilingual-bicultural supervision, 126–127
Billing, 255
Blumberg Analysis System, 137, 298t, 330
Body movements and postures, 166
Boone-Prescott Content and Sequence Analysis System, 298t, 316
Bottom-up information processing, 213, 214

t = table; f = figure

SUBJECT INDEX

Brainstorming, 218t, 220t
BRS (Bibliographic Research Service), 265
Bug-in-the-ear feedback system, 169
Bug list, 218t, 220t
Burnout, 45-46
Buzz sessions, 219t, 220t

CAFET (Computer-Aided Fluency Establishment Trainer), 266
CAI (Computer Assisted Instruction), 266, 267
Career data bases, 254
Career development, 42-45
CARF (Commission on Accreditation of Rehabilitation Facilities), 7
CAS (Conversation Analysis System), 298t
CASE (Comprehensive Assessment and Service Evaluation), 18, 296
Case Staffings, 66-67, 70t
CASLPA (Canadian Association of Speech-Language Pathology and Audiology), 6, 19
CAT (Conversation Assessment Technique), 298t
Categorical supervisors, 21
Causal attributions, 163, 303
C-BAM (Concerns-Based Adoption Model), 75
  Levels of Use (LoU) Instrument, 75
  Stages of Concern (SoC) Instrument, 75
CCC (Certificate of Clinical Competence), 7, 21, 74
CCTV (closed circuit television), 169-170
CFY (Clinical Fellowship Year), 5, 7, 74
Change, 74-78, 207
Channels of communication, 102, 301
Charts (notations, unit notes), 233
Checklists (graphs, audiograms, profiles, test forms, diagrams), 177, 234
Chi-square research design, 318, 319f
Chronemics, 166
Clarity of verbal behavior, 168
Classifications of supervisors, 21
Clinical Data Manager, 256
Clinical education. *See* Educator Role/Domain
Clinical Fellows, 5, 7
Clinical literacy, 229, 277
  professional, legal, ethical considerations, 231
Clinical reporting, 231-236
  clinical report reading, 232
  clinical report writing, 232, 237-239t, 240t, 241t, 242t, 243t
  forms of clinical reporting, 233-234
    anecdotal records (logs and journals), 234

charts (notations, unit notes), 233
checklists (graphs, audiograms, profiles, test forms, diagrams), 234
diagnostic or initial evaluation reports, 233
discharge summaries (disposition or transfer statements, end-of-therapy reports), 233
intervention plans (therapy plans, IEPs, service delivery plans, care plans, therapeutic records, unit records, operational management data, problem-oriented charts), 233
professional letters, 234
progress reports (end-of-term reports, interim summaries), 233
session plans (lesson plans, progress notes, daily entries, flow charts), 233
third-party payment reports (insurance forms, federal and state government agency forms), 233
developing clinical writing, 234-236
  formula writing, 235
  self-analysis, 236
oral reporting, 232, 236
Clinical Supervision (Colleagueship), 57
Clinical supervisors, 21
Clinical Theory of Instruction, 58
Clinician Role (Clinical Domain), 7, 8, 21, 23t, 48, 85-89, 86-87t, 96, 121, 144t, 157, 184, 217, 221-222t, 230, 254, 264, 276, 283, 316, 334-337t
Clock hours, 252-253t
Clock Hours Program, 252
Closed system, 56, 103
CLSA (Computerized Language Sample Analysis), 254, 255
Codes (registers) of communication, 104
Cognitive complexity, 106, 327
Cognitive dissonance, 75
Cognitive mediators, 216
Cognitive styles, 32, 43-44t, 215
Cognitivism, 27, 63f
Cohesion (cohesive harmony), 118
Collaborative consultation, 58
Colleagueship (Clinical Supervision), 57
Commitments, 330
Committee on Supervision of Speech-Language Pathology and Audiology, 6, 22, 230
Communication, 96
Communication analysis, 135-142
  analysis tools, 137

interaction analysis, 137-139
interview analysis, 139
organizational communication audit, 139
personal analysis, 135
Communication competence and incompetence, 142-144, 277
Communication Dynamics model, 219, 219t, 220t
Communication impaired personnel, 305
Communication Style Measure, 39, 43-44t, 105
Communication styles, 39, 43-44t, 63t, 105-106
Competence and competencies, 6, 21-22, 23t, 279-280, 281-282t, 287-289, 296, appendix A
   clinical, 280t
   equation, 22
   interpersonal, 280t
   profiles, 280t
   supervisor, 280t
Complementarity in communication, 98
Computerized library card catalog, 265
Computer applications in supervision, 251-268
   concerns, 268-269
   research, 265-266
CONAN (Conover Analysis System computer program), 254, 255
Concepts, 211
Conceptual Blockbusting model, 218, 218-219t, 220t
Conditions of Learning, 191
Conferences, 123-125, 126t, 255, 296
   AP/O (Advanced Planner/Organizer), 125
   direct/indirect, 59, 63f, 64f, 124-125, 323f, 328, 329, 330
   entry phase, 125
   feedback, 169, 296
   group, 125
   guidelines, 126t
   individual, 125
   research on, 124-125, 328-331
Confidentiality, 231, 268-269
Conflict communication, 42, 43-44t, 63f, 128-135
Conflict intervention, 133
   tactics, 134
   techniques, 134-135
Confluence, 106, 119
Confrontation, 133
Congruence, 106, 119
Conover Analysis System, 139, 254, 298t
Connoisseurship, 289

Consequences in assessment, 286
Content and Sequence Analysis System (Culatta and Seltzer), 137, 298t, 316, 323, 324f, 328, 330, 331
Content-related knowledge, 211
Contexts of intellectual functioning, 212
Contexts of supervision (see worksite profiles), 85-91, 86-87t, 90t, 222t
Contextual grid (Reddin's 3-D Theory), 39
Contrived situation responses, 177
Convergent thinking, 212
Conversational competence, 106-107, 114
Correlational research design, 320-321, 320f, 322f
CoRT (Cognitive Research Trust) Thinking Program, 218
Council of College and University Supervisors of Practicum in Schools, 5
Creative problem managing benefits, 212-213
Creativity, 211-212
Criterion cutoff in decision making, 191, 191f, 192f, 194f, 195f
Critical observation, 133-134
CSMI (Cognitive Style Mapping Instrument), 32
CSRS (Child Services Review System), 20
Culatta & Seltzer Content and Sequence Analysis System, 137, 298t, 316, 323, 324f, 328, 330, 331
CUSH (Computer Users in Speech and Hearing), 269
CUSPSPA (Council of University Supervisors of Practicum in Speech-Language Pathology and Audiology), 6, 18-19, 221t, 264, 265, 276, 316, 338
   first national conference, 6
   Research Net, 18, 265, 338
Cyberphobia, 269

Data base, 258-264, 259t, 262t, 263t, 265
deBono's Thinking Course, 218
Decision analysis, 185-198
Decision axis, 191-192, 191f, 192f, 194f, 195f
Decision criteria, 191
Decision making, 184, 198-200, 205, 277
Deductive reasoning, 215-216
Demographics of Communication Disorders supervisors, 18
Deville's Leadership Model, 39
Diagnostic or initial evaluation reports, 233
Diagnostic Supervision, 58

SUBJECT INDEX

Differences-focused reasoning, 215
Differential supervision, 47, 69-74, 72-73t
Discharge summaries (disposition or transfer statement, end-of-therapy reports), 233
Discourse abstraction, 118
Discoursive-nondiscoursive communication, 96
Discrete-continuous communication, 96
Discrete event records, 177
Dispositions, 22, 142, 155, 217
Divergent thinking, 212
DO IT!, 219, 221t
Domains of supervision. (*See* Roles and PREAC), 7, 8, 19-21, 23t, 48, 85-89, 86-87t, 96, 144t, 157, 184, 217, 221-222t, 229, 230, 254, 255, 264, 276, 283, 316, 334-337t
Domain-specific knowledge, 211
Duration of observation, 173
Dyadic supervision, 64, 220t, 283-285, 284f, 289
   comparison of dyadic and group supervision, 65t

ECCO (Episodic Communication Channels in Organization), 139
Ecological narratives, 196
Editing, 245-246
  competence for supervisee, 246
  competence for supervisor, 245
  self-editing, 236
  symbols, 246
Educational Beliefs System Inventory, 27, 43-44t
Educational Practice Belief Inventory, 27, 43-44t
Educator Role (Educational Domain), 7, 8, 20, 23t, 48, 85-89, 86-87t, 96, 121, 144t, 157, 184, 217, 221t, 230, 254, 255, 264, 276, 316, 334-337t
Electronic bulletin boards, 265, 338
Element formula writing, 235, 244
Environment in observation, 167
Equifinality, 56, 207
ERIC (Educational Resources Information Center), 265
Essentialism, 25, 63f
Evaluation-feedback cycle, 276, 289, 303-304
Evaluation-feedback process, 286-304
Evaluation in supervision, 275, 285-289, 288t
  formal, 286-289
  naturalistic, 289
  patterns, 290-291t
Existentialism, 26, 63f
Expansion, 100, 101, 105
  Elaborated, 100, 101, 105
  Restated, 100, 105
Experimentalism, 25, 63f

Facial expressions and eye movements, 166
Factor analysis, 322
Feedback, 169, 289-302, 329
  how, 296-302
    valence, 301, 302
  what, 296
  when, 295
  where, 295-296
  who, 291-295
Field notes, 176
Field supervisors (off-campus supervisors), 21
File (computer), 255
  managers, 260
  transfers, 264
First order change, 74
Five-Minute Think, The, 218t, 220t, 221-222t
Flanders Interaction Analysis System, 298t
Foci. (*See* styles of supervision), 58-60
Formal evaluation, 286-289
Formal logic, 213
Forms of supervision, 64-69
  dyadic, 64
  group, 64-69
Formula writing, 235
Frequency of observation, 173
Functions of communication, 102-103

Game theory in conflict, 132
Genderlect, 107-111, 108-110t, 111t
Generic supervisors, 21
Genuine communication, 96
Gestalt theory of problem managing, 207, 214
Gestures, 166
Goal revision, 211
Goals and issues in conflict management, 132
Goals and objectives, 236, 244-245, 281-283, 285t, 286, 292
  for the client, 244
  for the supervisee, 244-245
  for the supervisor, 142-144, 143-144t, 245
Goal state (outcome), 210, 212
(GPS) General Problem Solver, 208
Grading, 252, 287, 303-304
Graphics (computer), 267
Graticule. (*See* priority graticule), 285, 285f, 286
GRE (Graduate Record Examination), 267

Group supervision, 48, 64-71, 65t, 70-71t, 220t, 283-285, 284t, 289, 292, 295, 330, 331
  models, 64-69
    Case Staffings, 66-67, 70t
    comparison of dyadic and group supervision, 65t
    In Absentia Supervision, 68, 71t
    Microteaching, 67-68, 70t
    Multi-, Inter-, Transdisciplinary Teams, 68-69, 71t, 292
    Quality Circles, 67, 71t
    Teaching Clinic, 64, 66, 70t, 330, 331
    Wholistic Supervision, 48, 68, 71t, 292, 295
Groupthink, 121
GST (General Systems Theory/Thinking), 56
Guided vs. solo observation, 174-175
Gustatory sense in observation, 167

Halo effect, 303
Heuristics, 208
High tech-high touch (computers), 266
Humanism, 27, 63f
Humanistic Supervision, 58
Human Relations theory of supervision, 57
Human Resources theory of supervision, 57
Humor in supervision, 113-114

IA (Interaction Analysis), 254
  reliability/validity of IA tools, 298
  research with, 332
  tools/instruments discussed, 298-299t
ICP (Interpersonal Communication Pacing), 47, 105, 119, 134, 318, 327
  Confluence, 119
  Incongruity, 119
  Nonverbal Mirroring, 119
  Verbal Matching, 119
Ideal Type Managerial Grid (Blake and Mouton), 33
Idealist inquiry mode, 35t, 63f
In Absentia Supervision, 68, 71t
Incongruity, 119
Incubation in problem managing, 208
Index of Adjustment and Values, 327
Inferences in observation, 164
Information processing, 190-191, 208-212, 214
Initial states (givens), 208, 212
InQ Questionnaire, 33, 43-44t
Inquiry modes, 33, 35-38t, 63f
  Analyst, 37t, 63f
  Idealist, 35t, 63f

Pragmatist, 36t, 63f
Realist, 38t, 63f
Synthesist, 34t, 63f
INREAL (INter-REActive Learning), 68, 99-101, 105, 115, 144t
  Reactive Language, 115, 117
    Expansion—Elaborated, 100, 101, 105
    Expansion—Restated, 100, 105
    Mirroring, 105, 106, 115
    Modeling, 101
    Parallel Talk, 105, 116
    Reaction Time Latency (RTL), 102, 105, 144t
    Self Talk, 105, 116
    S.O.U.L. (Silence, Observation, Understanding, Listening), 99, 105
    Verbal Monitoring and Reflecting—Imitated, 99, 105
    Verbal Monitoring and Reflecting—Restated, 99, 105
Instructive language, 117
Intent/force of communication, 103
Interaction network, 38f
Interactional arhythmia, 119
Interactional synchrony, 106
  confluence, 106, 119
  congruence, 106, 119
  ICP (Interpersonal Communication Pacing), 47, 105, 119, 134, 318, 327
  incongruity, 119
  INREAL (INter-REActive Learning), 68, 99-101
  mirroring, 105, 106, 115-116, 119
  pacing and leading, 105, 115, 117, 318, 327
  postural synchrony, 119
  verbal matching, 119
  vocal convergence, 119
  vocal synchrony, 119
Interactive video disks, 172
Intermediate states (subgoals), 208
Internal brainstorming, 218t, 220t
Interpersonal communication, 39, 43-44t, 114
  entry phase, 115
  styles, 105, 129-130, 130f
Intervention in conflict, 133
Intervention plans (therapy plans, IEPs, service delivery plans, care plans, therapeutic records, unit records, problem-oriented charts, operational management data), 233
Interview Analysis System, 139, 298t
Interviewing, 122-123
Intrapersonal communication, 114

SUBJECT INDEX

Intuitive-receptive cognitive style, 215
IPA (Interaction Process Analysis), 38, 140–141f, 298t
ISCRS (Individual Supervisory Conference Rating Scale), 298t, 299t, 300, 320, 320f, 322, 323f, 331
ITEM (INREAL Training Evaluation Model), 299t
ITEM-ICP (INREAL Training Evaluation Model-Interpersonal Communication Pacing), 298t
ITMMS (Integrative Task-Maturity Model of Supervision), 58

JCAH (Joint Commission on Accreditation of Hospitals), 7
Job descriptions, 42, 276, 277, 279, 286, 292
Johari Window, 135–136, 136f

Kinesics, 166
Kolb's Model of Experiential Learning, 32

LAN (Local Area Network), 258
Language, 96–97
  nonverbal, 97, 165–167, 338
  verbal, 97, 168
Lateral thinking, 209, 210t, 212, 218, 218t, 220t
Lateral Thinking: Creativity Step by Step, 210
Leadership styles, 33, 39, 63f
Learning styles, 29–30
Lecture forum, 219t, 220t
Life scripts, 106
Lifelong learners communication, 127–128
Linear-intuitive communication, 96
Lingquest 1: Language Sample Analysis, 254, 255
Listening, 98–101, 232
Live observation, 168–169
Logical concepts, 211
LoU (Levels of Use) instrument, 75

4M (Me-values, Mates-values, Moral-values, Mankind-values), 218t, 220t
Macrofocus in observation, 163, 164t, 174
Management Style Assessment, 39
Managerial Grid (Ideal Type) (Blake and Mouton), 33
Marginal personnel, 304–305
Matching and modeling (see pacing and leading), 105, 115, 117, 318, 327
Matrix Management, 283–286, 284f, 285f, 287, 288f
Maximax decision making strategy, 197

MBTI (Myers-Briggs Type Indicator), 31, 30–31t, 43–44t
McCrea's Adapted Scales, 137, 299t, 328
McSAT (Multiple Choice Self-Assessment), 300
Medline, 265
Mesolect style of communication, 105
Metacognition, 209, 221–222t
Metacommunication, 98
Metamodel (Meta-Analysis), 105, 118
Metaphor in supervision, 118
Microcomputer Assisted Study Partner in Anatomy and Physiology of the Speech and Hearing Mechanism, 266, 267
Microcomputers (see computers), 251–269
Microfocus in observation, 163, 164t, 174, 177
Microteaching, 67–68, 70t
Minimax decision making strategy, 197
Minority language, multicultural communication (personnel), 126, 305
Mirroring, 105, 106, 119
Modeling, 101, 105
Models of supervision, 57–58
Modem, 258, 338
Modes of observation, 168–172
Modified Hill Cognitive Style Mapping Instrument, 32, 43–44t
Molar Model of Supervision, 58
Molyneaux-Lane Interview Analysis, 139, 266
Morphogenesis, 56, 207
Morphostasis, 56, 207
M.O.S.A.I.C.S. (Multidimensional Observation System for the Analysis of Interaction in Clinical Supervision), 124, 137, 138, 255, 299t, 320, 320f, 329, 331
Motivation, 216
Multivariate analysis research design, 322–323, 324f

Narrative data recording, 176–177
NATS (National Association of Teachers of Speech), 3
Natural concepts, 211
Naturalistic evaluation, 289
Neoscientific Management theory of supervision, 57
NESPA (National Examination in Speech-Language Pathology and Audiology), 267, 287
Networking, 266
Nine Mind Tests, 33, 43–44t
NLP (Neurolinguistic Programming), 105, 117–118

Nonparametric statistics, 318-319
Nonparticipant observation, 168-169
Nonstandard American English, 126
Nontraditional communication (learners), 125-128
Nonverbal language (behavior, communication, language), 97, 165-167, 338
Numeric therapy data, 256, 256f

Objects and artifacts in observation, 167
Observation competence, 155-158, 276-277, 297t
Observation modes, 16, 168-171, 297t
　audiotape recording, 170-171, 297t
　closed circuit television (CCTV), 169-170, 297t
　interactive video disks, 170
　live observation, 168-170, 297t
　telecommunication, 170
　videotape recording, 171-172, 297t
　written plans, 172
Observation of nonverbal behavior, 165-167
Observation of verbal behavior, 167-168
Observation (prearranged vs. spontaneous), 173-174
Observation reactivity, 303
Observation recording systems, 175-178
Observation reliability, 298
Observation (systematic), 172-175
OCD (Organization Communication Development), 139
Oculesics, 166
Off-campus supervisors (field supervisors), 21
Olfactory sense in observation, 166
On-campus supervisors, 21
Open system, 56, 103
Operations of intellectual functioning, 212
Operators (procedures), 208
Optimal decision, 195-197
Oral reporting, 232, 236
Oratio's Supervisory Transactional System, 137, 299t
Organizational communication, 121
Organizational communication audit, 139
Organismics in observation, 167
Outcomes in decision making, 185, 190, 198

Pacing and leading. (*See* interactional synchrony), 47, 105, 106, 115, 116, 117, 119, 134, 318, 327
Pacing Identification Form, 319f
Panel discussion, 219t, 220t
Paralinguistics, 166, 338

Parallel Talk, 105, 116
Parametric statistics, 319-324
Participant observation, 168-169
Pattern Recognition, 255, 299t
PDP (Professional Development Plans), 276, 277, 279, 286, 292
Pedagogy learning style, 29-30, 127-128
Peer supervision, 290t, 292, 305-306
Pentagonal Model of Communication Disorders Supervision, 8, 23, 96
Performance records, 177
Personal analysis, 26-42, 43t, 135
Personal growth research, 333
Personal Supervision Characteristics Profile, 42, 43t, 142, 144t
Personality types, 30-31t, 31-32, 43-44t
Philosophical orientations of learning, 25-26, 28t, 63f
　essentialism, 25, 28t, 63f
　existentialism, 26, 28t, 63f
　experimentalism, 25, 28t, 63f
Photographic records, 176
PISCO, 218t, 220t, 221t
Planning, 209-211, 277
Policies and procedures, 277, 278t
Portfolio development, 289
Positivity bias, 303
Power in conflict, 131
PPE (Program Planning Evaluation), 20, 296
Practicum Evaluation Procedure (Klevans and Volz), 298t
Pragmatics in communication, 104-105
Pragmatist inquiry mode, 36t, 63f
PREAC, 7, 8, 19-21, 23t, 48, 85-89, 86-87t, 96, 121, 144t, 157, 184, 217, 221-222t, 229, 230, 254, 255, 264, 283, 316, 338, 334-337t
Prearranged vs. spontaneous observation, 173-174
Primary supervisors, 21
Priority graticule, 285, 285f, 286
Proana 5, 138, 144t, 255, 299t
Probability, 184, 185-187, 198
　objective, 185
　subjective, 185, 186
Problem managing, 206-207, 277
　application to supervision, 219-222, 220t, 221-222t
　obstacles, 214-217
　programs, 217-221

SUBJECT INDEX

Problem Managing *(Cont.)*
  theories of management, 207-214
    strategies, 217-219, 218-219t, 221-222t
    sustaining, 221
  three stages, 217
Problem solving, 206
Problem space, 208
Problems, 206
Process analysis, 120
Products of intellectual functioning, 212
Professional communication, 121-122
Professional letters, 234
Professional Role (Domain), 7, 8, 19, 23t, 48, 85-89, 86-87t, 96, 121, 143t, 157, 184, 217, 221t, 229, 254, 255, 264, 278, 283, 316, 334-337t
Progress reports (end-of-term reports, interim summaries), 233
Prosthetics (computers), 268
Protective Motivation Theory, 76-78, 77t
Proxemics, 166
PRS (Primary Representational System), 105, 115
Psychoanalytic descriptions, 176
Psychological orientations of learning, 27, 28-29t, 63f
  behaviorism, 27, 28-29t, 63f
  cognitivism, 27, 28-29t, 63f
  humanism, 27, 28-29t, 63f

Qualitative research, 124, 176-177, 316-318, 317f, 333, 337t
Quality Circles, 67, 71t
Quantitative research, 124-125, 318-324, 319t, 320t, 321t, 322t, 323t, 324t, 333, 334-335t
Quantity of verbal behavior, 168
Question types, 111-113, 144t
  broad or open-ended, 112
    divergent, 112
    evaluative, 112-113
  effective strategies, 113
  narrow or closed-ended, 111
    cognitive-memory, 112
    convergent, 112
  problems with using, 113
  use in supervision, 113
Questionnaire research, 335t

Rate of verbal behavior, 168
Rating systems, 175-176

Readiness states of supervisees, 47, 74, 283-286, 289
Realist inquiry mode, 38t, 63f
Reasoning, 213, 215-216
Record (computer), 255
Record keeping (computer), 252-264
Recording systems, 175-178
  checklists, 177
  narrative data, 176-177
  ratings, 175
  tallying, 178
  timing, 177-178
Reddin's 3-D Theory, 39
Reflective thinking, 217, 219t, 220t, 222t
Registers (codes) of communication, 103-104
Relational data base, 260
Research considerations, 331-333
  analysis of data, 333
  anonymity of data, 332
  personal growth research, 333
  protection of human subjects, 331-332
  reliability of data, 332
  tools, 332
  training of coders, 332
Research methodology and designs, 124-125, 176-177, 316-324, 333
  books, 337t
  qualitative, 124, 176-177, 316-318, 317f, 333, 337t
  quantitative, 124-125, 318-324, 319, 320t, 321t, 322t, 323t, 324t, 333, 334-335t
  questionnaires, 333, 335t
  single subject, 333, 334t, 338
  thought papers, 333, 335-337t
Research questions, 339
Researcher identification, 338
Researcher Role (Research Domain), 7, 8, 19-20, 23t, 48, 85-89, 86-87t, 96, 121, 143t, 157, 184, 217, 221t, 230, 254, 255, 264, 278, 283, 316, 334-337t
Rhetorical sensitivity, 106, 327
Risk in decision making theory, 184, 197
  maximax strategy, 197
  minimax strategy, 197
Roles of supervisors (Professional, Researcher, Educator, Administrator, and Clinician), 7, 8, 19-20, 23t, 48, 85-89, 86-87t, 96, 121, 144t, 157, 184, 217, 221-222t, 229, 230, 254-255, 264, 283, 316, 338, 334-337t

Rosental effect, 303
RTL (Reaction Time Latency), 102, 105, 144t
Rule-governed reasoning, 215

SALT (Systematic Analysis of Language Transcripts), 254
Schema theory, 213–214
Schemata, 213
Scientific Management Theory of supervision, 56
Second order change, 74–75, 135, 143
Secondary supervisors, 21
Self talk, 105, 116
Self-confrontation, 133, 159, 162t
Self-editing, 236
Self-supervision, 302
Semantic mediators (networks), 211
Sensitizing concepts, 317, 317f, 328
Session plans (lesson plans, progress notes, daily entries, flow charts), 233
Sign test research design, 318, 319f, 338
Signal Detection Theory, 192–195
    correct rejection, 193
    decision matrix, 193, 193f
    false alarm, 192, 193, 193f, 196
    hit, 192, 193, 193f, 196
    miss, 192, 193, 193f
    signal, 192
    target, 192
Silence, 101–102, 167
Similarities-focused reasoning, 215
Simulations and role-playing, 217–218
Single subject research design, 334t, 338
Situation or environment in observation, 167
Situational Leadership model, 58
Skills, 22, 142, 155, 217
Skill-Streaming the Adolescent, 21
Sleight Clinician Anxiety Test, 326
Slot filler formula writing, 235, 244
Small group communication, 120–121
SOC (Stages of Concern) instrument, 75
Sociological descriptions, 176
Software (computer), 260–264
S.O.U.L. (Silence, Observation, Understanding, Listening), 99, 105
Special Children in Regular Classrooms, 218
Special Net, 265
Speech Act Theory, 96
Spreadsheets, 255, 255f

STACS (Supervisor-Teacher Analogous Categories System), 299t
Staff supervisors, 21
Standardized situation responses, 177
States of nature, 185, 187–188, 198, 199f
Static descriptors, 177
Stress, 45–46
Structure in conflict, 132
Structure-of-Intellect model of intellectual functioning, 212
STYLES of Communication Disorders supervision, 39, 60–64, 63f, 220t, 283, 284f, 289, 290, appendix B
    definition, 60
    STYLE I, 39, 63f, 128, 220t, 283, 284f, 290, appendix B
    STYLE II, 39, 63f, 128, 220t, 284f, 290, appendix B
    STYLE III, 39, 63f, 128, 220t, 284f, 290, appendix B
    STYLE IV, 39, 63f, 124, 128, 220t, 284f, 288, 290, appendix B
Styles of supervision, 58–60
    clinical disposition-interpersonal disposition, 59, 60f, 61f, 62f, 63f, 64f
    clinical skill-interpersonal skill, 59, 60f, 61f, 62f, 63f, 64f
    direct-indirect, 59, 63f, 64f, 124–125, 323f, 328, 329, 330
    goal-directed, 60
    goal-oriented, 59
    instructive-communicative, 59, 63f, 64f
    mutually directed, 60
    product concern–people concern, 59
    professional competence, 59
    self-directed, 60
    supervisee-oriented, 59
    supervisor-oriented, 59
    task oriented–relations oriented, 59, 63f, 64f
    unilateral-bilateral, 59, 60f, 61f, 62f, 63f, 64f, 290
SUPERnet, 18, 265, 338
SuperPILOT, 266
Supervisees, 46–47, 72–73t, 124
Supervision
    as art, 8
    as science, 8
    assumptions, 7–9
    components, 7

SUBJECT INDEX

Supervision *(Cont.)*
  concepts, 7
  constituents, 7
  contexts, 7
  definition, 9
  developmental timeline, 4f
  differential, 47, 69–74, 72–73t
  domains. (*See* Roles and PREAC), 7, 8, 19–21, 23t, 48, 85–89, 86–87t, 96, 121, 144t, 157, 184, 217, 221–222t, 229, 230, 254, 255, 264, 283, 316, 338, 334–337t
  first dissertation, 5
  first major research, 5
  forms, 64–69
    dyadic, 64, 220t, 283–285, 284f, 289
    group, 64–69, 220t, 283–285, 284t, 289
  history of, 3–6
  in businesses, 87t, 88, 90t, 221t
  in college and university training programs, 85–87, 86t, 90t, 221t
  in community speech-language and hearing centers, 87t, 89, 90t, 221t
  in medical settings, 86t, 88, 90t, 221t
  in schools, 87–88, 86t, 90t, 221t
  Pentagonal Model, 8, 23, 96
  specialty area, 78–79
  Speech-Language Pathology vs. Audiology, 78
  tasks and competencies, 6, 21, 22, 23t, 230, 296, appendix A
  theories of, 56–58
    Human Relations Supervision, 57
    Human Resources Supervision, 58
    Neoscientific Management, 57
    Scientific Management, 56
  training in, 24–42
    education vs. training, 25, 25f
    first program, 6
    human dimensions, 26–42
    importance of, 24–25
    theoretical dimensions, 25–26
  Trigonal Model, 7, 8, 17, 42, 48, 96
  types (STYLES + forms), 69, 220t, 280, 283, 289
SUPERvision, 18, 264
Supervision Hours Summary Form, 292, 293–294t
Supervision Style Index, 39, 43–44t
Supervision training (preparation), 24–42
Supervisors, 21–23
  classifications, 21
  competencies, 6, 21–22, 23t, 279–280, 280–282t, 287–289, 296, appendix A
  dispositions, 22, 142, 155, 217
  skills, 22, 142, 155, 217
  demographics, 18
  word first used, 5
Symmetry in communication, 98
Synectics, 217, 219t, 221t
Syntality, 121
Synthesist inquiry mode, 34t, 63f
Synthesized reasoning, 25
System for Analyzing Supervision-Teacher Interaction (Blumberg), 137, 298t, 330
Systematic observation, 172–175
  duration, 173
  focused, 174
  frequency, 173
  guided vs. solo, 174
  prearranged vs. spontaneous, 173–174
Systematic-preceptive cognitive style, 215
Systems, 56, 103, 207

t-test research design, 321, 321f, 322f
Tactile communication, 166
Tallying, 178
Tasks of supervision, 6, 21–22, 23t, 230, 279–280, 281–282t, 287–289, 296, appendix A
Teaching Clinic, 64, 66, 70t, 330, 331
Teams, 68–69
  interdisciplinary, 68, 71t, 292
  multidisciplinary, 68–69, 71t, 292
  transdisciplinary, 69, 71t, 292
TEC Framework, 218t, 221t
Technology, 277
Telecommunications, 170, 264–265
Television and supervision, 159
Theories of Supervision, 56–58
Third party payment reports (insurance forms, federal and state government agency forms), 233
Thought papers, 316–318, 335–337t
Timing, 177–178
Titles or names, 168
Top-down information processing, 213, 214
Transactional Analysis in conflict, 132–133
Trigonal Model of Communication Disorders Supervision, 3, 8, 17, 42, 48, 96

Types of supervision (STYLE + form), 69, 220t, 280, 283, 289

Underwood Category System for Analysis of Supervisor-Clinician Behavior, 137, 144, 299t
Univariate analysis, 320
UTD Competency Based Evaluation System, 299t, 317
Utility in decision making, 184, 185, 188–189, 198

Valence in communication, 301
Value in decision making, 184, 185, 188–189, 198
Values Clarification, 218
Verbal and Nonverbal Interpersonal Communication Pacing Facilitation Program, 105, 143
Verbal (behavior, communication, language), 97, 168
Verbal matching, 119
Vertical thinking, 208, 210t, 217, 219
Video disks, 172, 267
Video resumes, 123
Videotape recording, 159, 160–161t, 171–172, 325, 330
Visi-Pitch, 266

Visual literacy, 158–165
VMR (Verbal Monitoring and Reflecting), 99, 105
  imitated, 99, 105
  restated, 99, 105
Vocal convergence, 119
Vocal synchrony, 119

W-PACC (Wisconsin Procedure for Appraisal of Clinical Competence), 58, 279, 280, 299t, 300, 325
WCI (Word Class Inventory), 255
Whole-Brain Thinking, 39, 218, 218t
Wholistic Supervision, 48, 68, 71t, 292, 295
Word processing, 252, 254
Worksite profiles, 85–91, 86–87t, 90t, 221t
  businesses, 87t, 88, 90t, 221t
  college and university training programs, 85–87, 86t, 90t, 221t
  community speech-language and hearing centers, 87t, 89, 90t, 221t
  medical settings, 86t, 88, 90t, 221t
  schools, 87–88, 86t, 90t, 221t
  supervision tasks relative to worksites, 89, 90t
Written plans, 172